Textbook of Epidemiology

Textbook of Epidemiology

Second Edition

Lex Bouter, PhD
Professor of Methodology and Integrity
Amsterdam University Medical Centers
Department of Epidemiology and Data Science
Vrije Universiteit Amsterdam
Faculty of Humanities
Department of Philosophy
Amsterdam, The Netherlands

Maurice Zeegers, MBA, PhD
Professor of Complex Genetics and Epidemiology
Department of Epidemiology
Maastricht University
Maastricht, The Netherlands

Tianjing Li, MD, MHS, PhD
Associate Professor
Department of Ophthalmology, School of Medicine
Department of Epidemiology, Colorado School of Public Health
University of Colorado Anschutz Medical Campus
Aurora, CO, USA

WILEY Blackwell

Contents

Preface

The first Dutch version of the *Textbook of Epidemiology* was published in 1988. Since then, it quickly became the most used epidemiology textbook in the Netherlands used by bachelor, master, and postgraduate students as well as a reference book for epidemiology professionals. Over time, higher education in the Netherlands has increasingly attracted students from abroad and consequently the curriculum partly switched to English. This textbook was thus translated, commissioned by the European Epidemiology Federation (EEF), and endorsed by Association of Schools of Public Health in the European Region (ASPHER).

This is the second English edition of our *Textbook of Epidemiology* and the first edition published by Wiley-Blackwell. In this edition, we revised all chapters extensively and added a new chapter on systematic reviews with a goal to improve clarity, international accessibility, and relevance. We harmonized core terminology and enriched the book with recent and broadly applicable examples. We also introduced knowledge assessment questions at the end of each chapter for users to check their grasp of the key points.

The author team has also changed since the first edition of the textbook. The current author team – Lex Bouter, Maurice Zeegers, and Tianjing Li – are indebted to all those who have contributed to previous versions of the book, including the former co-authors Martien van Dongen and Gerhard Zielhuis. We are grateful for Gowri Gopalakrishna and Marino van Zelst who revised the chapter on outbreak investigations; Sander van Kuijk who provided useful comments to many chapters; and Magdalena Schellenberg-Konopka and Colina Simons who helped us improve Chapter 7. We thank Rachel Haley who drafted the self-assessment questions and provided edits to draft chapters. Specific administrative support for this book was provided by Erika Bemelmans.

We hope that a wide range of readers, including those in clinical medicine, public health, and allied health professions, will find our book useful, either as textbook in their formal epidemiology training, to immerse themselves single-handed in the principles of epidemiology, or to refresh their knowledge on specific methodological topics. Please also take a look at the website of the book (www.textbookepidemiology.org), where you can find enrichment materials, short bios of the authors, and corrections. We would also be grateful for your feedback and suggestions, which can help improve the contents of future editions of the book.

Lex Bouter
Maurice Zeegers
Tianjing Li

About the Companion Website

This book is accompanied by a companion website:

www.wiley.com/go/Bouter/TextbookofEpidemiology

The website includes:
- Weblinks
- Author bios
- Contact form

Epidemiology

Textbook of Epidemiology, Second Edition. Lex Bouter, Maurice Zeegers and Tianjing Li.
© 2023 John Wiley & Sons Ltd. Published 2023 by John Wiley & Sons Ltd.
Companion website: www.wiley.com/go/Bouter/TextbookofEpidemiology

1.1 What is epidemiology?

1.1.1 Definition

When a new infectious disease (such as COVID-19) is discovered, epidemiologists work with other scientists to find out who has it, why they have it, and what can be done about it. Epidemiology is the study of the distribution (frequency, pattern), and explanatory factors (causes, risk factors) of health-related states and events (health outcomes) in specified populations at a particular time. Using a COVID-19 outbreak as an example, epidemiologists identified the source of the outbreak by conducting field investigations in the community and health facilities in Wuhan, China. They collected specimens from the nose and throat for lab analyses. These field investigations informed those who were infected, when they became sick, and where they had been just before they became sick, which ultimately led to the identification of the likely source. Epidemiologists monitor and track the disease by using surveillance systems that report data on new cases of infection, symptoms, hospitalizations, treatments, deaths, and demographic information. Epidemiologists further investigate the disease to find out how contagious COVID-19 is, how to test for the presence of infection, what risk factors for severe illness are, what the natural and treated course of the disease on average is, and which treatments are most effective. Finally, epidemiologists contribute to developing guidance for preventive actions (e.g. face-mask wearing and social distancing) to slow the spread of the disease and lessen its impact.

Following on from the above, we can characterize epidemiology as follows:

- Health outcomes are the main focus of epidemiological research.
- Epidemiology is the study of health outcomes in human populations.
- Epidemiologists usually look at health outcomes in relation to other phenomena. These are factors suspected to have influenced the development of the health outcome in question (etiological factors), to give an indication of the presence of a particular health outcome (diagnostic factors), to be associated with the course of the health outcome (prognostic factors), or to mitigate the impact of the health outcome (interventions).
- The application of epidemiological study findings is meant to improve the wellbeing of the population.

Case 1.1 Scurvy and citrus fruits

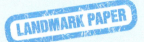

James Lind, a Scottish ship's doctor, carried out an inventive experiment on scurvy patients in 1747. Scurvy (or scorbutus) is a disease characterized by bleeding gums, internal bleeding, stiff limbs and rough skin, among other things. It was very common in those days among crews of ocean-going ships. Long after Lind made his observations, it was found that scurvy is caused primarily by a deficiency of vitamin C (ascorbic acid), which is needed to synthesize collagen, a substance that strengthens blood vessels. James Lind selected 12 cases in the same stage of the disease on his ship. In addition to the common diet all participants received as their primary source of nutrition, he compared six "treatments": two patients were prescribed cider, two elixir of vitriol, two sea water, two a mixture of nutmeg and a commonly used medicine based on garlic and mustard seed, and two were given two oranges and one lemon a day. Only the patients who were given the orange and lemon treatment experienced a rapid cure. The mechanism by which scurvy can be cured and prevented using citrus fruit was not known at that time. However, it did not present an obstacle to taking effective measures. It took many years for citrus fruit to be introduced as a prophylactic for this dreaded disease on ships. Nearly 50 years later (1 year after Lind's death), the Admiralty of England made issue of lemon juice compulsory in its navy. As a nod to Lind's pioneering work, the Institute of Naval Medicine includes a lemon tree in its crest.

1.1.2 Health outcomes

The basic variable in epidemiology, and in any epidemiological study, is a health outcome. Epidemiologists are interested in the extent to which diseases or more generally health outcomes occur (i.e. their frequency) among the population. This defines the object of epidemiological research, namely health outcomes in human populations. The word "disease" needs to be interpreted broadly in this context: it can mean a broad variety of medical conditions, both infectious and non-infectious, acute and chronic, somatic and mental. In this context "health outcome" can refer to all sorts of phenomena on a continuum from full health to death from a condition. It can also refer to a disability, injury due to trauma, quality of life, or a physiological measure. As there is no term that encompasses all these aspects, we generally use the phrase "health outcome" – or simply "outcome" – in this book. Chapter 2 provides more detail on measuring various aspects of health. For the purpose of epidemiological research, we need to define the health outcome of interest as precisely as possible so as to enable us to detect relationships with explanatory factors.

1.1.3 Frequency measures

Epidemiology is the study of health outcomes and explanatory factors in humans. Animal experiments and observations in cell or organ cultures do not fall into the domain of epidemiology. Although the measurements are usually carried out on individuals, the results of epidemiological research always relate to groups of people. As the disease frequency for a group can be interpreted as the mean disease risk for each member of the group, the knowledge gained from epidemiological research is valuable not only at the group level (for public health) but also at the individual level (in healthcare). Epidemiologists ascertain whether each individual has the health outcome and then count the number of individuals with the health outcome in the group as a whole, thus yielding the epidemiological fraction.

$$\frac{\text{Number of cases}}{\substack{\text{Total number of persons in the group} \\ \text{from which these cases are taken}}}$$

This fraction provides the basis for all epidemiological measures of frequency (see Chapter 2). For example, we refer to incidence when counting new cases of a disease in a group at risk of contracting that disease (the at-risk population). Prevalence, on the other hand, relates to the number of existing cases of the disease. Incidence is also a measure of risk: it indicates the average risk of developing the health outcome during the specified period.

Health and disease are not equally distributed among the population; and it is this fact that lends epidemiology its raison d'être. The purpose of epidemiology is first and foremost to identify differences in health outcomes between populations. The distribution of a health outcome among the population becomes clear when we investigate the differences in frequency between groups of people at different times, in different places, and with different characteristics. Differences in time can manifest themselves between seasons or over years or decades. Differences between geographical areas can relate to continents, countries, regions of a country, urban versus rural areas, or districts of a town or city. Examples of individual characteristics that can be associated with differences in disease frequency are age, sex, genetic predisposition, occupation, and lifestyle characteristics such as smoking, drinking, and physical activities. Categorizing the population into subpopulations based on time, place, or individual characteristics gives us an understanding of the distribution of the disease risk, and enables us to identify risk periods, risk areas, or at-risk groups. Identifying the distribution pattern of a health outcome falls under the domain of descriptive epidemiology. The branch of epidemiology that aims to identify causal factors underlying the distribution of a health outcome is known as analytical epidemiology.

1.1.4 Explanatory factors

In addition to the health outcomes, epidemiology studies the factors related to the occurrence of health outcomes. These factors fall into three categories: etiological, diagnostic, and prognostic. The term "explanatory factors" is used in this book as a generic term for these factors. Individuals can be exposed to several factors either at the same time or successively. Epidemiologists are interested first and foremost in factors that are causally responsible or co-responsible for the development of a disease (etiological factors or risk factors) or that influence the course of the disease (prognostic factors). They may also look for factors that distinguish people who have a particular disease from those who do not have it (diagnostic factors).

The factors that influence the development or course of a disease or a health outcome can be broadly divided into three categories: genetics, lifestyle, and environment. Genetic properties and biological characteristics of genetic origin are important factors, but they are as of yet, very difficult to manipulate. Interventions to influence the risk of disease are more likely to be available for environmental and lifestyle factors to which people are exposed voluntarily or involuntarily (e.g. diet, smoking, alcohol, drugs, sexual habits, microorganisms, environmental, and occupational exposures). Preventive, diagnostic, and therapeutic interventions can also be regarded as explanatory factors of disease and prognosis, for example, screening programs and various medical and paramedical interventions such as smoking cessation programs, physical activities for weight loss, or surgical and pharmaceutical therapies for a condition.

1.1.5 Epidemiological function

Epidemiology contributes to medicine and public health by discovering what factors are associated with a health outcome, how strong the link is, and what contribution these factors make to the occurrence of the health outcome. Usually, multiple exposures are involved in every health outcome at all stages. This can be expressed as follows:

$$P(O) = f(F_i)$$

This epidemiological function states that the occurrence of the health outcome (O) is a mathematical function of a series of k factors (F_i, where $i = 1, ..., k$). In this equation, the health outcome is the dependent variable or outcome variable. The factors are the independent variables in the formula. Various measures of association can be used to express the strength of the relationship between the occurrence of the factor and the health outcome. The most important measures of association will be discussed in Chapter 3.

Although an epidemiological study usually focuses on one single explanatory factor of a health outcome, if we want to gain a good understanding of the relationship between that explanatory factor and the outcome, we will almost always need to include other factors in the study design, measure them and take them into account when analyzing the data.

The presence of these other factors can affect the association. We know, for example, that if we want to examine the effect of alcohol consumption on road accidents, we need to take the driving behaviors (e.g.

speed and seatbelt use) into consideration, as the effect of alcohol is stronger for higher speed. In other words, the effect of alcohol on road accidents is modified by speed (effect modification). If we want to study the effect of exercise behavior on cardiovascular disease outcomes, we must not forget to adjust for the effect of healthy diet: people who are more active may also eat a healthier diet. Unless we include these extraneous factors, we cannot be certain whether the observed effect of exercise is actually due to healthy diet (confounding). More information on effect modification and confounding will be given in Chapter 5.

Case 1.2 Cannabis use and depression

In 2015, the United Nations Office on Drugs and Crime estimated the annual prevalence of cannabis use worldwide at around 2.8%–4.5%. This frequency varies between countries, with the highest prevalence (>10%) in Canada, the US, and Australia, and a prevalence between 2.5% and 10% in most European countries. With around 182.5 million users globally, cannabis ranks first among illicit drug use. Research has linked cannabis use to the development of depression. Most of these studies showed an increased risk of depression among cannabis users after adjusting for other possible risk factors for depression (confounding variables). There is also evidence of a dose–response relationship, since the risk of depression increases with higher levels of cannabis use.

Recently a US-cohort study was performed to study the effect of reducing cannabis use on depressive symptoms in young female adults. This cohort study included 332 young women of different ethnicities between the ages of 18 and 24 who had used cannabis at least three times in the previous three months. At baseline, and after three and six months of follow-up, the study participants filled out the Beck Depression Inventory-II questionnaire, which measures depression on a continuous scale with higher scores indicating more severe depressive symptoms. After controlling for alcohol use – which has been shown to be associated with depression – the results showed a significant reduction in depressive symptoms in participants who had stopped using cannabis. This reduction was more pronounced initially among moderately or severely depressed women compared to minimally depressed women. This cohort study supports the view that cannabis use may be a cause of depression. Since the research focused only on young women, the results may not be generalized to men directly. It may be worthwhile to study the existence of effect modification by sex in a mixed population. Before using these insights in the treatment of depressive patients who are also cannabis users, the effect of advice to stop using cannabis needs to be studied in a randomized trial (see Chapter 10).

1.1.6 The empirical cycle

The epidemiological function is a formal expression of the research question. The question whether cannabis use in humans increases the risk of depression (Case 1.2) can be represented by the following function:

$$P(depression) = f(cannabis use)$$

How do epidemiologists come up with a research question? Research questions do not just arrive unbidden; often casual observations lead investigators to tackle a particular topic. Researchers' curiosity can also be aroused by results of previous research or reports of other people's results, and they will feel the need to confirm such results (verification), dispute them (contradiction), refute them (falsification), or make them more specific (elaboration). Often, they will feel the need to improve on weaknesses in the design and conduct of previous research. Subsequent studies on similar research questions will gradually increase our understanding of that particular aspect of reality. This is referred to as the empirical cycle. In its simplest form, the empirical cycle is shown in Figure 1.1.

Researchers start with a theory, a statement or coherent series of statements intended to have universal validity. In some cases, the theory is being handed down, but it is usually based partly on observations of phenomena, which do not by definition have to be systematic. Sometimes they come from incidental encounters of the researchers. Usually

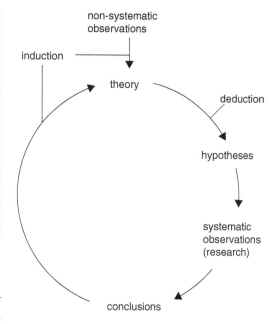

Figure 1.1   The empirical cycle.

systematic observations form the basis for theoretical explorations: results of previous research into the same topic conducted by the researchers themselves or other researchers. This previous research is by no means always epidemiological in nature. Incorporating these systematic and nonsystematic observations into a theory is no simple matter; it calls for a good deal of creativity and originality. This process of developing a more abstract, universal summary of reality from observations is known as induction. According to inductive reasoning, a new theory applies not only to the cases observed but also to all similar cases. To find out whether this is true, researchers carry out new, systematic observations. If the new observations tally with the expectations, confirmation is obtained that we are on the right track with our theory.

Another way of developing a theory is to try to prove that it is incorrect. This idea was introduced in the twentieth century by the philosopher of science Karl Popper (1902–1994) (Figure 1.2) and now forms a cornerstone of empirical science. It is impossible to confirm anything with certainty, but it is possible to falsify it. Popper therefore stated that every scientific theory must be falsifiable. Falsifiability means that we can prove that some proposition, statement, or theory is wrong. To do

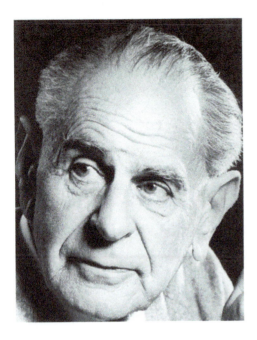

Figure 1.2 Kari Popper (1902–1994), philosopher of science and founding father of the falsifiability theory. Source: LSE Library / Flickr / Public domain.

this, we first need – taking the theory as our starting point – to formulate hypotheses, statements that can or cannot be refuted based on real-world observations.

This process of going from an abstract theory to one or more hypotheses for testing is known as deduction. In effect, the deduction process corresponds to translating a general research idea into one or more research questions. In contrast to what Figure 1.1 suggests, not every systematic study is designed to test a hypothesis, there is also research of a more exploratory nature. Exploratory research is conducted mainly on new and relatively unexplored problems, with the aim of generating promising hypotheses. The findings from this type of research also contribute to scientific theory.

As we have said, empirical research is needed to test a hypothesis or explore a new problem area. The phases of empirical research are as follows:
1. Formulate the research question
2. Draw up a study design:
   - Select the study population (specifying the sampling framework, the sampling procedure, the subpopulations to be compared, and the inclusion and exclusion criteria)
   - Decide what to measure, when to measure, and how to measure
   - Design a statistical analysis plan that addresses the research question.
3. Conduct the research (carry out the observations and collect data).
4. Analyze the results:
   - Tabulate the frequency and distribution of the variables measured (univariate analysis, descriptive in nature)
   - Examine relationships between the variables (bivariate and multivariate analysis, either descriptive, or explanatory).
5. Interpret the results and draw conclusions.

The empirical cycle can therefore be expanded as shown in Figure 1.3. The results of a single study can rarely make or break a theory or hypothesis. A theory represents current knowledge on a particular subject at a particular time. Plenty of research is usually needed before a theory can gain a satisfactory empirical basis. In effect each study means a fresh circuit of the empirical cycle, or rather the empirical spiral, working toward an ever-better description of reality. See also Figure 1.4.

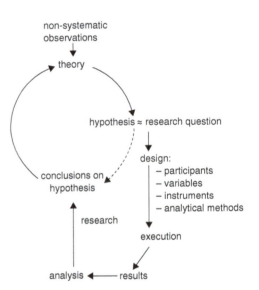

Figure 1.3 Research as an element in the empirical cycle.

FOKKE & SUKKE

KNOW WHAT SCIENCES IS ALL ABOUT

VERY IMPRESSIVE, COLLEAGUE...

BUT DOES IT ALSO WORK IN THEORY?

RGvT

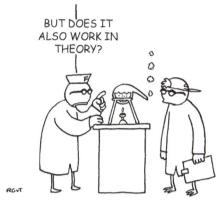

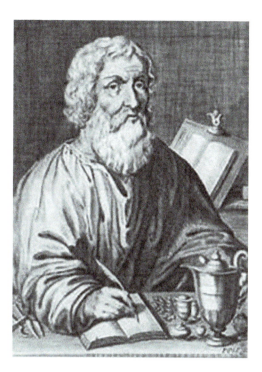

○ **Figure 1.4** Fokke and Sukke on the empirical cycle.

1.2 Developments in epidemiology

1.2.1 Historical examples

○ **Figure 1.5** Hippocrates (circa 470–430 BC), epidemiologist *avant la lettre. Source: Welcome Images / Wikimedia Commons / CC BY 4.0.*

As an epidemiologist *avant la lettre*, Hippocrates (circa 470–430 BC) stressed the importance of describing cases of disease meticulously (○ Figure 1.5). Hippocrates demonstrated in his *book On Airs, Waters and Plac*es that health and disease are determined by all sorts of observable environmental factors. Subsequently, for more than two millennia, ideas on disease remained related to humoral pathology (water, earth, fire, and bile), with scarcely any attention being paid to empirical observation. Not until the end of the seventeenth century was the Hippocratic approach re-adopted, for example by the Italian clinician Bernardino Ramazzini (1633–1714), who stressed the importance of asking patients about their medical history, nutritional habits, and working conditions. He even demonstrated the added value of comparing similar cases and looking for patterns. The idea of recording, counting, and analyzing causes of death dates from the same period. The London physician John Graunt (1620–1674) is regarded as the founding father of this type of descriptive epidemiology (○ Figure 1.6).

The advent of empirical research, introduced by Galileo Galilei (1564–1642), William Harvey (1578–1657) and others, laid the foundation for the further

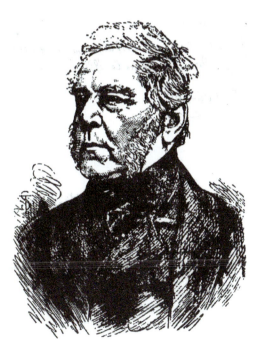

○ **Figure 1.6** Captain John Graunt (1620–1674), founding father of descriptive epidemiology. Source: John Graunt / Wikimedia Commons / Public domain.

development of epidemiology. The systematic record-ing and analysis of causes of death yielded a wealth of information, on the basis of which researchers such as William Farr (1807–1883) presented impressive and highly relevant reports to the British Minister of Health. John Snow (1813–1858) studied the causes of cholera (see Case 1.3), presenting one of the first clear examples of the epidemiological approach (◻ Figure 1.7).

In the eighteenth and early nineteenth century great progress was made in statistics, whose influence also grew in medical science. An important person in this regard is the French physician Pierre Louis (1787–1872), who introduced the "numerical method" in medicine and demonstrated with statistics that blood-letting was ineffective and even harmful. Empirical medical research became popular in the first half of the nineteenth century, an era with major developments in biology, pathology, and public health, and the first clas-sifications of diseases as well. The German scientist Rudolf Virchow (1821–1902) played a vital role here,

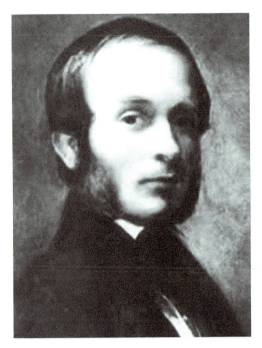

◻ **Figure 1.7** John Snow (1813–1858), one of the founding fathers of analytical epidemiology. Source: Thomas Jones Barker / Wikimedia Commons / Public domain.

being not only an eminent pathologist but also a great advocate of a vigorous approach to public health prob-lems. The work of the Frenchman Louis Pasteur (1822–1895) and the German Robert Koch (1843–1910) in the field of microorganisms uncovered the causes of many infectious diseases, including tubercu-losis, which was widespread at that time. Thanks to Koch we have a first set of criteria for causality in epi-demiological research. Around 1900, epidemiology was virtually synonymous with the epidemiology of infectious diseases. The epidemiological approach rose in popularity in the mid-twentieth century for the study of chronic conditions.

Present-day epidemiology has been highly influ-enced by the studies into the relationship between smoking and lung cancer carried out around World War II. Following initial reports of a possible link in the late 1930s, three studies published in 1950 showed that smoking is likely to be causally linked to the risk of lung cancer. One of these studies was car-ried out by Richard Doll and Austin Bradford Hill, two researchers who continued their studies into the harmful effects of smoking on health during subse-

---

Case 1.3 Cholera and drinking water

The London physician John Snow is often named as one of the founding fathers of epidemiology. A cholera epidemic broke out in the London district of Soho in 1848, and 500 residents of a single neighborhood died of the disease within 10 days. Snow started surveying the cholera cases system-atically. He suspected that there was a connection with drinking water, as none of the monks at a nearby monastery – who drank no water, only beer – had cholera. Snow then compared the water supply provided by the Southwark and Vauxhall Company with that provided by the Lambeth Company. He concluded that the victims must have mainly used the water pump in Broad Street. At Snow's insistence the pump was sealed off and the cholera epidemic ended. Only years later did it become clear that cholera is actually caused by a bacterium, but for Snow this was not an obstacle to taking adequate preventive action. Close study of his writings demonstrates that he was guided by an explicit theory about the etiology of cholera despite the fact that the biological mechanism was far from understood.

BRITISH MEDICAL JOURNAL

LONDON SATURDAY SEPTEMBER 30 1950

SMOKING AND CARCINOMA OF THE LUNG
PRELIMINARY REPORT

BY

RICHARD DOLL, M.D., M.R.C.P.
Member of the Statistical Research Unit of the Medical Research Council

AND

A. BRADFORD HILL, Ph.D., D.Sc.
Professor of Medical Statistics, London School of Hygiene and Tropical Medicine ; Honorary Director of the Statistical Research Unit of the Medical Research Council

Figure 1.8   Doll and Hills' famous article on smoking and lung cancer.

quent decades. In 1964, they published the results of a major study among British physicians that clearly showed a causal relationship (□ Figure 1.8) (see also Case 4.5 in Chapter 4). It is no coincidence that soon afterwards (in 1965) Hill published a revised set of criteria for causality, which were applicable both to infectious diseases (as were Koch's criteria mentioned above) and non-infectious diseases (see Chapter 6). From the particularly heated debate about the relationship between smoking and lung cancer in the 1950s and 1960s we can infer that lack of understanding of the exact mechanisms of disease is both a strength and a weakness of the epidemiological approach. This convincing epidemiological example has certainly raised interest in the contribution of epidemiology to the solution of many other public health problems.

In addition, clinicians became interested in the potential of epidemiology for solving diagnostic, prognostic, and treatment problems. This development gained a major boost from the publication in 1972 of the book "Effectiveness and Efficiency: Random Reflections on Health Services," in which Archie Cochrane (1909–1988) ardently advocated the systematic use of randomized controlled trials (RCTs) to assess the efficacy of interventions (□ Figure 1.9). Present-day epidemiology can be regarded as the combination of classic observational epidemiological methods with experimental study designs rooted in statistical theory developed since the 1930s.

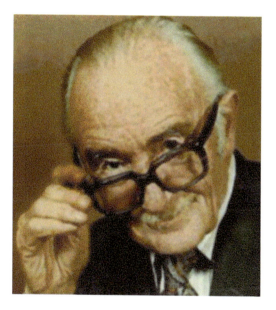

Figure 1.9   Archie Cochrane (1909–1988), who introduced the use of randomized controlled trials in epidemiology. Source: Cardiff University Library, Cochrane Archive, University Hospital Llandough.

1.2.2   Epidemiology today

Modern epidemiology has two key purposes: the development of epidemiological research methods and the production of biomedical knowledge by the application of these methods. Both have gained in strength enormously since World War II. By comparing recent and early editions of medical handbooks, you will discover what an enormous contribution epidemiology has made to our knowledge and understanding of the distribution of, explanatory factors of, and intervention options for major diseases, including ischemic heart disease, asthma, various types of cancer, and HIV/AIDS. The first book on epidemiological methodology was published in 1960; nowadays there are enough such books to fill a large bookcase. Novel study designs and data analysis methods have been developed over the past few decades to meet the needs of epidemiological practice. The rapid developments in science and information technology are also contributing to the development of the field, in particular:

- The incorporation of modern molecular biology techniques in epidemiological research, enabling not only phenotypes but also genotypes to be studied on a large scale. New developments in immunology, molecular biology, and genetics are being incorporated in epidemiological research: for example, using biomarkers (e.g. protein adducts containing exogenous toxins) instead of questionnaires to measure exposure. The study of individual genetic susceptibility will contribute to identifying the most vulnerable groups.
- Progress in clinical medicine, with a host of new diagnostic and treatment options and the adoption of evidence-based medicine.
- The rise of e-epidemiology – the use of digital media such as the internet, wearables, and mobile phones in epidemiology: for example, data collection through portable devices, recruitment through social media, predicting flu epidemics by analyzing Google search behavior and Twitter activity, and measuring air quality, personal physical activity, and food intake using personal wearables. These new methods have many advantages and are increasingly being seen as fully fledged alternatives to traditional methods. Nevertheless, we need to evaluate the internal and external validity of the findings they produce, safeguard privacy, and manage ethical issues related to new ways of recruiting participants and collecting data.
- Data have grown in variety, volume, and velocity. Big data, when properly tackled using epidemiological

methods have the potential to revolutionize how we identify and intervene on the explanatory factors of population health.

- Increasing awareness that human health depends to a large extent on the quality of the physical and social environment. That quality has deteriorated precisely due to human action; epidemiology is relevant for identifying and tackling the public health problems.
- Recently, the issues of health equity, social, and racial justice have been brought to the forefront of public health. Health equity is when all members of society have a fair and just opportunity to be as healthy as possible. This requires removing obstacles to health such as poverty, discrimination, and their consequences. Epidemiology can contribute to identifying important health disparities and implementing interventions, practices, and policies to reduce inequities.

1.3 Developments in the discipline itself

Specialization is growing in epidemiology, just as in every maturing scientific discipline. Content and methodological development are growing fast with separate attention being paid to improving methods for exposure monitoring, measurement quality, dose–response models, longitudinal designs, and so on. Epidemiologists are also specializing in specific topic areas, either focusing on a particular category of diseases (e.g. cancer epidemiology, infectious disease epidemiology, or the epidemiology of aging), a particular category of explanatory factors (e.g. nutritional epidemiology, genetic epidemiology, or pharmacoepidemiology), a particular application (e.g. clinical epidemiology or forensic epidemiology), or a particular method (e.g. prediction modeling, systematic reviews, or machine learning). These types of specialization are an inevitable consequence of the successful development of the discipline, but they also entail the risk of losing sight of the wood for the trees, with few scholars still being able to tackle a complex public health problem using a general approach, and not enough results of epidemiological research finding their way into healthcare practice.

Case 1.4 The third-generation oral contraceptive pill and the risk of venous thrombosis

Soon after the first oral contraceptives (OCP) were introduced in 1960, there were reports of increased risk of thrombotic events, resulting in the development of new types of contraceptive pills with a lower estrogen content (but containing more progestogens). The first-generation OCP was followed by a second and then a third generation, the aim being to reduce the risk of arterial thrombosis. An increased risk of venous thrombosis remained, however. The World Health Organization concluded in 1998 that users of modern oral contraceptives (containing 30–40 µg of estradiol) are at a three to six times higher risk of venous thrombosis than similar women who are not on the pill. It should be noted, however, that the absolute risk is still low, from less than one case of venous thrombosis per 10,000 person-years in women not using the pill to 3 to 6 cases per 10,000 person-years in women using it. A host of epidemiological studies – both cohort studies and case–control studies – have meanwhile been published comparing the risk of venous thrombosis from "third-generation" OCP with that from second-generation OCP. These show that venous thrombosis is 1.5–4.0 times more frequent in users of third-generation pills than in users of second-generation pills. The risk of venous thrombosis is highest in the first few years of using this type of pill, approximately one case per 1,000 in the first years of use. This is thought to be due to the progestogens in the third-generation OCP having an adverse effect on certain blood coagulation factors. The advice, based on these findings, is not to prescribe a third-generation OCP to new users of oral contraceptives.

Case 1.5 Prediction of live birth after IVF treatment

In-vitro fertilization (IVF) is a complex and costly assisted reproductive technology that involves a substantial emotional and physical burden for women and their families. Unfortunately, IVF treatment does not guarantee success. Couples would therefore like to know their prior probability of success before starting IVF treatment. The prediction models predict pregnancy followed by live birth after IVF are based on old data, and the model predictions often underestimate the clinical outcomes. These models include among other things the age of the women, previous pregnancies, and the use of donor cells. However, other factors associated with pregnancy outcome in women undergoing IVF, such as body-mass index (BMI), ovarian reserve, and ethnicity are not included in these models. Recently, data from a cohort study among 9915 women in the UK and Ireland derived and validated a novel prediction model of live birth for women undergoing IVF. The model includes age, duration of infertility, BMI, antral follicle count, previous miscarriage, previous live birth, cause of infertility and ethnicity. While the average probability of success in the cohort was 31.5%, individual predictions ranged between 18% and 41%, with overall good validity. This prediction model can be used to create a user-friendly decision aid to inform couples and their physicians about the likelihood of a successful pregnancy. The application of this new prediction model can increase the quality of the decisions and may reduce the number of unsuccessful IVF treatments.

Recommended reading

Bonita, R., Beaglehole, R., and Kjellstrom, T. (2006). *Basic Epidemiology*, 2e. Geneva: World Health Organization.

Carneiro, I. and Howard, N. (2005). *Introduction to Epidemiology*, 2e. Maidenhead: Open University Press.

Celentano, D.D., Szklo, M., and Gordis, L. (2019). *Gordis Epidemiology*, 6e. Philadelphia, PA: Elsevier. (Chapter 1).

Holland, W.W., Olsen, O., and du V Florey, C. (ed.) (2007). *The Development of Modern Epidemiology: Personal Reports from Those Who Were There*. Oxford: Oxford University Press.

Morabia, A. (2004). *A History of Epidemiologic Methods and Concepts*. Basel: Birkhäuser Verlag.

Szklo, M. and Nieto, F.J. (2019). *Epidemiology: Beyond the Basics*, 4e. Burlington, MA: Jones & Bartlett Learning. (Chapter 10).

Source references (cases)

Lind, J. (1957). *A Treatise of the Scurvy in Three Parts. Containing an Inquiry into the Nature, Causes and Cure of that Disease, Together with a Critical and Chronological View of What Has Been Published on the Subject*. London: A. Millar (Case 1.1).

LevRan, S., Roerecke, M., Le Foll, B. et al. (2014). The association between cannabis use and depression: a systematic review and meta-analysis of longitudinal studies. *Psychol. Med.* 44: 797–810. (Case 1.2).

Moitra, E., Bradley, J.A., and Stein, M.D. (2016). Reductions in cannabis use are associated with mood improvement in female emerging adults. *Depress. Anxiety* 33: 332–338. (Case 1.2).

Frost, W.H. (1936). *Snow on Cholera.* New York: The Commonwealth Fund (Case 1.3).

Vandenbroucke, J.P., Rosing, J., Bloemenkamp, K.W.M. et al. (2001). Oral contraceptives and the risk of venous thrombosis. *N. Engl. J. Med.* 344: 1527–1535. (Case 1.4).

Dhillon, R.K. (2016). Predicting the chance of live birth for women undergoing IVF: a novel pretreatment counselling tool. *Human Repr.* 31: 84–92. (Case 1.5).

Knowledge assessment questions

1. Are the following statements true or false?
1.1 Health outcomes are always binary (i.e. diseased or non-diseased).
1.2 Prevalence is a proportion.
1.3 Incidence is calculated using the number of new cases in the numerator.
1.4 All explanatory factors can be modified.
1.5 Deduction is the process by which one goes from theory to one or more hypotheses for testing.

2. Epidemiology, as defined in this chapter, would include which of the following activities? (select all that apply)
   A. Describe the demographic characteristics of persons with colorectal cancer in Denver, Colorado.
   B. Prescribe anti-hypertensive drugs to treat a patient with high blood pressure.
   C. Compare the demographic characteristics, family history, and environmental exposures of those with and without newly diagnosed glaucoma.
   D. Conduct a randomized study to compare two different surgical procedures for hip fractures.

3. John Snow's investigation of cholera is considered a model for epidemiological field investigations because it included a: (select all that apply)
   A. Biologically plausible hypothesis.
   B. Comparison of a health outcome among exposed and unexposed groups.
   C. Multivariate statistical modeling.
   D. Known biological mechanism.
   E. Recommendation for public health action.

Frequency

Textbook of Epidemiology, Second Edition. Lex Bouter, Maurice Zeegers and Tianjing Li.
© 2023 John Wiley & Sons Ltd. Published 2023 by John Wiley & Sons Ltd.
Companion website: www.wiley.com/go/Bouter/TextbookofEpidemiology

2.1 Definition of health outcomes

As the previous chapter made clear, epidemiology studies the frequency of health outcomes in human populations, usually in relation to one or more explanatory factors. In formal terms, this means estimating the epidemiological function.

$$P(O) = f(Fi)$$

The health outcome (O) is thus examined as the mathematical function of a set of k explanatory factors (F_i, where i = 1, . . ., k), often expressed as a linear relationship, although it could be any other kind of mathematical function. We shall go into the epidemiological function in more detail in subsequent chapters. This chapter focuses on the left-hand side of the equation, the outcome studied. This side of the equation is typically health-related, such as the occurrence of disease and the preservation or restoration of health or quality of life.

This chapter examines various measures of frequency used in epidemiology: prevalence, incidence, mortality, and some derived measures. The estimated frequency of an outcome in a population will depend directly on how the disease or health is defined and measured. Many different definitions of "health" can be found in the literature, the most familiar one being that of the World Health Organization (WHO): "A state of complete physical, mental and social well-being and not merely the absence of disease or infirmity."

In this definition, health is synonymous with well-being and defined in positive terms. This definition emphasizes that being "healthy" is more than simply the absence of disease. Health can also be viewed as dynamic and evolving. For example, health may refer to an individual's successful response to changing stresses and challenges from the environment. Seen in this way, ill health or disease is the result of going beyond an individual's limits of adaptability. This can be due to overload or reduced physical or psychological capacity. The concept of health is generally regarded as comprising a somatic, a mental, and a social component.

In epidemiological research, the term "health," "disease," or more generally "outcome" needs to be defined in a measurable form. The concept needs to be made specific and measurable for which there are three dimensions. The objective dimension focuses on the organic level ("disease," as in: I have a disease), insofar as that can be determined, for example, on the basis of a diagnosis made by a physician. The subjective dimension concerns the individual level ("illness," as in: I feel ill). This dimension pertains to people's perception of their own health, and closely relates to quality of life. The third dimension relates to the social level ("sickness," as in: I act sick). This dimension relates to behavior, for example, in the form of sickness absenteeism or use of healthcare facilities and resources.

When designing a research study, researchers typically select one particular dimension of health to focus. Measurements of health at the individual level can also be aggregated at the group level to give an impression of the health of the population. A specific measure of this dimension of health, or of a particular aspect of that dimension at the group level, is referred to as a health indicator. ◻ Figures 2.1 and 2.2 show examples of health indicators. Researchers and public health professionals consider numerous health indicators: infant mortality, number of confirmed COVID-19 cases, occurrence of diabetes, number of appendectomies, admissions to psychiatric hospitals, and use of sedatives are just a few examples.

2.2 Definition of disease

A disease is a pathophysiological response to internal or external factors. At a glance, it may seem that a particular disease is either present or not. This binary view is useful, both for medical research and in clinical practice. However, disease cannot usually be characterized dichotomously: the thresholds between disease and no disease are not always clearly defined. Instead, disease often manifests as a complex pattern of signs and symptoms. As such, a wide variety of severity is often found in a patient population. Also, individual patients usually go through various stages of severity as time passes.

We refer a disease pattern that changes over time as the course of a disease. ◻ Figure 2.3 shows a simplified outline of the course of a disease. In reality, many signs and symptoms will manifest differently in different patients. A diagnosis, therefore, is a crude simplification of the complex phenomena and is by no means fully objective. For this reason, diagnostic criteria must be standardized and made

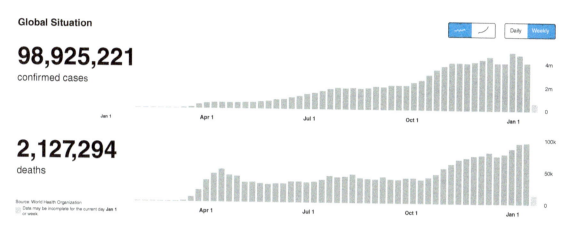

Figure 2.1 Confirmed coronavirus disease (COVID-19) cases and deaths reported to the World Health Organization (WHO) as of 26 January 2021.
Source: https://covid19.who.int.

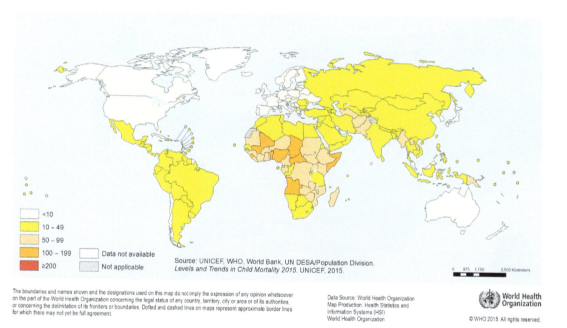

Figure 2.2 Under-five mortality rate, 2015.
Source: https://childmortality.org/.

specific and measurable, so that it is clear what is meant by a particular disease. The International Classification of Diseases (ICD), currently in its 11th revision (revised in January 2022), holds an important role in this process. What epidemiological researchers need is a detailed description of the diagnostic criteria used, ideally based on international standards.

Indicators of health are also reported in epidemiological studies. Investigators may measure, for example, limitations on activities, utilization of healthcare resources, sickness absenteeism, or

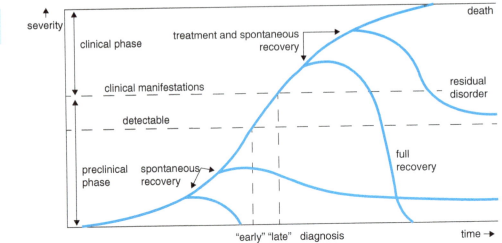

□ **Figure 2.3** Various possibilities for the course of a disease.

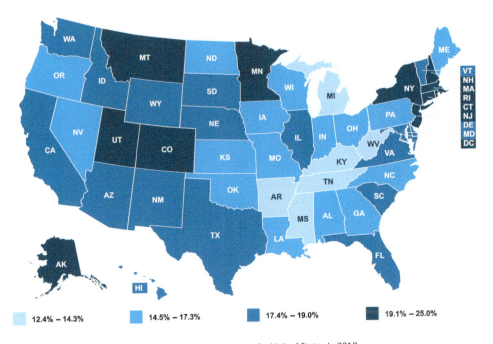

□ **Figure 2.4** Adult self-reported excellent health status in the United States in 2018.
Source: Kaiser Family Foundation's State Health Facts. https://bit.ly/3bRvQy3.

self-rated health to quantify disease. An example of the latter is □ Figure 2.4, which shows the percentage of people reporting having excellent health in the United States in 2018. The percentages of the population that reported excellent general health were higher in states coded in the darker color than states coded in the lighter color at the time of the survey.

Limitation of daily activities is a useful measure of the severity of a chronic condition in epidemiological research. Many standardized and validated instruments have been developed for this purpose, in the form of interviews, questionnaires, and observation scales, for example, those that focus on activities of daily living (ADL).

Many instruments also exist for measuring health-related quality of life, ranging from disease-specific (applicable to particular conditions and/or patient groups) to generic. These generic questionnaires can be applied across the board to all health problems, regardless of nature and severity. The most commonly used are the SF-36 (Medical Outcomes Study 36-Item Short Form Health Survey) and EQ5 (EuroQol-5) for measuring quality of life.

Indicators of disease or illness can relate to utilization of healthcare resources at the population level. Relatively poor health will be associated with increased demand for and use of resources. Utilization of medical care can be expressed in terms of frequency of use or in monetary terms. Another example of an indicator of illness is recorded sick leave, the idea being that the higher the absenteeism, the more illness is expected. In principle, this argument can apply to an individual or to the workforce of a particular industry. Sickness absenteeism is difficult to interpret, however, and probably not a particularly valid indicator of health, as there are many reasons for absenteeism that have nothing to do with the occurrence of disease (labor disputes, for instance). Many people who feel ill may also want to carry on working as long as they can, and therefore do not take sick leave.

2.3 Disease frequency: existing or new cases of disease

Epidemiologists focus on the occurrence of phenomena related to health in groups of people, namely the frequency with which particular health outcomes occur. They ascertain whether each individual has the outcome and then count the number of individuals with the outcome in the group as a whole. The two most commonly used measures are prevalence and incidence.

Prevalence is a proportion. It is defined as the number of persons with an outcome present in the population at a specified time, divided by the number of persons in the population at that time.

$$Prevalence = \frac{\begin{array}{c} No.\ of\ persons\ with\ an \\ outcome\ present\ in\ a \\ population\ at\ a\ specified\ time \end{array}}{\begin{array}{c} No.\ of\ persons\ in\ the \\ population\ at\ that \\ specified\ time \end{array}}$$

Incidence, on the other hand, relates to the number of persons developing an outcome during a specified period of time. The number of new cases is then divided by the number of persons who are at risk of developing the outcome during that period of time.

$$Incidence = \frac{\begin{array}{c} No.\ of\ new\ cases\ in\ a \\ population\ during\ a\ specified \\ period\ of\ time \end{array}}{\begin{array}{c} No.\ of\ persons\ who\ are\ at\ risk \\ of\ developing\ the\ outcome \\ during\ that\ period\ of\ time \end{array}}$$

2.4 Populations

Before delving into the various measures of frequency used in epidemiological research in more detail, let us first consider the types of population that can be identified and the importance of the concept of time.

2.4.1 Closed and open populations

Populations can be closed or open. Closed populations add no new members over time and lose members only due to death. Open populations may gain new members over time through immigration or birth, or lose members with time due to emigration or death.

The membership in an open population depends on a particular state and ends once the individual is no longer in that state. The population at risk is open to new members and the duration of membership is variable.

Examples of open populations:
1. Residents of Cape Town.
2. COVID-19 patients aged 65 or older in London.
3. Students at the Johns Hopkins University.

Unlike those of a closed population, the characteristics of an open population do not necessarily change with time. For example, the age structure of an open population may remain relatively constant, whereas a closed population always ages over time. The same can be true of the other characteristics of an open population. An open population of this kind is referred to as stable. The assumption that an open population is stable underlies the measures of frequency discussed below, and also the measures of association that we shall consider in Chapter 3. Different individuals will contribute to the experiences of an open population to varying degrees, as different people come and go.

2.4.2 Cohort

The term most commonly used for closed populations is a cohort, which refers to a group of persons with permanent group membership. Membership of a cohort is determined by a single defining event. "Once in a cohort, always in a cohort" is a succinct description of this principle. Although members of a cohort may be lost to follow-up (e.g. people move away from the study area or refuse to continue with the study), those lost to follow-up remain a member of the initial cohort. With this definition, the members of any cohort constitute a closed population along the time axis in which the defining event is taken as time zero (t_0).

Examples of cohorts:
1. Women recruited for a research study.
2. COVID-19 patients who have been treated with remdesvir.
3. All employees of WHO as of January 1, 2021.

For each individual there is a time (t_0) when he or she enters the cohort: this may be the same calendar time for every member of the cohort (as in Example 3), but this need not be the case (as in the other examples). The point at which events occur in a cohort is usually expressed in relation to t_0, i.e. in terms of follow-up time rather than calendar time. In case of a complete follow-up from t_0 to the end of the study, we know exactly what happened to each cohort member (in terms of outcomes of interest).

2.5 The concept of time

Time is a crucial concept when studying frequency of health outcome. Let us illustrate this with a few scenarios.

Measures of frequency, especially measures of incidence, are also measures of risk: they indicate the likelihood of people in the group developing the outcome of interest. Although the term "risk" or "likelihood of disease" is easy for most people to understand, it is often used carelessly. For example, if we read in the press that 60-year-old women have a 2% likelihood of dying of cardiovascular disease, it is impossible to interpret this number, as there is no indication of time. A 2% mortality risk for 60-year-old women would be very high if it relates to the next 24 hours, the next week or even the next year, whereas 2% would be very low if it relates to the mortality risk from cardiovascular disease during the remainder of life. Estimates of risk are impossible to interpret without an indication of time.

Obviously, the longer the time period the higher the risk of death. The theoretical value increases from 0% for a very short interval to 100% for a very long interval. This argument is just as true of any other risk. The way a disease risk changes with age can also differ markedly in different populations or for different conditions. The annual risk of chickenpox, for instance, rises sharply during the first few years of life but decreases substantially after childhood, whereas the risk of cardiovascular disease only starts to rise sharply in middle age.

If we follow a cohort over time to ascertain the frequency of an outcome, we have to contend with the problem that some of the cohort members will die from other causes or more generally, experience another event or outcome that would prevent them from developing the outcome of interest. This "competing risks" phenomenon will be negligible if the follow-up period is short, but it will cause problems of interpretation if we follow the cohort over a long period.

One solution to the problem of incomplete follow-up of the cohort is to sum up the time each individual contributes to the cohort. If a population is followed for 30 years and an individual in that population dies after 5 years, that person has contributed five person-years to the follow-up of the cohort. Other persons will have contributed more or fewer years, up to a maximum of 30. Using person-time in the dominator will yield incidence density (ID), a concept that we shall examine in detail in Section 2.6.2 of this chapter.

Epidemiological studies sometimes focus on an outcome that can occur more than once in an individual over the years: contraction of common cold, migraine headache, and urinary tract infection, for example. Researchers then need to decide whether to include only the first disease episode or also the second and any subsequent episodes. The information in the denominator then presents a challenge: which person-years of the individual cohort members count in such cases and which do not? Generally speaking, it is a good idea to apply the "at risk" concept and only count the person-time when the person was actually at risk of developing the outcome of interest. We should not count women's person-time when studying prostate cancer, for example.

If risks are expressed in terms of person-time, it is critical that time is precisely defined. Suppose we measure a disease frequency of 47 cases in a population of individuals who have together contributed 1580 person-months to the follow-up in the study. The disease frequency is then 47 per 1,580 person-months, i.e. 0.03 cases per person-month. We could just as well have expressed the disease frequency in person-years: 47 cases per 132 person-years, i.e. 0.36 cases per person-year. If we compare numbers of this kind across populations, but fail to consider the time units (which may not even be stated), we may well come to the wrong conclusions.

Sometimes, researchers are interested not in the disease frequency, but in the time to a particular event (e.g. the time to cancer relapse in a study of breast cancer). In such cases, the reciprocal of the disease frequency per unit of person-time, under certain assumptions, is what's called waiting time to an event. In the example above, with a disease frequency of 0.03 cases per person-month, the mean waiting time will be 1/0.03 = 33 months.

As these examples demonstrate, we need to be careful when using the concept of time in epidemiological research. This has given rise to various measures of disease frequency and derived measures. We need to include the relevant time dimension in every calculation and interpretation. Another take-home message is that measures of frequency provide little information without an understanding of how the study was designed and how the outcome data were collected.

2.6 Measures of outcome frequency

2.6.1 Prevalence: existing cases

The proportion of the population where a particular outcome is present at a particular time is referred to as the prevalence of that outcome. For example, the prevalence of influenza is the percentage of influenza

cases at a particular time in the population of interest, regardless of whether we are looking at a cohort or an open population. Prevalence implies a cross-section of the population, a snapshot. The snapshot may be taken at any specified time point.

By way of illustration, ◘ Figure 2.5 shows the occurrence of a condition in a cohort of 10 persons in six years from t_0. This is a nonfatal condition that can occur more than once in the same person. The prevalence of the condition in question is 40%, 20%, and 20% in years 2, 4, and 6, respectively.

Similarly, we can study the prevalence cross-sectionally of an open population except that, in this case, the total number of persons in the population can differ from one moment to the next. ◘ Figure 2.6 shows an open population: here, the prevalence of the disease in question is 43%, 25%, and 75% in years 2, 4, and 6 respectively.

In addition to point prevalence, another type of prevalence is period prevalence, the proportion of the population that had the outcome of interest during a particular period. The important aspect is that every person represented by the numerator had the outcome of interest at some time during the period specified. In ◘ Figure 2.5, for instance, 70% of the cohort had the condition in question at least once during the first four years of the follow-up period. If we examine in a cross-section of a population whether a particular outcome has ever been present in an individual up to that time, that is referred to as the lifetime prevalence. An example is the percentage of a company's workforce who have ever had an industrial accident by the time they reach retirement age.

If we need to calculate the period prevalence in an open population, we first have to calculate the mean number of persons in the population in that period. In ◘ Figure 2.6, for instance, the period prevalence from years 4 to 6 year is 5/6 = 83%. As we can also see from ◘ Figures 2.5 and 2.6, the point prevalence of a condition will depend on both the number of new cases that develop as time passes and the mean duration of the condition. Prevalent cases constitute a heterogenous group: on one hand, they have survived the condition so far, but also have not been cured. Because of this selection effect, prevalent cases are less suited to study the causes of diseases (etiological epidemiology). When it comes to determining the demand for healthcare services and the burden on available resources, however, prevalence is usually just what we need.

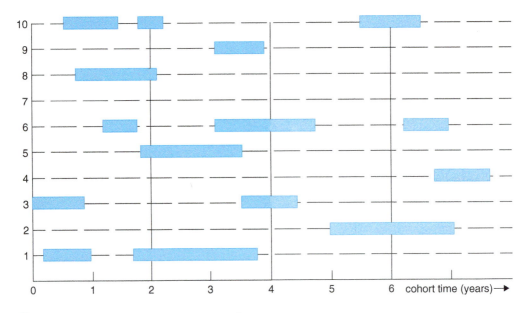

Figure 2.5 Prevalence of a condition in a cohort of 10 persons.

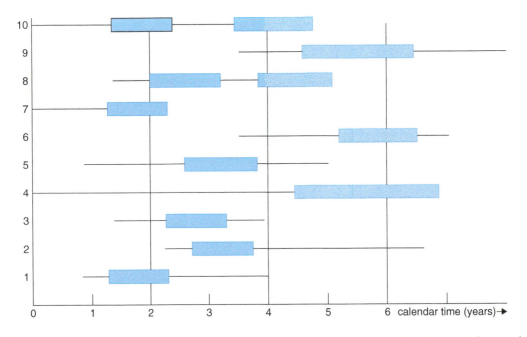

Figure 2.6 Prevalence of a condition in a dynamic population of 10 persons. Animation of measures of disease frequency. Source: Bas Verhage. http://bit.ly/1tGnFSv.

$$\text{Period prevalence in an open population} = \frac{\begin{array}{c}\textit{No. of cases present}\\\textit{in a population during}\\\textit{a certain time period}\end{array}}{\begin{array}{c}\textit{Mean no. of the}\\\textit{population}\\\textit{(average between start}\\\textit{and end of the period)}\end{array}}$$

2.6.2 Incidence: new cases

Epidemiologists usually prefer to ascertain the frequency of new cases of a disease. This entails following a population for some time and identifying new cases that occur during that period. Incidence refers to the occurrence of new cases of disease in a population over a specified period of time. We can study the incidence of first heart attacks, for example, as well as that of second or subsequent heart attacks. Incidence is by definition estimated in populations where all members are, in principle, candidates for or are at risk of the event. We can only track down the incidence of first heart attacks in a population of individuals who have not yet had a heart attack. Similarly, we could study the incidence of second heart attacks in a population who have had a heart attack and survived it.

The relationship between incidence and prevalence

There is a dynamic relationship between incidence and prevalence. The prevalence in a population increases when there are more new cases added (through incidence) or when people with the condition live longer. The prevalence decreases when the disease is cured, or people die more rapidly. Curing a disease and death have the same effect on prevalence: they reduce the number of individuals with the disease in the population and thus lower prevalence. As an example, the incidence of HIV in the United States has been reduced by more than two-thirds since the height of the HIV epidemic in early 1980s. However, the prevalence of people living with HIV in the United States has increased steadily between 1980 and 2010 because of effective anti-virus treatment (◘ Figure 2.7).

Prevalence does not take into account the duration of disease. When the prevalence is low (less than 10%) and in a "steady state" situation (the prevalence is constant because the incidence is in equilibrium with cure and mortality), we can estimate the prevalence from the product of the mean disease duration and the ID (described in ◘ Figure 2.7):

Prevalence = Incidence density × Duration of disease

From this equation, we can infer that higher prevalence of a condition in a population (in comparison to another) may not because the risk of getting the disease is higher, but because affected people survive longer or recover slower.

Cumulative incidence

Calculating the cumulative incidence (CI) essentially involves following all the members of a cohort for a period of time. The period could, for instance, be 1, 5, or 10 years from time t_0, which is usually a different calendar time for different members of the cohort. At time t_0, all members of the cohort are by definition at risk for the outcome of interest, i.e. susceptible to the condition in question and hence as yet free from it at t_0. The CI comprises the proportion of cohort members (at t_0) who develop the condition during the follow-up. It is therefore a proportion with minimum

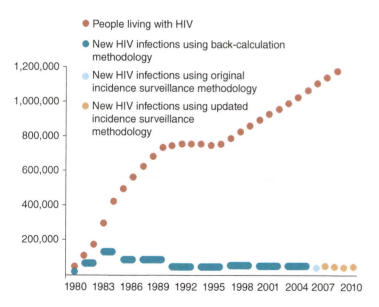

◘ **Figure 2.7** HIV prevalence and incidence in the United States, 1980–2010. Source: https://bit.ly/3Afd0ZZ.

2

and maximum values of 0 and 1 (0% and 100%), respectively.

$$Cumulative \atop incidence = \frac{No.\ of\ new\ cases\ in\ a\ population \atop during\ a\ specified\ time\ period}{No.\ of\ persons\ at\ risk\ in\ the\ population \atop at\ the\ start\ of\ that\ period}$$

In order to interpret a CI, we need to know the length of period to which it relates. A problem with interpretation is the implicit assumption that there will not be any competing diseases or causes of death. This assumption is usually unjustified, especially in the case of long follow-up periods.

The proportion of the cohort still at risk for developing the outcome under consideration will eventually fall right down to zero, at which point, it would be pointless to continue calculating CI. For this reason, the ID instead of CI is often used as the measure of frequency in long-term cohort studies. The length of the period to which the CI relates can be either variable or fixed, depending on how the end is defined. Here are some examples of both:

Variable period:
1. Lifetime incidence of prostate cancer.
2. Hospital mortality of patients with a heart attack.

Fixed period:
1. Five-year incidence of second heart attack in persons with a non-fatal first heart attack.
2. Ten-year survival rate following successful surgery of women with metastatic breast cancer affecting the axillary lymph nodes.

Note that the CI can also be regarded as the individual risk of a member of the cohort at time t_0 of developing the outcome of interest during the follow-up period. If the CI of second heart attacks within five years is 10%, that is the average risk of having a second heart attack after having (and surviving) the first heart attack in the next 5 years. Note that this is the average risk, which needs to be modified if relevant characteristics of the individual are taken into consideration. The risk will be substantially higher, for instance, if we know that the person is a persistent heavy smoker aged 75 with high blood pressure.

Incidence density

If we cannot follow every person over time, we have to fall back on an open population to ascertain the risk at

which new cases occur. In an open population, the occurrence of the event itself is one of the mechanisms by which individuals are removed from the population at risk. For example, persons who have already been admitted to a hospital with a heart attack no longer form part of the open population of persons who would be admitted to that hospital in the event of a heart attack. Incidence in an open population is expressed not in relation to the number of members at a particular time (as in the case of a cohort) but in relation to the total person-time at risk that is observed (usually expressed in person-years). The resulting measure is referred to as the ID, incidence rate or hazard rate. The dimension is 1 per year (year^{-1}) and its value will be between zero and infinity.

The ID is calculated by dividing the number of new cases by the number of person-years observed: for example, identifying 15 cases of bladder cancer in an open population where 5,000 person-years are observed yields an ID of 0.003 per year. We cannot tell from this calculation whether an average of 100 persons were followed for an average of 50 years or an average of 500 persons for an average of 10 years. ID is a measure of the speed at which new cases of the disease occur in the population. Note that people are only at risk of the condition under consideration for relevant person-time: the ID of sports injuries is expressed per 100 sports hours and that of accidents at work per 1,000 working days, for instance.

$$Incidence\ density = \frac{No.\ of\ new\ cases \atop during\ a\ specified\ time\ period}{No.\ of\ person-time\ at \atop risk\ during\ the\ same \atop time\ period}$$

ID cannot be translated directly into an individual risk during a particular period. Given certain assumptions, however, it is possible to calculate the CI (for a hypothetical cohort) from the ID in an open population. Assuming that the ID is constant over the period in question, in the case of short-time intervals, the CI can be estimated from the product of the ID and the duration of the time interval.

Many health statistics are incidence figures based on an open population. Recorded frequencies of events are usually expressed in relation to demographic statistics (e.g. number of residents of a region by age and gender at a particular time). Examples are the annual incidence of syphilis in

Berlin; the monthly incidence of influenza among those aged 65 or over in Melbourne; the annual incidence of breast cancer in women aged over 40 in India. With statistics of this kind, it is not clear whether all the recorded events actually occurred in the open population for which the incidence is calculated. For example, patients who live elsewhere could end up in a hospital by chance (while traveling or on holiday) or intentionally (because the hospital specializes in treating the condition in question). The size and structure of the population can also fluctuate. An open population is usually not completely stable, and we have to rely on the quality of available demographic data.

2.6.3 Mortality: a special type of incidence

Mortality is the incidence of death, so everything we have said earlier about calculating the CI and ID also applies to the corresponding mortality. Analytical epidemiology uses both CI and ID, depending on the study design. In descriptive epidemiology, questions are often but not always formulated in terms of CI.

$$\text{Cumulative incidence of mortality} = \frac{\text{No. of deaths in a population during a specified time period}}{\text{No. of persons in the population at the start of the period}}$$

Mortality is probably the most commonly used indicator of public health; the argument being that when mortality is low the population must be healthy. This argument, however, is not always correct. The validity of mortality as a health indicator depends on the type of health problems under consideration. Conditions that are not often fatal but can cause substantial long-term impairments and disabilities cannot be characterized fully using this indicator. Another reason for the popularity of mortality as a health indicator at the aggregate level is that recording deaths is relatively reliable and straightforward. Many countries have been doing this for considerable time. Comparing mortality is often the only way to compare the health of different countries. Various measures of mortality can be found in publications on descriptive epidemiological research and health statistics, some of which are described below.

Crude mortality

A crude mortality describes the number of deaths during a period (usually one year) in a population. It is usually expressed per 100,000 persons. These numbers can be calculated for different periods and different populations. ◻ Table 2.1 shows an example. The crude mortality in index population A is $(50+4)/(10{,}000+1{,}000)$ = $54/11{,}000$ = $491/100{,}000$. The crude mortality in index population B is $(5+40)/(1{,}000+10{,}000)$ = $45/11{,}000$ = $409/100{,}000$. The crude mortalities in the two index populations are different; however, it is misleading to compare these two numbers directly because the age distribution between the two populations is different.

Other types of age-specific mortality are shown in ◻ Table 2.2. These too are calculated over a particular period and expressed, e.g. per 10,000 or

◻ **Table 2.1**   Example of direct standardization of mortality (expressed per 100,000 per year).

Age		Index population A	Index population B	Standard population
Young	Deaths	50	5	55
	Size	10,000	1,000	11,000
Old	Deaths	4	40	44
	Size	1,000	10,000	11,000
Total	Deaths	54	45	99
	Size	11,000	11,000	22,000
Crude mortality rate		491/100,000	409/100,000	450/100,000
Standardized mortality rate		450/100,000	450/100,000	450/100,000

2

Table 2.2   A selection of age-specific measures of mortality, as defined by the World Health Organization

Perinatal mortality	Stillbirth or death to live births within the first 7 days of life after a pregnancy duration of at least 22 completed weeks
Neonatal mortality	Death occurring during the first 4 weeks after birth
Early neonatal mortality	Death between 0 and 6 days after birth
Late neonatal mortality	Death between 7 and 27 days after birth
Infant mortality	Death occurring within the first year of life
Under-five mortality	Death occurring within the first 5 years of life
Post neonatal mortality	Death between 1 and 59 months
Adolescent mortality	Death between 10 and 19 years

100,000 persons. The WHO regards the age-specific mortality in the first year of life shown in ▢ Table 2.2 as a good indicator of the quality of healthcare as a whole, especially in low-income countries. Maternal mortality is also often used. It captures the risk of deaths among women due to complications during pregnancy or soon after delivery. Maternal mortality is not an age-specific but a cause-specific mortality.

Age-specific mortality
Mortality is usually specified for particular age groups. 5, 10, and 15-year age groups are generally used, depending on the size of the population for which they are calculated and the purpose.

Direct and indirect standardization
To compare the health of different populations with different age structures, we will need to aggregate the age-specific mortalities for each of the populations into a single number. This is in effect what happens when we calculate a standardized mortality (i.e. standardized for age). There are two ways of standardizing.

Direct standardization for age involves applying the age-specific mortality of the population in question (the index population) to the age distribution of a selected standard population. The result is the expected mortality in the standard population had the age-specific mortality for the index population been applied. The example in ▢ Table 2.1 compares two index populations using one common standard population. Here, the standard population has simply been calculated as the sum of the two populations.

The expected number of deaths in the standard population based on the age-specific mortality in index population A is $(50/10,000 \times 11,000) + (4/1,000 \times 11,000) = 99$. The standardized mortality in this population is therefore: $99/(11,000 + 11,000) = 450/100,000$. The standardized mortality for population B is calculated similarly: $(5/1,000 \times 11,000) + (40/10,000)/(11,000 + 11,000) = 450/100,000$. After standardizing for age, the difference in mortality between two populations disappears completely in this example.

When comparing different countries or regions within a country, the combined population is usually taken as the standard population, as in ▢ Table 2.1. When studying trends over time, the demographic structure at the start or in the middle of the period for which the mortality is compared are usually taken as the standard. Standardization can, in principle, be applied to other factors besides age, but this is no longer common practice, as the multivariable analysis has enabled simultaneous adjustments for differences in multiple factors.

In order to carry out direct standardization, we need to have sufficient numbers of events in each age group in the index population. The numbers must not be too small, as this will make the estimates of the expected numbers of death too imprecise. This was not a problem in the example in ▢ Table 2.1, but it often is a problem in practice. An alternative way of comparing mortalities in two populations is to apply the age-specific mortality found in the standard population (which is usually sufficiently precise) to the age structure of an index population. The result is the expected mortality in the index population if the age-specific mortality figures for the standard population were to apply. This method is referred to as indirect standardization.

Using the numbers in ◻ Table 2.3, we can take a male population in 2014 as the standard population. Based on the number of deaths in that year in each age group we calculate the mortality per 100,000 men for each group. These mortality figures are shown in column 2 of ◻ Table 2.3. Column 3 of the table shows the numbers of men in each age group in the index population for 2012. Multiplying the mortality figures with the numbers in columns 2 and 3, we arrive at column 4, the number of deaths for each of these age groups that we could have expected in 2012, had the mortality for 2014 been applied. The sum of these numbers 9,263 is the total number of deaths expected for 2012 if the mortality were the same in that year as in 2014 (the indirect standardized mortality). The crude mortality in 2012 was 13,319. The crude mortality in the index population divided by the indirect standardized mortality gives us the standardized mortality ratio (SMR). The SMR in the example is 13,319/9,263 = 1.44.

◻ **Table 2.3** Example of indirect standardization of mortality (expressed per 100,000 per year).

Age (years)	Mortality per 100 000 men in 2014	Number of men in 2012	Number of deaths expected for 2012
0–24	0.1	2,990,488	3
25–29	0.8	552,556	4
30–34	4.7	444,516	21
35–39	15.5	402,241	63
40–44	37.8	387,333	147
45–49	71.5	365,953	262
50–54	132.2	335,549	444
55–59	249.2	303,004	755
60–64	381.1	269,132	1,026
65–69	630.0	223,720	1,409
70–74	940.3	164,614	1,548
75–79	1,378.2	111,897	1,542
80–84	1,793.8	63,661	1,142
85+	2,550.3	35,207	898
Total	156.2	6,649,871	9,263

This SMR is indicative of 44% "excess mortality" in the index population compared with the standard.

In principle, indirect standardized mortality, and therefore SMRs, for different index populations should not be compared, as they relate to different populations. If the differences in age structure are not too big, however, the resulting error will remain within bounds.

Cause-specific mortality

As an indicator, mortality is far too rough and not suitable for epidemiological research into the causes and effects of disease. Mortality is therefore often provided separately for different causes, either standardized for age or not. Such figures are usually based on the records of causes of death that are required in many countries. We have already mentioned one example of cause-specific mortality, namely maternal mortality. Other examples are cancer mortality, mortality due to road accidents, and mortality from suicide. How useful such cause-specific mortalities are will depend on the validity and reliability of the records on the cause of death. In many cases, the cause of death is not immediately obvious. First, the correct diagnosis is not always made before death, and autopsies are rarely carried out. Second, the primary cause of death recorded is often the result of complex reasoning. The condition that caused the series of events resulting in death needs to be determined, and this determination is not straightforward, especially in the elderly, who often suffer from multiple chronic conditions (comorbidity). The International Classification of Disease, or a simplified version thereof, is generally used when recording causes of death.

Case fatality

The case fatality is the proportion of the incident cases with a particular condition who die of that condition during a period.

$$\frac{Case}{fatality} = \frac{No.\ of\ deaths\ from\ the\ condition}{No.\ of\ incident\ cases\ of\ a\ condition}$$

This measure reflects the combination of the severity of the condition and the efficacy of the healthcare provided. The case fatality is highly dependent on the severity of the condition and how cases are ascertained. As an example, although the case fatality of home births is lower than that of hospital deliveries, concluding that giving birth at home is safer, this is flawed because the anticipated childbirth-related complications are indications for hospital delivery. In other words, women who deliver at hospitals are at higher risk of childbirth-related complications on average than those who deliver at home. In another example, the case fatality for COVID-19 is likely over-estimated because many asymptomatic cases are not identified.

In effect, the case fatality is the cause-specific mortality among the incident cases of the condition. The case fatality is expressed as a CI of cause-specific mortality, but the period to which it relates is not always clearly specified. Take the case fatality of heart and lung transplants, for instance: this can, in theory, relate either to mortality due to the operation itself or to mortality from complications in the operating room, during subsequent hours or days, during the stay in hospital, during the year after the operation, or during the entire remainder of life. As this example shows, case fatality is not always easy to interpret.

Proportional mortality

The proportional mortality is the proportion of total mortality in a population due to a particular condition.

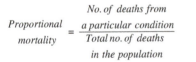

$$\begin{matrix} Proportional \\ mortality \end{matrix} = \frac{\begin{matrix} No.\,of\ deaths\ from \\ a\ particular\ condition \end{matrix}}{\begin{matrix} Total\ no.\,of\ deaths \\ in\ the\ population \end{matrix}}$$

It can be expressed not only in relation to deaths due to all causes but also in relation to a subset of all causes. For instance, mortality from prostate cancer can be expressed either in relation to total deaths or in relation to total deaths from cancer. Proportional mortality figures are difficult to interpret because differences in estimates can be due to differences in the frequency and fatality of the condition under consideration as well as the frequency and fatality of all other conditions. For example, the proportional mortality due to accidents is approximately 40% for one to four-year-olds and approximately 2% for 70–75-year-olds. However, far more elderly people than children die due to accidents. Because of such possible misinterpretations, cause-specific mortality is generally preferred.

Life expectancy

Life expectancy is the mean number of years of life expected at birth. It is calculated based on the age-specific mortality for the successive age groups at the time of birth. If the age-specific mortality improves as a result of improvements in healthcare, the mean life expectancy calculated at birth will be an underestimate. Likewise, the remaining life expectancy at any age can be calculated by applying the age-specific mortality following that age. Interestingly, a man who had a life expectancy of 83 years at birth may have a further life expectancy of 24 years at age 65. The reason for this is that, by the age of 65, he has already survived 65 years, thus increasing the likelihood of living a longer life.

Survival

The complement of the case fatality is survival: the proportion of individuals with a particular condition who are still alive after a certain period. Common examples are the 5-year and 10-year survival of cancer patients after treatment. Here again, there is a strong dependency on the disease spectrum: lung cancer patients who are diagnosed through annual X-ray exams have a far better five-year survival than those who are referred to a pulmonologist with symptoms, for example.

We can draw a survival curve, which plots survival against time since diagnosis or some other logical starting point. ◘ Figure 2.8 shows an example of

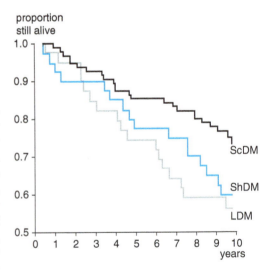

◘ **Figure 2.8** Survival curves for patients with Diabetes Mellitus (DM) by disease duration. ScDM: patients detected by means of screening. ShDM: patients with a short disease duration of 6.2 years or less. LDM: patients with a long disease duration of over 6.2 years.

survival curves for patients with diabetes with different duration of disease. We can use the survival curve to read off the surviving proportion for any time period. Survival is the converse of the CI of mortality.

There are various methods for estimating survival curves. The method described by Kaplan–Meier is often used in epidemiology. This involves recalculating the proportion of "survivors" each time a member of the cohort dies or experiences the event of interest. The advantage of the survival curve approach is that it shows not only the proportion of individuals with outcome of interest at a particular time but also the time trajectory (in this case of mortality, but it can also be used for other outcomes such as disability, cure, or pregnancy).

Quality-adjusted and disability-adjusted life years

We can also consider quality of life as a health metric. To do this, we assign a value to years of life expected: this weighting factor, or utility, usually ranges from 0 to 1. A utility of 0.75 (3/4) suggests that we regard four years of life spent in the state at issue as interchangeable with three years of life in full health. This enables us to calculate life expectancy adjusted for quality, expressed as quality-adjusted life years (QALYs). Various methods have been developed to estimate utility, which is beyond the scope of this book. The QALY concept is gaining popularity for use at the aggregate level, e.g. for cost-utility analyses.

In public health, similar measures are used, for example, healthy life expectancy and disability-adjusted life years (DALYs). DALYs is a measure of the number of years lost due to ill-health: it is the sum of the number of years lost due to death (lost years of life) and the healthy years "lost" due to living with a disease. We can use DALYs to compare diseases in terms of their effect on public health, as they are calculated based on four important factors: the number of people suffering from the disease, the severity of the disease, mortality from it, and the age at which death occurs. To account for the severity of the disease, weighting factors are used to "weigh" the years spent with the disease. For example, a weighting factor of 0.5 for a particular disease means that 1 year of life with that disease is regarded as equivalent to 0.5 years lost due to premature death.

There are other variations on this theme. Healthy life expectancy is the mean number of years of life that people can expect to spend "in good health." This measure of health combines life expectancy and quality of life in a single number, using indicators for such as life expectancy in good self-rated health (Healthy Life Expectancy [HLE]), disability-free life expectancy (DFLE), and life expectancy in good mental health (Mental Health Lived Experience [MHLE]).

2.7 Continuous measures of health outcomes

The outcome in epidemiological research is often expressed on a dichotomous scale (e.g. disease versus no disease). The distribution of an outcome in the population can then be described simply based on the numbers or proportion of people with the outcome. Many aspects of health and disease, however, are not measured on a dichotomous scale but on a continuous scale. For example, blood pressure, lung function, hearing loss, cognitive function, severity of pain, and quality of life would all be measured continuously. Each of these variables could easily be reduced to a dichotomous variable (e.g. hypertension yes/no, quality of life good/poor). However, there can be valuable information in a continuous scale. In such cases, the continuous variable should be incorporated into the epidemiological function as the outcome variable: the left-hand side of the function is then not the frequency of the outcome (calculated as a proportion or a rate) but the mean (or other measures of central tendency) of the variable in question. The form of the function also changes and becomes a linear model instead of a logistic model (see Chapter 3). Case 2.1 gives a simplified example of a linear regression function of this kind and how it can be used to study the association between various prognostic factors and outcome (change in functional limitations) in people with acute or chronic low back pain.

The distribution of a continuous outcome can be summarized in two measures, one for the central value around which the observed results cluster and one for the spread in the observations.

Examples of measures of central tendency:
- mean, i.e. the sum of all the measured values divided by the number of values
- median, i.e. the value at which 50% of the measurements are higher and 50% are lower
- mode, i.e. the measured value that occurs most frequently.

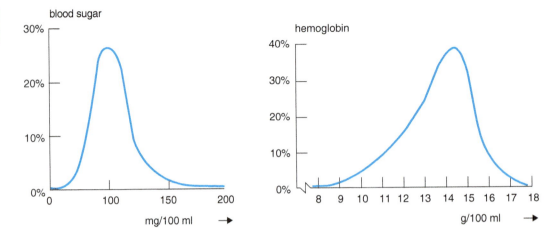

Figure 2.9 Examples of frequency distributions of clinical parameters in the general population: blood glucose and hemoglobin.

Examples of measures of spread:

- standard deviation (SD): a measure of how far each individual observation is from the mean
- interpercentile range: an area marked by two values containing a certain percentage of the observations
- range: the distance between the largest and smallest measures.

Which measures of central tendency and spread to use will depend on the scale on which the variable is measured and the shape of the distribution.

Figure 2.9 shows an approximation of the distribution of two biological measures – blood glucose and blood hemoglobin. Although the natural distribution of many clinical measures approximates the normal distribution (the Gaussian curve), it rarely coincides precisely. The normal distribution is a theoretical distribution with unique statistical properties, the most important of which is symmetry: i.e. a fixed percentage of the observations are in the area between one, two, or more SDs from the mean value (X ± 1 SD = approx. 68%; X ± 2 SD = approx. 95%; X ± 3 SD = approx. 99%). Many biological variables, however, including blood glucose and hemoglobin, have a distribution that is unimodal (one peak value) and asymmetrical (skewed due to an excess of high or low values).

A prerequisite for using a continuous variable as the outcome in many epidemiological studies and analysis are that it should roughly follow a normal distribution. Skewed distributions can often be "normalized" by applying a transformation to the original scale, either a logarithmic transformation (ln = natural logarithm), a root transformation or some other type of transformation, depending on shape of the distribution.

Case 2.1 Predicting Symptoms in People with Acute Versus Chronic Low Back Pain

A study by Grotle et al. investigated whether there were differences in factors predictive of unfavorable symptoms in people with acute low back pain and people with chronic low back pain. The outcome measure was the score after 12 months on the Roland Morris Disability Questionnaire (RMDQ, range 0–24), a 24-item questionnaire that measures the severity of functional limitations due to back pain. The outcome was treated as continuous and the association with various prognostic factors was examined using linear regression analysis. The study was carried out on participants recruited from general practices in Staffordshire in England, of whom 258 reported transient (acute) low back pain and 668 chronic low back pain. A number of potential prognostic factors were examined. ◻ Table 2.4 shows the results of analyzing two factors: the presence of radiating pain (below the knee) and a high score for fear of pain.

The epidemiological function will have looked like this:

$$RMDQ_{12m} = \beta_0 + \beta_1 \left(F_x \right)$$

where F_x represents the presence or absence of certain explanatory factors, which is often coded as 0 for participants without that factor (i.e. who do not report radiating pain or score low for fear of pain) and as 1 for participants with that factor. The intercept (β_0) indicates the outcome – the RMDQ score after 12 months – for participants without that factor. The regression coefficient (β_1) indicates the difference in outcome between people with the factor and those who without.

From the table, we can read off that the difference for radiating pain is 3.18 points (confidence interval 1.85–4.51) among participants with acute back pain and 3.60 points on the RMDQ (confidence interval 2.61, 4.59) in the case of chronic back pain. The confidence interval captures the uncertainty about the estimates, which will be introduced in Chapter 5. The presence of radiating pain at the time of inclusion, then, based on this analysis, is associated with more severe functional limitations after 12 months, and this association is approximately equally strong among participants with acute and participants with chronic low back pain. The association is statistically significant because the confidence interval does not include the null value of no difference.

However, the investigators state that various factors could confound this association. The difference in limitations could be explained partly by the fact that people with radiating pain also have a higher pain score at baseline, or that they are older, or that more of them are women. The investigators have therefore expanded the epidemiological function to adjust for potential confounding by age, gender, and severity of pain at baseline:

$$RMDQ_{12m} = \beta_0 + \beta_1 \left(F_x \right) + \beta_2 \left(age \right)$$
$$+ \beta_3 \left(gender \right) + \beta_4 \left(pain\ score\ at\ baseline \right)$$

The adjusted regression coefficient β_1 indicates the difference in outcome taking the influence of these confounders into account. ◻ Table 2.4 shows that the association between radiating pain and functional limitations after 12 months is much smaller and no longer statistically significant in participants with acute as well as in participants with chronic low back pain. The difference is less than 1 point on the RMDQ and the confidence interval now covers zero.

The same analysis was carried out on "fear of pain." Even after adjusting for confounding, this factor was still found to be statistically significantly associated with the severity of limitations after 12 months, although the differences after adjustment were smaller. Fear of pain was found to be a stronger prognostic factor in the case of participants with acute low back pain (adjusted difference of 1.73 on the RMDQ) than in the case of those with chronic low back pain (adjusted difference of 1.03).

◻ Table 2.4 Analysis of the prognostic factor "radiating pain" and "fear of pain."

Prognostic factor	Acute low back pain (n = 258)		Chronic low back pain (n = 668)	
	Crude regression coefficient (β_1)	Adjusted[a] regression coefficient (β_1)	Crude regression coefficient (β_1)	Adjusted[a] regression coefficient (β_1)
Radiating pain	3.18 (1.85, 4.51)	0.82 (−0.46, 2.10)	3.60 (2.61, 4.59)	0.73 (−0.09, 1.55)
Fear of pain	3.46 (1.93, 4.99)	1.73 (0.31, 3.15)	2.97 (1.77, 4.18)	1.03 (0.04, 2.02)

[a]Adjusted for age, gender and severity of back pain at the time of inclusion.

2

Recommended reading

Celentano, D.D., Szklo, M., and Gordis, L. (2019). *Gordis Epidemiology*, 6e. Philadelphia, PA: Elsevier. (Chapters 3 and 4).

Rothman, K.J., Lash, T.L., VanderWeele, T.J., and Haneuse, S. (2021). *Modern Epidemiology*, 4e. Philadelphia: Wolters Kluwer. (Chapter 3).

Szklo, M. and Nieto, F.J. (2019). *Epidemiology: Beyond the Basics*, 4e. Burlington, Massachusetts: Jones & Bartlett Learning. (Chapter 2).

Source Reference (Case 2.1)

Grotle, M., Foster, F., Dunn, K., and Croft, P. (2010). Are prognostic indicators for poor outcome different for acute and chronic low back pain consulters in primary care? *Pain* 151 (3): 790–797.

Knowledge assessment questions

1. The figure below shows the number of COVID-19 deaths in Sweden, by age groups (as of February 2, 2021). (Source: https://bit.ly/3K0AC96)

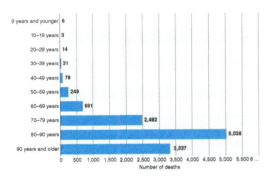

1.1 Which age group has the highest number of deaths?
1.2 Based on this figure, can you tell which group has the highest mortality?
1.3 What additional piece(s) of information will you need in order to calculate age-specific mortality?
1.4 What additional piece(s) of information will you need in order to calculate age-specific case fatality?
2. Which of the following is NOT a proportion? (Select the one best answer)
   a. Prevalence
   b. Incidence density
   c. Proportional mortality
   d. Case fatality
3. A South Korean university releases a report that they have seen a dramatic rise in depressive symptoms among students in recent years. They have observed a total of 1800 students reporting depressive symptoms in 2019, with 780 students reporting newly developed symptoms in 2020. If the enrollment at the start 2019 was 35,007 (and there are no drop outs or new admissions), what was the cumulative incidence of new cases reporting depressive symptoms in 2020?

4. Investigators successfully recruited 35 individuals at risk for flu into their study but lost five individuals to follow up after two weeks and four more at week 4. Five cases of flu have been reported at the end of week 6. Calculate the incidence density (also known as incidence rate) of the flu outbreak using appropriate person-time measures.
5. The figure below shows the age distribution of disabilities in the United States (US) in 2016. Which of the following statement(s) is/are correct? (Select all that apply)(Figure source: https://bit.ly/2EL1msH)

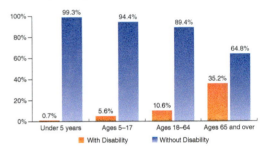

   a. The percentage of people with disabilities is highest among those aged 65 and over
   b. There is an age-related increase in the risk of disabilities
   c. The percentage of people with disabilities increases with age
   d. Most individuals with disabilities are aged of 65 and over
6. The table below gives information on two towns – Dragonstone and Winterfell – in the year 10,000 BCE.

Age group (years)	Dragonstone Population	# of deaths	Winterfell Population	# of deaths
0–20	4,000	350	6,000	400
21–40	5,000	500	10,000	700
41+	3,000	150	12,000	1,000

6.1 What is the crude mortality in Dragonstone in 10,000 BCE?
6.2 Using the direct adjustment method and the combined populations of Dragonstone and Winterfell as the standard population, what is the age-adjusted mortality in Dragonstone in 10,000 BCE?
6.3 There were 40 deaths observed among the silversmiths at King's Landing. Using the indirect method and the data below, calculate the standardized mortality ratio (SMR) for silversmiths with the combined population as the comparison population.

Age group (years)	Combined population Population	# of deaths	Age-specific number of silversmiths
0–20	10,000	750	100
21–40	15,000	1,200	200
41+	15,000	1,150	150

Association

Textbook of Epidemiology, Second Edition. Lex Bouter, Maurice Zeegers and Tianjing Li.
© 2023 John Wiley & Sons Ltd. Published 2023 by John Wiley & Sons Ltd.
Companion website: www.wiley.com/go/Bouter/TextbookofEpidemiology

3

3.1 The epidemiological function describes the association between health outcomes and explanatory factors

As we have seen in previous chapters, the epidemiological function expresses the question being addressed by an epidemiological study mathematically. The epidemiological function links the outcome to one or more other explanatory factors:

$$P(O) = f(F_i)$$

Case 3.1 gives a classical example of an epidemiological function and how it can be used.

Chapter 2 focused on the left-hand side of the equation, the outcome. This chapter looks at the relationship between the left- and right-hand sides of the equation. Let us now consider the relationship between specific explanatory factors (F_i) and the outcome P(O).

Let us first consider the various kinds of explanatory factors and the various types of epidemiological functions. When these explanatory factors help us to estimate disease probability, we call these risk factors; other explanatory factors could be prognostic or diagnostic.

In epidemiological research, as we saw in Chapter 2, the outcome studied is usually an aspect of health, and the presence or absence of disease or a stage of disease is

Case 3.1 Risk Factors for Cardiovascular Disease

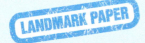

The Framingham Heart Study, named after the small town of Framingham in Massachusetts in the United States, is one of the first large-scale epidemiological studies of cardiovascular disease. The Framingham Heart Study, which began in 1949, has become a classic example in epidemiology. The entire adult population in Framingham was invited to take part in regular health checks. Their blood pressure, serum cholesterol, body weight and height were measured annually or biennially. The study also collected data on various lifestyle and behavioral factors (smoking, alcohol consumption, etc.). These data were linked to data from local hospitals and death records.

The study participants were followed for decades. The data below relate to the first 12 years' follow-up of the cohort of 2,187 men and 2,669 women, aged 30–62, who did not have coronary heart disease at the time of the first health survey.

Over the 12-year period, 258 men and 129 women developed coronary heart disease (CHD), representing a cumulative incidence of 11.8% for the men and 4.8%

for the women. A logistic regression analysis was used to link disease frequency to various risk factors. This function looks as follows:

$$P(O) = \frac{1}{1 + e^{-(b_0 + b_1 x_1 + b_2 x_2 + b_3 x_3 + \ldots + b_k x_k)}}$$

To put it into words, the probability of suffering CHD P(O) can be estimated based on a mathematical logistic equation with a constant b_0 and a combination of various factors x_i, weighted by their associated coefficients b_i. ◻ Table 3.1 shows the various explanatory factors with their coding and regression coefficients separately for men and women. Using the formula and the table we can calculate, for example, that a 60-year-old woman with a serum cholesterol level of 250 mg/100 ml, systolic blood pressure of 140 mmHg, relative weight of 140 kg, a hemoglobin level of 120 g/l, and who smokes one pack of cigarettes a day but whose ECG is normal has an 85% risk of CHD within 12 years. A 40-year-old woman who has not smoked and weighed 70 kg but otherwise displays all the same characteristics, would have a 44% risk of CHD within 12 years. Try to calculate this for yourself, using the formula and data in the table.

thus often regarded as the resultant of one or more risk factors acting upon the individual. In etiological research risk factors can be divided into three categories, broadly speaking: behavior, biology and environment. ◻ Table 3.2 gives a few examples from each of these categories.

If we wish to prevent the development of a disease, we need to know the risk factors of the disease, and what these are will differ from one population to another. In low-income countries and regions, the main risk factors that can be modified are malnutrition, unsafe sex, and poor hygiene, whereas in high-income countries, smoking, being overweight, and a lack of physical activity are predominant risk factors of diseases (see ◻ Table 3.3). Whether a risk factor can be modified and whether this will actually reduce the risk needs to be determined by research, and research of

this kind is vital to effective prevention. This will be discussed in Chapters 6 and 10.

Sometimes explanatory factors are used solely to identify individuals and groups who are at increased risk of a health problem, leaving aside the question of whether the given factor is causal. A familiar example is the relationship between socioeconomic position and disease. Although socioeconomic position does not cause disease, it's strongly associated with the causal factors of health problems. A description of socioeconomic health differences can therefore help identify the neighborhoods or groups within a population that are most in need of healthcare. Another example of the use of explanatory factors is in life insurances, where the amount of premium payable is increasingly geared to the applicant's profile in terms of his or her "risk profile."

◻ **Table 3.1** Risk factors of cardiovascular disease and associated weights in the Framingham Heart Study.

Risk factor	Unit of measurement	Coefficient for men	Coefficient for women
constant	–	$b_0 = -10.90$	$b_0 = -12.59$
x_1 = age	years	$b_1 = 0.071$	$b_1 = 0.076$
x_2 = serum cholesterol	mg/100 ml	$b_2 = 0.011$	$b_2 = 0.006$
x_3 = systolic blood pressure	mmHg	$b_3 = 0.017$	$b_3 = 0.022$
x_4= relative weight	100 × weight/standard weight	$b_4 = 0.014$	$b_4 = 0.005$
x_5 = hemoglobin	gram/l	$b_5 = -0.084$	$b_5 = 0.036$
x_6 = cigarette smoking	0 = none, 1 = < 1 pack per day, 2 = 1 pack per day, 3 = > 1 pack per day	$b_6 = 0.361$	$b_6 = 0.077$
x_7 = abnormality on ECG	no = 0, yes = 1	$b_7 = 1.046$	$b_7 = 1.434$

◻ **Table 3.2** Examples of risk factors of health and disease.

Behavior	Smoking	Drinking	Exercise	Diet	Medication
Biology	Blood pressure	DNA	Cholesterol	Age	Sex
Environment	Occupational exposure	Social support	Socioeconomic position	Residential environment	Access to care

Table 3.3 Ranking of the main modifiable determinants of disease for low-, middle- and high-income countries in 2004.

	Risk factor	Deaths (millions)	Percentage of total		Risk factor	Deaths (millions)	Percentage of total
World				**Low-income countries**			
1	High blood pressure	7.5	12.8	1	Underweight in children	2.0	7.8
2	Smoking	5.1	8.7	2	High blood pressure	2.0	7.5
3	High blood sugar	3.4	5.8	3	Unsafe sex	1.7	6.6
4	Physical inactivity	3.2	5.5	4	Contaminated water	1.6	6.1
5	Overweight and obesity	2.8	4.8	5	High blood sugar	1.3	4.9
6	High cholesterol	2.6	4.5	6	Smoke in the home	1.3	4.8
7	Unsafe sex	2.4	4.0	7	Smoking	1.0	3.9
8	Alcohol consumption	2.3	3.8	8	Physical inactivity	1.0	3.8
9	Underweight in children	2.2	3.8	9	Poor breastfeeding	1.0	3.7
10	Smoke in the home	2.0	3.3	10	High cholesterol	0.9	3.4
Middle-income countries				**High-income countries**			
1	High blood pressure	4.2	17.2	1	Smoking	1.5	17.9
2	Smoking	2.6	10.8	2	High blood pressure	1.4	16.8
3	Overweight and obesity	1.6	6.7	3	Overweight and obesity	0.7	8.4
4	Physical inactivity	1.6	6.6	4	Physical inactivity	0.6	7.7
5	Alcohol consumption	1.6	6.4	5	High blood sugar	0.6	7.0
6	High blood sugar	1.5	6.3	6	High cholesterol	0.5	5.8
7	High cholesterol	1.3	5.2	7	Low fruit and vegetable consumption	0.2	2.5
8	Low fruit and vegetable consumption	0.9	3.9	8	Air pollution	0.2	2.5
9	Smoke in the home	0.7	2.8	9	Alcohol consumption	0.1	1.6
10	Air pollution	0.7	2.8	10	Exposure at work	0.1	1.1

3.2 Measures of association for dichotomous outcomes

Many measures of association in epidemiology are based on comparing the occurrence of a health outcome (incidence, prevalence: see Chapter. 2) between two categories of a dichotomous explanatory factor. This can be simply visualized in a two-by-two table, also known as a contingency table (see ◘ Table 3.4).

Table 3.4. A two-by-two table.

	With the outcome (or cases)	Without the outcome (or controls)
Exposed	a	b
Non-exposed	c	d

More complex situations in etiological epidemiology will be considered in Chapters 4 and 6, and the way in which the association between diagnostic or prognostic factors and a health outcome is quantified will be discussed in Chapter 9.

3.2.1 Attributable risk

◻ Figure 3.1 shows a cohort divided into two levels of explanatory factor F (F_1 and F_0). It also shows how cumulative incidence (CI) and incidence density (ID) can be calculated for both subgroups. The obvious way of quantifying the effect of the risk factor on the outcome is to subtract one incidence from the other, thus yielding the attributable risk (AR). If the persons in which the factor is present (F_1) and in which it is absent (F_0) are comparable in all other respects, this is the additional risk that is attributable to the explanatory factor at issue.

$$AR = I_1 - I_0$$

For the sake of simplicity, the examples in this chapter are based on the assumption that there is a causal relationship (see Chapter 6).

Suppose that a study on serum cholesterol levels and cardiovascular mortality shows that the AR is 26 per 10,000 per 10 years. This means that, among persons with a high cholesterol level, 26 per 10,000 will die of a cardiovascular condition within 10 years due to their high cholesterol level. In other words, within this group, the cardiovascular mortality over 10 years would have been 26 per 10,000 lower if everyone had had a low cholesterol level (instead of a high one). The attributable risk is also known as the risk difference (RD). When calculating the AR, the risk can be measured either as the CI or the ID, thus yielding the cumulative incidence difference (CID) and the incidence density difference (IDD).

If the factor studied is an intervention, the reciprocal (1/AR) can also be used to derive another measure of association: this expresses the average number of persons who need, on average, to be treated in order to achieve the desired outcome (e.g. cure) in one person. This measure is referred to as the number needed to treat (NNT = 1/AR). An NNT of 385 (=10,000/26) in the above example means that, on average, 385 persons with a high cholesterol level would need to be treated successfully for 10 years in order to prevent one case of cardiovascular mortality.

◻ Table 3.5 shows among other things how the AR can be calculated based on CIs and IDs. The CID is dimensionless and applies to a specified period. The IDD is usually expressed per year. The shorter the follow-up period and the rarer the condition under consideration, the closer the CID and IDD will approximate each other numerically. It is standard practice to subtract the lowest risk from the highest so that AR is always a positive number.

3.2.2 Relative risk

Another way of representing the effect of an explanatory factor on the disease outcome is by dividing the risk in the group where the factor is present by that in the group where it is absent, thus yielding the relative risk (RR):

$$RR = \frac{I_1}{I_0}$$

An RR of cardiovascular mortality of 2 for persons with a high cholesterol level compared with persons with a low cholesterol level means that persons with a high cholesterol level run a risk of cardiovascular mortality that is twice as high. When calculating the RR, the risk can be measured either as the CI or the ID. The terms risk ratio and rate ratio are both

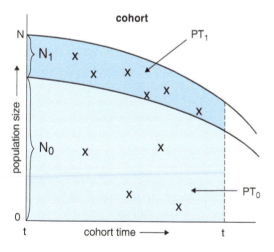

◻ **Figure 3.1** Incidence in exposed and non-exposed persons in a cohort study. $CI_1 = n_1/N_1$; $ID_1 = n_1/PT_1$, $CI_0 = n_0/N_0$; $ID_0 = n_0/PT_0$. CI: cumulative incidence; ID: incidence density; n: number of new incident cases (x); N: population size; PT: observed person-time (area under the curve); 1: in exposed persons; 0 in non-exposed persons.

◻ Table 3.5 Calculating measures of association in a cohort study.

	O	$\bar{O}$	
F	n_1	N_1	$CI_1 = n_1/N_1$
$\bar{F}$	n_0	N_0	$CI_0 = n_0/N_0$
	n_T	N_T	$CI_T = n_T/N_T$

$$RR = \frac{CI_1}{CI_0} = CI$$

$$AR = CI_1 - CI_0 = CID$$

$$EF = \frac{CI_1 - CI_0}{CI_1} = 1 - 1/CIR$$

$$PAR = \frac{CI_T - CI_0}{CI_T} = \frac{p(CIR - 1)}{p(CIR - 1) + 1}$$

$$p = N_1 / N_T$$

	O	PT	
F	n_1	PT_1	$ID_1 = n_1/PT_1$
$\bar{F}$	n_0	PT_0	$ID_0 = n_0/PT_0$
	n_T	PT_T	$ID_T = n_T/PT_T$

$$RR = \frac{ID_1}{ID_0} = IDR$$

$$AR = ID_1 - ID_0 = IDD$$

$$EF_e = \frac{ID_1 - ID_0}{ID_1} = 1 - 1/IDR$$

$$PAR = \frac{ID_T - ID_0}{ID_T} = \frac{q(IDR - 1)}{q(IDR - 1) + 1}$$

$$q = PT_1/PT_T$$

O: disease (cases)
$\bar{O}$: no disease (controls)
F: with explanatory factor
$\bar{F}$: without explanatory factor
N: cohort/subcohort size
n: number of incident cases
PT: observed person-time
1: in exposed persons
0: in non-exposed persons
T: in the total population
p: proportion of exposed persons
q: proportion of exposed person-time
CI: cumulative incidence
ID: incidence density
CIR: cumulative incidence ratio
IDR: incidence density ratio
CID: cumulative incidence difference
IDD: incidence density difference
RR: relative risk
AR: attributable risk
EF: etiological fraction
PAR: population attributable risk

abbreviated as RR, although strictly speaking they should be referred to as the cumulative incidence ratio (CIR) and incidence density ratio (IDR), respectively. As a result, these terms are often treated – not entirely correctly – as synonymous. ◻ Table 3.5 shows how the RR can be calculated from CIs and IDs. Both the CIR and the IDR are dimensionless. Here again, the shorter the follow-up period is and the rarer the condition under consideration, the more the CIR and IDR will approximate each other numerically.

The RR can have values between zero and infinity, where usually $0 < RR < 1$ suggests a protective effect and $RR > 1$ a harmful effect; $RR = 1$ means that there is no evidence of association between a factor and the outcome. There is symmetry between RR > 1 and RR < 1, as any risk factor can be turned into a protective factor by removing it and vice versa. In the previous example, for instance, the risk of cardiovascular mortality was halved by reducing the high cholesterol level.

3.2.3 Hazard rate ratio

Another term for ID is hazard rate. It measures the probability of occurrence of an outcome at a point in time. The ratio between two hazard rates, the hazard rate ratio, is thus quite simply the IDR already mentioned. The reason for devoting a separate section to this is that hazard rate ratios are useful for comparing two survival curves.

If we imagine a survival curve as a linear descending line, the rate at which the line descends is determined by the hazard rate. We assume here that the hazard rate is approximately constant and therefore yields the mean, the ID. If we then want to compare the mean hazard rate of a population in which a factor is present with a population in which it is absent, we calculate the hazard ratio, which indicates the ratio between the rates at which the two curves fall. The Cox proportional hazards model for the statistical analysis of these survival curves is based on the hazard rate and hazard ratio. Anyone who wants to find out more about this should to read a book on survival analysis.

3.2.4 Odds ratio

Odds is the ratio of the probability of an event occurring to the probability of an event not occurring. It is a term taken from English horse racing. For example, if the horse "Jumping Jack" is likely to win 20% of the time and lose 80% of the time, the odds of winning are 1 : 4. An odds ratio (OR) is the ratio of two odds. In a cohort study (see Chapter 4), OR is expressed as the odds that an outcome will occur given a particular exposure, divided by the odds of the outcome occurring in the absence of that exposure. Using the notations in ◻ Table 3.4.

$$OR = \frac{a/b}{c/d} = \frac{ad}{bc}$$

Although ORs can be used in any type of study design, they are most commonly used in case–control studies (see Chapter 4). In a case–control study, we first identify the cases (a group known to have the outcome) and the controls (a group known to be free of the outcome). We then look back in time to learn which participants in each group had the exposure, comparing the odds of exposure among the cases to the odds of exposure among the controls.

$$OR = \frac{a/c}{b/d} = \frac{ad}{bc}$$

Note that ad/bc represents the OR in both cohort and case–control studies. OR is also known as the cross-product ratio – the ratio of the products of both diagonal cells in a two-by-two table (◻ Table 3.4). For the same reason, the OR of exposure from a case–control study equals the OR of outcome.

In a case–control study, only the OR can be calculated as a measure of association, whereas in a cohort study, both the RR and the OR are valid measures of association. This is because a case–control study does not characterize the entire population from which the cases have been collected. It is not possible to determine incidences and thus calculate the RR or the AR. However, when the following three conditions are met, the OR obtained in a case–control study is a good approximation of the RR in a population:

1. When the cases studied are representative, with regard to history of exposure to explanatory factors, of all people with the outcome in the population from which the cases were drawn.
2. When the controls studied are representative, with regard to history of exposure to explanatory factors, of all people without the outcome in the population from which the controls were drawn.
3. When the outcome being studied is rare, by which is usually meant a frequency of less than 5% in the source population. When the rare disease assumption is not met OR must not be misinterpreted as RR.

The third condition can be explained mathematically. When the outcome is infrequent, very few

3

persons exposed and unexposed to the explanatory factor studied will actually develop the outcome.

$$\frac{\left(\dfrac{a}{a+b}\right)}{\left(\dfrac{c}{c+d}\right)} \approx \frac{\left(\dfrac{a}{b}\right)}{\left(\dfrac{c}{d}\right)} = \frac{ad}{bc}$$

In epidemiological studies, ORs are often estimated using logistic regressions. When a logistic regression model is fitted, the regression coefficient represents the change in the log odds of the outcome per unit change in the value of the exposure. The exponential function of the regression coefficient is the OR associated with a one-unit change in the exposure.

3.2.5 Etiological Fraction

Various other measures of association can be derived from the RR and AR. The AR divided by the risk in the group in which the explanatory factor is present yields the proportion of risk actually attributable to the presence of the explanatory factor. This measure, which is only relevant if the RR is greater than 1, is referred to as the etiological fraction (EF).

$$EF = \frac{I_1 - I_0}{I_1} = 1 - \frac{1}{RR} = \frac{RR-1}{RR}$$

An EF of 48% for cardiovascular mortality and high cholesterol level, for instance, means that among people with high cholesterol, 48% of the cardiovascular mortality is attributable to high cholesterol. In other words, in this group the cardiovascular mortality would be 48% lower if everyone had a low cholesterol level (instead of a high one). Translating the EF to an average patient with high cholesterol who died of a cardiovascular condition, we could say that the likelihood that death was actually caused by the high cholesterol level is 48%. As the interpretation of the EF applies to individuals with a specific risk factor, this measure is sometimes used when describing causality in individuals, for example, when determining industrial or medical liability.

🔲 Table 3.5 shows how the EF can be calculated from both CI and ID. The EF is dimensionless and is expressed as a proportion (0–1) or percentage (0%–100%). The value will be zero if there is no association and higher, the stronger the association between the risk factor and the outcome.

3.2.6 Population attributable risk

It is also possible to calculate the population attributable risk (PAR):

$$PAR = \frac{I_T - I_0}{I_T}$$

The total population is a mix of people with and without the explanatory factor of interest. The risk of the disease in the total population is the weighted average of the risk in the group with the explanatory factor (proportion: p) and risk in the group without the explanatory factor (proportion: $1-p$), respectively. Using incidence as an example:

$$I_T = pI_1 + (1-p)I_0$$

Thus, the value of the PAR is dependent not only on the value of the RR but also on the prevalence of the explanatory factor in the population (p). The PAR can therefore also be expressed as follows:

$$PAR = \frac{pI_1 + (1-p)I_0 - I_0}{pI_1 + (1-p)I_0}$$
$$= \frac{RR-1}{(RR+1)/(p-1)}$$
$$= \frac{p(RR-1)}{p(RR-1)+1}$$

A PAR of 33% for cardiovascular mortality and high cholesterol level, for instance, means that in the population of interest (which contains both persons with low and persons with high cholesterol), 33% of the mortality is attributable to the fact that part of the population has high cholesterol. In other words, in this population, the cardiovascular mortality would be 33% lower if everyone had low cholesterol. As the interpretation of the PAR applies to an entire population, this measure is sometimes used when setting regional or national public health priorities.

☐ Table 3.5 shows how the PAR can be calculated, again from CI and ID. Note, however, that in the alternative method of computation, using the CI approach, p is the proportion of persons in which the explanatory factor is present, whereas in the ID approach, q is the proportion of person-time in which the explanatory factor is present. The PAR is again a dimensionless number that is expressed as a proportion (0–1) or percentage (0%–100%). The value zero indicates the absence of any association. The stronger the association, the higher the value.

As already explained, the OR generally gives a good approximation of the RR when the outcome is rare. Based on this assumption, an EF and a PAR can also be calculated in a case-control study, by analogy with the formulas used to do this in a cohort study based on the IDR and CIR (see ☐ Table 3.5). To calculate the PAR, we need not only the OR but also an estimate of the prevalence of exposure. This is estimated based on the prevalence in the control group, assuming that the control group is representative of the total population in terms of exposure.

The calculation of a PAR can be extended for a combination of risk factors, in which case, the numerical value indicates the proportion of the disease attributable to the combination of factors under consideration:

$$\text{Combined PAR} = 1 - (1 - \text{PAR}_1)(1 - \text{PAR}_2)(1 - \text{PAR}_3)\ldots$$

3.2.7 Potential impact fraction

The potential impact fraction (PIF) measures how much of the incidence could be avoided by reducing the presence of an explanatory factor in the population by means of a preventive measure. If this causes the incidence to fall from I_t to $I_{t'}$, the PIF is:

$$PIF = \frac{I_t - I_{t'}}{I_t}$$

Unlike the PAR, this epidemiological measure allows for the situation that a preventive intervention usually reduces the presence of the explanatory factor in only part of the population. Therefore, using the PIF avoids overestimating the potential effects of a preventive measure. The PIF can also be calculated on the basis of the RR (CID or IDR) and the proportion of the total population with the explanatory factor before and after the intervention at issue:

$$PIF = \frac{I_t - I_t'}{I_t}$$

$$= \frac{\left[p_a \times RR_a \times I_0 + (1 - p_a) \times I_0\right] - \left[p_a' \times RR_a \times I_0 + (1 - p_a') \times I_0\right]}{p_a \times RR_a \times I_0 + (1 - p_a) \times I_0}$$

$$= \frac{(p_a - p_a') \times (RR_a - 1)}{p_a \times (RR_a - 1) + 1}$$

Where:

- I_t: incidence of the disease in the total population before the intervention
- I_t': incidence of the disease in the total population after the intervention
- P_a: proportion of the total population in which explanatory factor "a" is present before the intervention
- P_a': proportion of the total population in which explanatory factor "a" is present after the intervention
- I_0: incidence of the disease in the total population if explanatory factor "a" is absent
- RR_a: relative risk of getting the disease for persons exposed to explanatory factor "a" compared with persons not exposed to it.

A majority of individuals may not directly benefit from an effective preventive intervention (vaccination, behavior change, legislation, infrastructure, screening) because they would not experience the outcome anyway. The problem is that no one can say in advance, or with hindsight, which individuals would have developed disease without the preventive intervention and therefore will benefit from it. This is known as the prevention paradox: the potential health benefit for each individual is small but, for the population as a whole, this small reduction in individual risk yields a substantial reduction in the number of cases. For example, the number of road traffic deaths has been reduced substantially by requiring all motor riders to wear a helmet, whereas even without this intervention, the vast majority of them would never have been involved in a serious road accident.

Case 3.2 Fluoride and Bone Fractures (Hypothetical Example)

Suppose we want to find out whether using additional fluoride in toothpaste or in tablet form during childhood reduces the risk of bone fractures by strengthening bone structure. We decide to investigate this question in primary school children. When primary school children see the school doctor, various data are collected routinely, including data on the use of additional fluoride. Over a period of a few years, all primary school children in a region who see their school doctors for the first time are included in the cohort. They are monitored for about five years while at primary school. During the follow-up period, the hospitals in the region record all cases of bone fractures in children in the age group concerned. Thirty-thousand children ultimately take part in the study, of whom 20,000 are additional fluoride users and 10,000 are non-users. □ Figure 3.2 shows the design of the study.

An analysis of the research question based on the information available on all the participants would yield the results shown in □ Table 3.6.

$RR_{F-/F+}$ = relative risk (CIR) of bone fractures in non-fluoride users compared with fluoride users:

$$= I_{F-} / I_{F+}$$
$$= (500 / 10,000) / (200 / 20,000) = 5$$

$AR_{F-/F+}$ = additional risk (CID) of bone fractures in non-fluoride users compared with fluoride users:

$$= I_{F-} - I_{F+}$$
$$= (500 / 10,000) - (200 / 20,000)$$
$$= 800 / 20,000 \text{ (in 5 years)}$$
$$= 4\% \text{ (in 5 years)}$$

NNT = number of children who need to use fluoride for five years to avoid 1 bone fracture:

$$= 1 / AR$$
$$= 1 / 0.04$$
$$= 25$$

EF_{F-} = proportion of the risk (CI) of bone fractures among non-fluoride users attributable to non-use:

$$= (I_{F-} - I_{F+}) / I_{F-}$$
$$= (500 / 10,000 - 200 / 20,000) / (500 / 10,000)$$
$$= 0.8$$
$$= 80\%$$

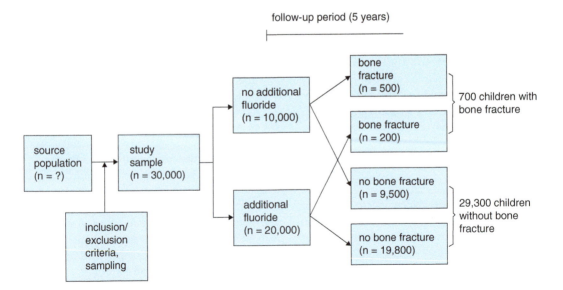

□ **Figure 3.2** Design of a cohort study into fluoride use and bone fractures.

$EF_T =$ proportion of the risk (CI) of bone fractures in the total population attributable to non-use of fluoride (by a third of that population):

$$= (I_T - I_{F+}) / I_T = (700 / 30,000 - 200 / 20,000) / (700 / 30,000)$$

$$= 0.57$$

$$= 57\%$$

Assuming that all study participants were monitored for precisely five years and that the bone fractures occurred uniformly over that period, the relevant measures of association can also be calculated from incidence densities:

$$ID_{F-} = 500 / \left[(10,000 \times 5) - (500 \times 2.5) \right]$$

$$= 0.01026 \text{ person / year}$$

$$ID_{F+} = 200 / \left[(20,000 \times 5) - (200 \times 2.5) \right]$$

$$= 0.00201 \text{ person / year}$$

$$RR_{F-/F+} = 5.10$$

$$AR_{F-/F+} = 0.00825 / \text{year}$$

$$NNT = 121 (= \text{number of children who need to use fluoride for 1 year to avoid 1 bone fracture})$$

$$EF_{F-} = 0.804 = 80.4\%$$

$$EF_T = 0.574 = 57.4\%$$

Table 3.6 Analysis of all subjects in the cohort study into fluoride use and bone fractures.

	Fracture	No fracture
F−	500	9,500
F+	200	19,800
	700	29,300

$I_1 = I_{F+} =$ (cumulative) incidence of bone fractures in fluoride users:

= 200/20,000 (in 5 years) = 1% (in 5 years)

$I_0 = I_{F-} =$ (cumulative) incidence of bone fractures in non-fluoride users:

= 500/10,000 (in 5 years) = 5% (in 5 years)

$RR_{F-/F+} =$ relative risk (CIR) of bone fractures in non-fluoride users compared with fluoride users:

$$= I_{F-} / I_{F+}$$

= (500/10,000):(200/20,000) = 5

3.3 Measures of association for continuous outcomes

Epidemiology examines the association between one or more factors and an outcome of interest. Some health outcomes, however, are expressed not as frequencies of a dichotomous variable but on a continuous scale, for example blood pressure, birth weight and quality of life. This section discusses the measures of association for continuous outcomes.

3.3.1 Difference of means

We introduced the central measures (mean, median, mode) and measures of spread (standard deviation, inter-percentile range, range) in Chapter 2. The obvious way of comparing means and standard deviations between two groups is to subtract one mean from the other and interpret the difference in the light of the two standard deviations. A large difference with a small spread is more impressive than a large difference with a large spread, and certainly more impressive than a small difference with a large spread.

Another measure for continuous outcome is the standardized mean difference (SMD):

$$SMD = \frac{M_1 - M_0}{SD_{1-0}}$$

where M_1 and M_0 are the means of an outcome for two groups and SD_{1-0} is the standard deviation of the difference of means between the two groups. This principle also forms the basis for the statistical procedures for comparing means: calculating a confidence interval for the difference of means, Student's t-test, one-way analysis of variance, simple linear regression etc. for which we refer to a statistics textbook for further explanations.

3.3.2 Correlation and regression

Sometimes we wish to link two continuous variables in a population to each other, for example, length of pregnancy and birth weight, salt consumption and blood pressure, or lung function and quality of life. In such cases, we start by drawing a chart, a scatter plot, and plotting one continuous variable against another. Each point in the scatter plot represents an individual in the population with its particular combination of values for the two variables. ◻ Figure 3.3 is an example of a scatter plot.

A scatter plot will often take the form of a flattened cloud with a lot of observations in the middle and not many at the ends. The density of the cloud is indicative of the correlation between the two variables: if the points form a (rising or falling) more or less straight line there is a strong correlation; on the other hand, if the points are completely spread out between the two axes of the chart and the cloud has no discernible structure, the two variables are likely unrelated. Every conceivable variation can occur between these two extremes (a non-horizontal straight line and an amorphous cloud). The closer the points are to an imaginary line, the stronger the correlation, and we can actually draw this line in such a way that it runs through the middle of the cloud in the direction indicated by the cloud. Some statistical measures are based on these principles.

- The correlation coefficient provides a measure of the density of the cloud: the closer the points are to the best fitted line, the higher the correlation coefficient is.
- A completely different measure is the regression coefficient, which quantifies the slope between the best fitted line (known as the regression line) and the x-axis. The steeper the slope, the stronger the association between a continuous variable and a continuous outcome is (see also Section 3.4).

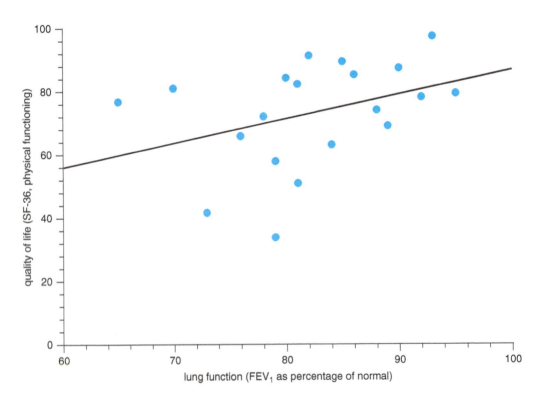

◻ **Figure 3.3** Scatter plot with regression line and calculated measures of association. Quality-of-life score = 10.86×lung function (FEV$_1$); Regression coefficient = 0.75; Correlation coefficient (Pearson's r) = 0.36.

Thus, the correlation coefficient is indicative of the extent to which the points can be represented by a line, whereas the regression coefficient is indicative of the slope of this line. Both these measures are important. Calculations of this kind are subject to several assumptions (e.g. a normal distribution of the two continuous variables and a straight line as the best fitted function).

3.4 Regression analysis

Epidemiological function $P(O) = f(F_i)$ describes the relationship between the outcome O and one or more explanatory factors F_i. This type of function can also be expressed as a mathematical regression equation. In its simplest form, a regression equation describes a linear relationship between a health outcome and a single explanatory factor:

$$P(O) = b_0 + b_1 F_1 \qquad (3.1)$$

Case 3.3 provides an example of a simple linear regression. The mortality rate from laryngeal cancer (O) is calculated and plotted for five levels of daily cigarette consumption (F_1). The regression line $P(O) = 1.15 + 0.282 \times F_1$ is an almost perfect fit with the data from the study on which ▢ Figure 3.4 is based.

It is not difficult to add a second exposure to this simple linear regression function:

$$P(O) = b_0 + b_1 F_1 + b_2 F_2 \qquad (3.2)$$

This too is a straight line, but in a three-dimensional space with the disease parameter O on the vertical y-axis and the two explanatory factors F_1 and F_2 on the horizontal x and z-axes (see ▢ Figure 3.5).

If we want to examine the joint and separate contributions that two (or more) explanatory factors to the outcome, we need multidimensional regression models of this kind. For example, daily alcohol consumption – also a risk factor for laryngeal cancer and associated with cigarette consumption – would be a worthwhile second explanatory factor to consider in the example in Case 3.3. By including both variables in the model, we can get a good idea of the separate contributions made by each of the explanatory factors to the occurrence of the disease.

Straight lines as described with formulas (3.1) and (3.2) will not be encountered very often in epidemiological research, as a straight line is likely to conflict with the range of possible values for the outcome studied. The incidence can never be negative, for instance, whereas a linear regression function as described in Case 3.3 may be inappropriate for this circumstance. Also, the disease frequency, expressed as a risk, is by definition limited to the values 0 and 1. For such situations, we use simple mathematical transformations of the probability of outcome variable (P_o) so that the regression function fits better with the actual data from epidemiological research.

Common transformations are the logarithmic regression function:

$$\ln(P_O) = b_0 + b_1 F_1 + b_2 F_2 + \dots \qquad (3.3)$$

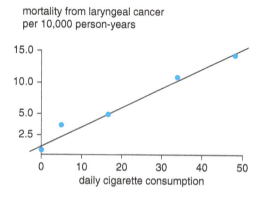

mortality from laryngeal cancer
per 10,000 person-years

▢ **Figure 3.4**   A 2D linear regression function.

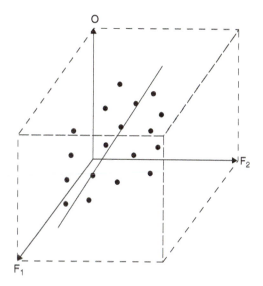

▢ **Figure 3.5**   A 3D linear regression function.

Case 3.3 Laryngeal Cancer and Smoking

Figure 3.4 shows the data from a study into the number of cigarettes smoked per day and the age-standardized mortality per 10,000 person-years for laryngeal cancer. The data fit a simple straight line, which is described mathematically as:

Mortality = 1.15 + 0.282*cigarettes.

The intercept (1.15) in Figure 3.4 represents the mortality from laryngeal cancer when nobody smokes. The regression coefficient (0.282) indicates that, in this model, the mortality rate per 10,000 person-years increases by 0.282 deaths when the average daily number of cigarettes smoked in the population increases by one. Assuming that no other variables are involved, the regression coefficient of 0.282 indicates the effect of cigarette-smoking on laryngeal cancer mortality. According to the model, a person who smokes two packs a day (50 cigarettes) has a mortality of 15.25 per 10,000 person-years on average. Compared with 10,000 person-years of non-smoking, 10,000 person-years of heavy smoking (two packs a day) result in approximately 14 additional cases of death from laryngeal cancer. We could also say that people who smoke two packs a day run 15.25/1.15 = 13.3 times as much risk of dying from laryngeal cancer compared with non-smokers.

and the logistic regression function:

$$ln\left(\frac{P_O}{1-P_O}\right) = b_0 + b_1F_1 + b_2F_2 + \dots$$

(3.4)

Note that the transformed Eqs. (3.3) and (3.4) are to some extent also linear functions, as the right-hand side of the equation describes a straight line when the y-axis is transformed. The regression functions described in this section are therefore referred to as generalized linear models.

A simple linear regression function is useful primarily in the case of a continuous normally distributed outcome. If the primary exposure variable is dichotomous (factor present: $F_1 = 1$; factor absent: $F_1 = 0$), interpretation is fairly simple.

The outcome in people with the factor present is:

$$P(O_1) = b_0 + (b_1 \times 1) = b_0 + b_1$$

For the persons with the factor absent, the outcome is:

$$P(O_0) = b_0 + (b_1 \times 0) = b_0$$

The effect of the factor on the outcome is then expressed simply by looking at the difference between the groups with and without the factor of interest:

$$P(O_1) - P(O_0) = (b_0 + b_1) - b_0 = b_1$$

The regression coefficient b_1 thus directly indicates the difference in outcome between the groups when the data fit a straight line.

Recommended reading

David, D., Szklo, M.M., and Gordis, L., 1934-2015. Epidemiology. (2019). *Gordis Epidemiology Celentano*, 6e. Philadelphia, PA: Elsevier. (Chapters 12 and 13).

Szklo, M.M. and Nieto, F.J. (2019). *Epidemiology:Beyond the Basics*, 4e. Burlington, Massachusetts: Jones & Bartlett Learning. (Chapters 3 and 7).

Rothman, K.J., Lash, T.L., VanderWeele, T.J., and Haneuse, S. *Modern epidemiology*, 4e. Philadelphia: Wolters Kluwer, [2021]. (Chapters 4 and 20).

Source References

Truett, J., Cornfield, J., and Kannel, W. (1967). A multivariate analysis of the risk of coronary heart disease in Framingham. *J. Chron. Dis.* 20: 511–524. (Case 3.1).

Rothman, K.J., Lash, T.L., and Greenland, S. (2012). Modern Epidemiology, 3e. Philadelphia: Lippincott: Williams & Wilkins. (Case 3.3).

(2009). *Global Health Risks: Mortality and Burden of Disease Attributable to Selected Major Risks*. Geneva: World Health Organization. (Table 3.3).

Knowledge assessment questions

A researcher in rural Ethiopia was investigating if exposure to guinea worm increases the risk for sepsis in children. He enrolled and followed a cohort of children from age 0–10, and documented their hospital visits and conditions. At the end of 10 years, of 1,298 children in the cohort, 370 were exposed to guinea worm and 25 experienced sepsis, while three children not exposed to guinea worm experienced sepsis.

1. Create a contingency table to model this relationship.

	Sepsis +	Sepsis -	Totals
Guinea worm +			
Guinea worm -			
Totals			**1,298**

2. What is the attributable risk of sepsis among those exposed to guinea worm in this study?
3. How many individuals would you have to treat for guinea worm to prevent one case of sepsis (NNT)? (Hint: round up for whole numbers of people.)
4. Calculate the relative risk of sepsis for children exposed to guinea worm compared with children not exposed to guinea worm.
5. Which of the following is a correct interpretation of the relative risk calculated above? (select the one best answer)
    a. Individuals with guinea worm are (100−answer 4) times more likely to have sepsis as compared to individuals without guinea worm.
    b. The population was (answer 4) times more likely to develop guinea worm over the course of 10 years.
    c. Individuals with guinea worm have (answer 4) times the risk of developing sepsis as compared to individuals without guinea worm.
    d. (answer 4) percent of the risk for sepsis in the population can be attributed to guinea worm

Investigators at the University of Paris wanted to look at the effect of passive smoking on hospitalization due to asthma symptoms. They recruited 1,025 restaurant workers with asthma in the city and asked them to report if their restaurant allowed individuals to smoke in their facilities. They then asked for participants to report whether in the previous six months they had been hospitalized because of their asthma symptoms. Of 1,025 participants, 700 reported they worked in restaurants that permitted smoking. 64 of these individuals reported hospitalization in the previous six months due to asthma symptoms, compared with 25 in the control group.

6. Complete the contingency table below. What are the odds for hospitalization for restaurant workers exposed to passive smoking?

	Hospitalized +	Hospitalized -	Totals
Passive smoking +			
Passive smoking -			
Totals			**1,025**

7. Calculate the odds ratio and 95% confidence interval of hospitalization due to asthma symptoms comparing those exposed to passive smoking with those not exposed to passive smoking.
8. What is the correct interpretation of the correct confidence interval above?
    a. The interval includes 1, thus the result is not statistically significant. There is insufficient evidence to conclude that passive smoking increases the odds of hospitalization due to asthma in this study
    b. The interval does not include 0, thus the result is statistically significant. There is sufficient evidence to conclude that passive smoking increases the asthma risk in this study odds of hospitalization due to asthma in this study
    c. The interval includes 1, thus the result is not statistically significant. Passive smoking reduces the odds of hospitalization due to asthma in this study
    d. The interval does not include 0, thus the result is not statistically significant

Study Design

Textbook of Epidemiology, Second Edition. Lex Bouter, Maurice Zeegers and Tianjing Li.
© 2023 John Wiley & Sons Ltd. Published 2023 by John Wiley & Sons Ltd.
Companion website: www.wiley.com/go/Bouter/TextbookofEpidemiology

4

4.1 Introduction: the research question determines the design

This chapter explains how epidemiological studies should be designed in order to find the link between an explanatory factor and a health outcome. A variety of research questions can be addressed: for example, investigating the influence of risk factors on the development of a condition (an etiological study); investigating the influence of prognostic factors on the course of a disease (a prognostic study); investigating the extent to which diagnostic tests give correct classifications (a diagnostic study); or assessing the effectiveness of preventive or therapeutic interventions (an intervention study). Choosing a study design to answer each type of research question has direct consequences for the validity of the results, and on the credibility of the conclusions that can be drawn from the study. In this chapter, we will describe the standard study designs and discuss threats to validity. We cannot adequately design and carry out an epidemiological study unless the research question has been formulated in advance and made specific and measurable. Getting off to a good start is half the battle!

4.1.1 Elements of a research question

The research question needs to be formulated in specific, measurable terms. PICO or its derivatives, such as PECO provides a useful guide here:
- **Population**: Which people and population are we talking about? What is the disease or condition of interest and the setting?
- **Intervention (or exposure to an explanatory factor)**: What is the intervention, diagnostic test, risk factor or prognostic factor that we want to link with the outcome?
- **Comparator**: To what intervention, diagnostic test, risk factor or prognostic factor do we want to make a comparison?
- **Outcome**: What health outcomes are we studying?

Examples of research questions for different types of study:
- Etiological study: In adults aged 65 or older (P), what is the risk of death (O) associated with COVID-19 in people with body mass index of 30 or higher (obese individuals) (E) compared with people with body mass index between 18 and 25 (individuals with normal weight) (C)?
- Prognostic study: What is the 10-year risk of death (O) in patients with bladder cancer (P) who stopped smoking (E) compared with those who continued to smoke (C)?
- Diagnostic study: Compared with a doctor's clinical opinion (C), does an abdominal CT scan (I) reduce the false negative diagnoses (O) in patients with appendicitis symptoms (P)?
- Intervention study: Is intensive glycemic control (I) more effective than conventional glycemic control (C) for reducing cardiovascular disease (O) in patients with type 2 diabetes (P)?

4.1.2 The research question can be expressed using the epidemiological function

Once we have formulated a research question, it is relatively easy to translate it into an epidemiological function. The epidemiological function expresses the research question in mathematical terms. The epidemiological function for the etiological research question in Section 4.1.1, for instance, could be:

$$P\left(death_{\text{in adults aged 65 or older with COVID-19}}\right)$$

$$= f\left(b_0 + b_1\left(\text{obesity vs. normal weight}\right)\right)$$

Opting for this formal notation has several advantages: it makes the research question quantifiable; it draws attention to elements in the research question that may not be entirely clear yet, and it provides an immediate guide to making the study question specific and measurable, including the data analysis plan.

4.1.3 Selection of the study population

The target population is a subset of the total population for which we wish to generalize the results (see ▣ Figure 4.1). It is not usually feasible to study the entire target population.

The source population, the population from which study participants are drawn, is a suitable subset of the target population that enables an answer to the research question applicable to the target population.

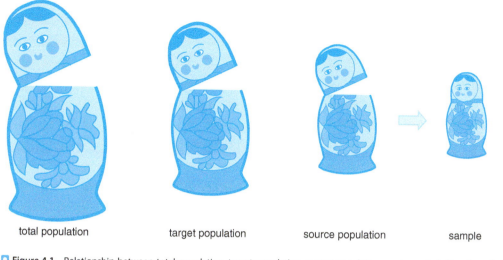

| total population | target population | source population | sample |

Figure 4.1 Relationship between total population, target population, source population, and sample (with acknowledgments to Martijn Boers).

The source population is not necessarily (or desirably) representative of the target population. The study sample, consisting of individuals that end up in a study, on the other hand, is statistically representative of the source population, so that the results in the sample are also valid for the source population.

In an etiological study, the representativeness has a twist to it, as we are always using study results observed in a specific time and place to say something about an abstract reality (this generalization process is referred to as "inference"). Our aim is to show that there is a causal link between an explanatory factor and a health outcome, regardless of any specific population. The goal is to find a study sample and setting that maximizes the chance of uncovering the link that we are looking for – assuming that it actually exists, of course. The study design must also ensure as much as possible that only the exposure of interest can be responsible for the outcome measured, not other factors (i.e. the internal validity of the design).

A suitable study sample in epidemiological research is characterized by:

- a clear contrast in the exposure under consideration (the presumed cause)
- maximum comparability of the study groups with and without the explanatory factor of interest in terms of other factors for the outcome being studied (potential confounders)
- maximum comparability of the study groups in terms of how the various variables are measured (information bias)

- maximum information to be obtained per participant (per unit of time or resources).

A clear contrast in the primary explanatory factor studied means that the study sample is selected in such a way that all the relevant levels of that factor are adequately represented. In many cases, we might focus on the effects of extreme values (maximum contrast). Sometimes, however, we might prefer an even distribution among the various levels of the explanatory factor of interest. For example, a researcher wishing to find out whether eating plenty of dietary fiber protects against appendicitis will ideally have a study population consisting mainly of people with very low or very high consumption of fiber-rich foods. Although most people's level of consumption will be fairly close to the population average, that category provides the least information for etiological research; extreme categories are far more informative and should ideally be adequately represented in the study sample. Some of the in-between categories can also be included in the study to give an idea of the entire range. Furthermore, the study groups being compared should have a similar distribution of all other factors that affect the occurrence of the disease (potential confounders) in each category of the explanatory factor of interest. This idea is discussed in Chapter 5.

The third criterion is to obtain measurements of comparable quality: a difference in outcome frequency between the categories of the explanatory factors studied must not be due to a difference in measuring procedures. Suppose, for example, that an occupational physician has made regular lung X-rays to study the lung cancer risk among butchers. The incidence of lung cancer found in this way cannot be compared with the incidence for lung cancer among patients seen at the regional cancer centers confirmed by biopsy; instead, we should compare the butchers with another category of employees that also had regular lung X-rays done by their occupational physician.

Lastly, the choice of study sample can improve the efficiency of the study. It is recommended to focus on subpopulations where the association being studied is the strongest; this is not necessarily the population with the highest disease frequency. ◘ Figure 4.2 illustrates this principle based on two subpopulations with different background risks I_0 for the disease being studied.

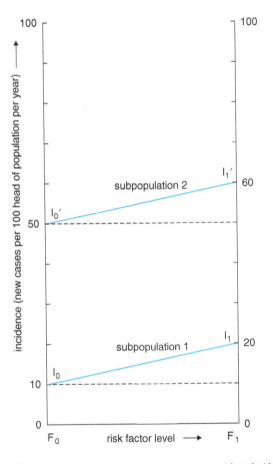

◘ **Figure 4.2** Disease incidences among persons with and without the risk factor in two subpopulations with different background risks of the disease being studied.

If these people, regardless of the background risk, have a 20% risk of developing the disease due to the primary risk factor (F_1), we can calculate the AR and RR for both subpopulations:

$$AR = CI_1 - CI_0$$

$$RR = CI_1 / CI_0$$

subpopulation 1

$$AR = 20 - 10 = \frac{10}{100} \text{ per year}$$

$$RR = 20 / 10 = 2.0$$

subpopulation 2

$$AR = 60 - 50 = \frac{10}{100} \text{ per year}$$

$$RR = 60 / 50 = 1.2$$

It shows that, with AR remaining the same, the RR will increase when the background risk decreases. This also explains why substantial differences in the strength of an association – expressed as RR – between an explanatory factor and outcome are sometimes found when it is studied in populations with different background risks.

In etiological research, we are looking for an undistorted picture of the effect of an explanatory factor, starting with the incidence in people among whom that factor is present. Ideally, we would want to compare this with the incidence in the theoretical situation where among these same people (in precisely the same circumstances) that the factor would be absent. This mirror image is called a counterfactual. A perfect counterfactual can never be achieved in practice; we always have to work with approximations, either by studying the same persons again at another point in time at which their explanatory factor status is different (and assuming that there have been no substantial other changes in the meantime), by including other comparable persons with a different explanatory factor status in the study, or by randomizing people to intervention and comparison groups (which in theory achieves a counterfactual groups at baseline).

4.1.4 Classifications of study designs

Study designs can be classified on the basis of their design characteristics (see ◘ Figure 4.3).

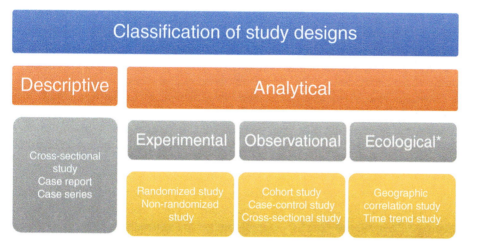

Figure 4.3 Classification of epidemiological study designs. *Unlike other study designs, ecological studies analyze aggregate data at the group or population level.

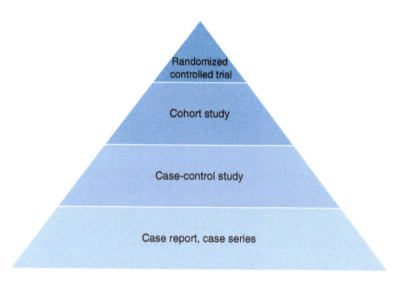

Figure 4.4 Hierarchy of evidence for drawing causal conclusions.

The first distinction is between descriptive and analytical studies. A descriptive study allows the researcher to describe the distribution of one or more variables, sometimes without a specific hypothesis. Some examples of the descriptive studies are population-based survey (e.g. census), case report, and case series.

In an analytical study, researchers try to establish an association between one or more explanatory factors with a health outcome or demonstrate an effect of an intervention. Among analytical study designs, we can broadly categorize study designs into experimental, observational, or ecological. Researchers allocate different levels of the explanatory factor (usually an intervention) to participants in experimental studies. A randomized experiment, or randomized controlled trial (RCT), is generally regarded as the study design with the highest evidential value for drawing causal conclusions (■ Figure 4.4), as it enables the researcher to exert maximum control over confounding and selection bias. RCTs are discussed in Section 4.2 and Chapter 10.

Note that in the evidence-based medicine paradigm, systematic reviews of RCTs are usually placed

4

on the top of hierarchy. Systematic review follows pre-specified methods to identify, appraise, and summarize all evidence out there that answers a well-defined research question. The evidence that a systematic review synthesizes can be of any study design. The method of conducting a systematic review is presented in Chapter 11. Systematic reviews take precedence over other types of research evidence, as it makes sense for decisions to be based on the totality of relevant evidence rather than individual studies or a subset of the evidence.

Case reports are often based on a single case, or only a small number of cases, and are therefore regarded as the study design with the lowest evidential value. Case series are better in that respect, but they are often small-scale and do not include a comparison group. Cohort studies and case–control studies, described below, do include a comparison group and usually have a substantial number of participants.

In the case of observational studies, the researcher does not allocate different levels of the explanatory factor of interest; instead, the distribution of various categories of the explanatory factor that happen naturally is taken. The researcher merely observes and tries to identify as neatly and efficiently as possible what is going on or has already happened, without actually intervening.

Observational studies can in turn be divided into cohort studies, case–control studies, and cross-sectional studies, which are discussed in Sections 4.3.1, 4.3.2, and 4.3.3. A cohort study is assembled on the basis of the exposure to an explanatory factor of interest. Groups with different exposure status at the start of the observation period are compared to see whether these differences are associated with differences in the occurrence of outcomes being studied (cohort study). In a case–control study, the study population is assembled on the basis of an outcome. Groups with different outcome status (usually cases versus controls) are compared in terms of the presence or absence of an explanatory factor at a relevant time in the past.

An ecological study examines the relationship between a health outcome and other phenomena based on aggregate data at a group or population level (e.g. average alcohol consumption per capita and annual mortality from laryngeal cancer per 100,000 head of population in UK). Two subtypes of ecological studies are time-trend studies (analysis of time series) and geographical correlation studies. We shall discuss these types of study in more detail in Section 4.3.4.

Study designs can also be cross-sectional and longitudinal in nature. In a cross-sectional study, the explanatory factor(s) and health outcome(s) are ascertained at the same time. Cross-sectional studies are not ideal for establishing causal relationships, as exposure to the explanatory factors needs to take place before the occurrence of the outcome: this can be achieved in a longitudinal study but not in a cross-sectional study. RCTs, cohort studies, and case–control studies are generally considered as being longitudinal.

Although the above classification suggests that there are fundamental differences between these study designs, the dividing lines between them are less clear cut than it might seem at first sight. For example, if we are interested in explanatory factors that remain constant over time (e.g. genes, sex, blood group, congenital enzyme deficiencies) – which can therefore be measured at the same time as the outcome without any problem – the dividing line between a cross-sectional study, a cohort study, and a case–control study becomes less clear.

4.2 Randomized experiment as the paradigm for establishing a causal relationship

Randomized experiment is the standard design for establishing causal effect. Careful design and meticulous application of the rules for experimental research based on Good Clinical Practice maximizes the internal validity. However, practical or ethical considerations often prevent an experiment being carried out (see ▢ Figure 4.5). Chapter 10 discusses further the practical aspects of experimental studies.

4.2.1 Randomized experiment

The basic structure of an experiment is shown in ▢ Figure 4.6. Participants in an RCT are recruited from the source population, restricted to a relatively homogeneous group (e.g. people in the same age

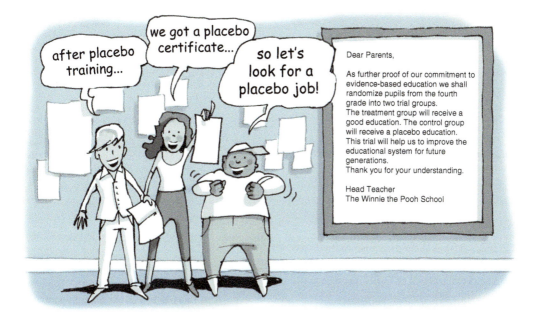

Figure 4.5 An RCT is not always ethically feasible (with acknowledgments to http://freshspectrum.com). Source: Courtesy of freshspectrum.com.

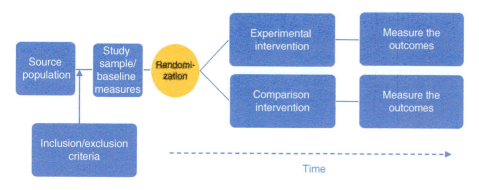

Figure 4.6 Design of a randomized controlled trial.

group, with the same disease or at the same stage of the disease). The researcher determines in advance how many participants will be needed to estimate the effect of the intervention with sufficient precision (i.e. sample size calculation). The candidates are checked to see whether they meet the inclusion and exclusion criteria and are told what the proposed experiment entails. They are then asked to consent to take part on a voluntary basis (informed consent).

The intervention being studied is allocated to the participants using a random procedure (randomization) which gives each participant a predefined chance of being assigned to the intervention or the comparison group. As a result of this random assignment, the intervention and comparison groups will be comparable on average in all respects at the start of the experiment. Randomization deals with all confounders (factors that may distort the relationship being studied, more to come in Chapter 5), both known, unknown and difficult-to-measure ones. The randomized experiment therefore meets one of the essential requirements for establishing causality, namely comparability of the study groups. Randomization does not guarantee

4

that the study groups will be completely equal; but when randomization is done properly, any differences between groups seen at baseline are due to chance.

Once the baseline measurements have been taken, the intervention is applied, according to a treatment protocol. Steps must be taken to ensure that participants adhere to the assigned intervention (compliance) and any non-compliance is recorded. The comparison group is given a comparison intervention consistent with the research question (the standard treatment, no treatment, a placebo, an active comparator, or a different dosage of the same treatment). A placebo (i.e. a control intervention that is indistinguishable from the real intervention in terms of appearance, taste, etc. but lacks the active ingredient) provides the best guarantee that the groups are comparable for co-interventions and outcome measurements. There are situations, however, where a placebo intervention is not feasible or ethically unacceptable, for example, when effective interventions already exist.

The use of a placebo intervention enables the trial participants and researchers to be blinded. Neither the participants nor the researchers would know which intervention is given to whom. This prevents them from possibly acting in a way that could undermine the experimental design. If the researcher or the participant knows which intervention is assigned, it can result in conscious or unconscious manipulation of the behaviors and observations. Sometimes, it is not possible to blind the participants and the treating professional, for example, when a surgical intervention is compared with a non-surgical intervention. It is usually possible, however, to have the outcome measured by someone else and blind this person carefully for the intervention assigned. This type of problem is further minimized by choosing outcomes or measurement instruments that leave little opportunity for subjective interpretation (e.g. mortality).

Although randomization produces trial groups that are comparable at the start of a trial, differences can develop along the way as a result of participants dropping out during the follow-up period (i.e. lost to follow up; attrition). When lost to follow-up is selective and is associated with factors that affect the outcome, the internal validity of the study is compromised. The problem is particularly serious if there are different reasons for being lost to follow up.

There are a number of variations on the basic RCT structure, which will be discussed in Chapter 10. The reporting of RCTs should follow the CONSORT guideline and its extensions, available from the EQUATOR network's website.

Case 4.1 A Randomized Dietary Experiment in Premature Infants

Infants born prematurely often experience problems after birth because of immature organ systems. One of these problems is dietary intolerance in the gastrointestinal tract; another is a greater risk of infection. These problems occur particularly in the first month of life. Before birth, fetuses receive amino acids that are important to the function of those organs, including glutamine, through the placenta. To investigate whether adding glutamine to the diet from Day 3 to Day 30 after birth has a beneficial effect on dietary tolerance (the primary outcome studied) and the occurrence of serious infections (one of the secondary outcomes), an RCT was conducted on premature children at increased risk of these problems (the inclusion criteria were a length of pregnancy of less than 32 weeks or a birth weight less than 1,500 g). Informed consent had been obtained from the parents. Infants who were at increased risk of these problems for other reasons were not included (the exclusion criteria included congenital abnormalities and genetic defects). The study, sponsored by a large baby food company, took place at a neonatal intensive care unit of a teaching hospital. It involved a total of more than 100 children. Although there was no evidence of difference in dietary tolerance between the two groups, far fewer serious infections occurred in the group of infants who were given glutamine (the intervention group) than the group given maltodextrin (the placebo group). The follow-up showed, among other things, by means of brain imaging, that the children in the intervention group had greater brain volume at the age of eight than the children in the control group. Statistical analysis was able to show that this effect was attributable to the reduction in the number of serious infections brought about by adding glutamine.

4.3 Observational study designs

Although the randomized experiment is the paradigm for establishing causal relationship in epidemiological research, experimental designs are often not feasible. Observational study designs, where the researcher has no influence over the distribution of the explanatory factor studies and instead, utilize a distribution that has come about in some other way, are more frequently encountered in epidemiology. We discuss the most common types of observational study designs below.

4.3.1 Cohort study

The basic structure of a cohort study is shown in ☐ Figure 4.7. Each of the main characteristics is discussed below.

Defining the study population
A cohort study has two or more groups sampled from the source population on the basis of absence or presence of the explanatory factor of interest. The outcomes studied have not yet occurred in any of the participants at the start of the study.

Exposure measurement
A cohort study examines the effects of an explanatory factor (usually a risk factor of the outcome). The participants are categorized into a minimum of two groups based on the measured values of the primary explanatory factor. Important to note, other explanatory factors should be measured in a cohort study, as the primary explanatory factor is often (due to lack of ran-

domization) associated with other explanatory factors for the health outcome. If we are studying the effects of alcohol consumption on cardiological outcomes, for instance, we need to realize that drinkers and teetotalers may well have different dietary habits, smoking habits, and exercise patterns. By measuring these other explanatory factors in all the participants, we can control the influence of these factors in the design or the analysis. For example, we can select only non-smokers for the study (restriction), or ensure that the percentage of smokers is the same among the drinkers and the teetotalers (matching), or adjust for the influence of these other factors in a regression analysis. These concepts are discussed in detail in Chapter 5.

Follow-up and outcome measurement
The follow-up period must be long enough for any effect of the primary risk factor to be able to manifest itself. By recording the number of incident cases with the health outcome (e.g. a disease) accurately, we can calculate the cumulative incidence (CI) or incidence density (ID) in each group. In the case of continuous outcome variables, for example, we calculate the mean value of the outcome at the end of the follow-up period, or the mean change in the value of the outcome from baseline.

In a cohort study, the outcome should ideally be measured by assessors who do not have prior knowledge of the participants' risk factor status (i.e. blinded outcome assessor). The need for blind measurements will depend on the nature of the outcome being studied and the type of measuring procedure. Blinding is more important in the case of subjective outcomes.

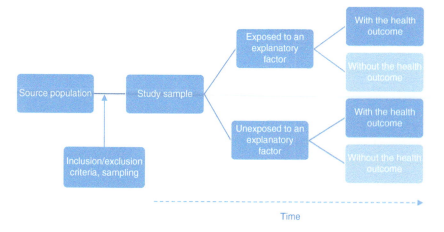

☐ **Figure 4.7** Design of a cohort study.

The evidential value of a cohort study is determined mainly by the following factors:

1. The explanatory factors and outcomes are measured at the individual level instead of at the population level.
2. Study participants are free from the outcome of interest at baseline. The outcome does not therefore play any role in the formation of the cohort (i.e. no selection bias: see Section 5.4.1).
3. The explanatory factors (as well as the confounders) are measured before outcome occurs. Any measurement errors in the factors are therefore independent of outcome (i.e. no differential misclassification of the exposure measurement: see Section 5.4.1).
4. In many cases, outcome status can be measured by blinded outcome assessors, so that any measurement errors are not related to risk factor status (i.e. no differential misclassification of the outcome measurement).

Cohort studies have some limitations:

1. Due to the absence of randomization, there are fewer opportunities for creating comparable groups as in an RCT. Confounding thus poses a serious threat to a cohort study. Any differences in these factors will have to be controlled for in the design or adjusted for in the statistical analysis – assuming that these factors have been properly measured.
2. A cohort study is not suitable for exploration; it can only be designed once well-founded hypotheses on the explanatory factors have been developed.
3. The classification of study participants according to explanatory factor status as the basis for assembling cohorts is a snapshot. For example, people who are exposed to a harmful factor conceivably constitute only a selective group, as many potential participants have already "dropped out" due to disease or death, and the remainder may be relatively immune to the disease (survival bias). This is less of a problem with new exposures to a harmful factor (e.g. new employees of a company), where cohorts have a comparable past risk factor status. Furthermore, after formation of a cohort, the explanatory factor pattern may change substantially, diluting the original contrast in explanatory factor status. Levels of the primary explanatory factor need to be monitored during the follow-up period.

4. A cohort study may not be efficient for studying outcomes that occur infrequently and those with a long preclinical phase. Cohort studies usually have large numbers of participants and long follow-up periods. For common conditions such as the common cold, hemorrhoids, or hypertension, small cohorts may suffice, especially if the association with the explanatory factor of interest is strong. Cohort studies do not always need to take a long time either. For a study of congenital abnormalities due to risk factors during pregnancy, the follow-up period is confined to a maximum of 9 months.

There are ways of maximizing information per study participant, and at minimum cost:

1. By ensuring there is sufficient contrast in the distribution of the primary explanatory factor. As explained in Section 4.1.3, the size of the study population can be reduced substantially by selecting persons at the most extreme levels of exposure to explanatory factors.
2. By using data that have been recorded in the past, it is sometimes possible to perform a historical cohort study. The distinguishing feature of a historical cohort study is that the researchers conceive the study after the explanatory factor status has been measured in the past. The researchers will determine outcome status of the cohort members and then find out the explanatory factor status of these individuals as recorded in the past. In practical terms, this means having access to records or databases that bring together relevant data on large groups of people: for example, company records with information on working conditions and explanatory factors. Based on these records, we can then check which participants subsequently developed the outcome. This type of study follows the basic design of a cohort study, except that the exposures of interest happened in the past. A historical cohort study is particularly useful to study the etiology of outcomes with a long preclinical stage. In those situations, a regular cohort study would take far too long to obtain enough incident cases of the outcome. As historical records containing enough individual-level information on the primary exposure and potential confounders are relatively rare, the opportunities for historical cohort studies are sparse. The opportunities for such studies

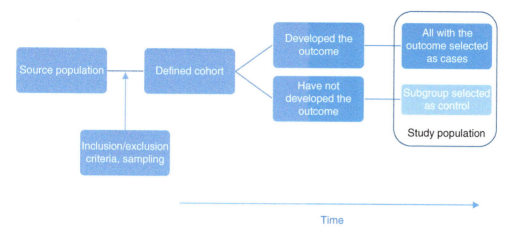

Figure 4.8 Design of a nested case–control study within a cohort.

have been substantially improved – at least potentially – with the introduction of large-scale storage of biological samples in biobanks (see Case 4.2). In addition, digital information is increasingly collected and stored in large volume via the Internet and social media. These data may contain records of demographic characteristics, diagnoses, and therapies on millions of people – anonymously or in encoded form. Using "big data" could make historic cohort studies very efficient, but lack of complete and valid data on explanatory factors and confounders, and the fact that the data cannot always be linked to outcomes, will often force researchers toward prospective cohort studies. In this book, we will use cohort studies to refer to both prospective and historical cohort studies for simplicity because the explanatory factors are measured before the outcomes, which is a key feature that distinguishes a cohort design from a case–control and a cross-sectional design.

3. By carrying out case–control analysis within a cohort study (nested case–control study). When studying a rare outcome, only a small portion of participants are likely to develop the outcome of interest during the follow-up period. Often, it is inefficient to include all the participants who are still healthy at the end of the follow-up period in the analysis. A more efficient approach can sometimes be adopted: collect and store the relevant explanatory factor data on all members of the cohort at the start of the study (if collection of data is feasible), but do not analyze and process them. Record all the new cases developing the outcome dur-

ing the follow-up period. Analyze only then the available data (risk factors, confounders) for these individuals with the outcome, along with data from a random sample of the original cohort, which could theoretically include people with the outcome (see Figure 4.8). Performing nested case–control study improves efficiency especially when:

- analysis of all explanatory factor data would be expensive or labor-intensive (e.g. processing dietary questionnaires, imaging interpretation, and biomarkers)
- the unprocessed data can be stored for a long time (e.g. frozen serum samples).

Cases 4.2 and 4.3 provide examples of cohort studies.

Case 4.2 UK Biobank, a Large Cohort Study in the United Kingdom (UK)

UK Biobank is a major national population cohort enabling longitudinal studies on a wide range of illnesses – including cancer, heart diseases, stroke, diabetes, arthritis, osteoporosis, eye disorders, depression and dementia. UK Biobank recruited 500,000 people aged between 40 and 69 years in 2006–2010 from across the UK to take part in this project. They have undergone many measurements, provided blood, urine and saliva samples for future analysis, and agreed to have their health status followed. Over many years, this biobank has built into a powerful resource to help scientists discover why some people develop particular diseases and others do not. UK Biobank is hosted by the University of Manchester and open to bona fide researchers anywhere in the world. In addition to information collected during the baseline assessment, participants wear wrist activity monitors and complete detailed web-based questionnaires on their diet, cognitive function and work history. A large number of the participants have undergone MRI body and DEXA bone scanning. All data, including genetic, biochemistry and imaging data, are being made available for research as they become ready.

Case 4.3 Ionizing Radiation and Risk of Death from Leukemia and Lymphoma in Radiation-Monitored Workers (INWORKS): An International Historic Cohort Study

To quantify the risks of leukemia and lymphoma after repeated or protracted low-dose radiation in occupational, environmental, and diagnostic medical settings, an international consortium set up a large-scale historic cohort study on leukemia, lymphoma, and multiple myeloma mortality among radiation-monitored adults employed in France, the UK, and the United States (US). The investigators assembled a cohort of 308,297 radiation-monitored workers employed for at least one year by atomic energy companies in France, by the Departments of Energy and Defense in the US, and by nuclear industries in the UK. The cohort was followed up for a total of 8.22 million person-years. All registered deaths caused by leukemia, lymphoma, and multiple myeloma were recorded. Poisson regression was applied to quantify associations between estimated red bone marrow absorbed dose and leukemia and lymphoma mortality. Radiation doses were very low (mean 1.1 mGy per year, SD 2.6). The excess relative risk of leukemia mortality (excluding chronic lymphocytic leukemia) was 2.96 per Gy (90% CI 1.17–5.21; lagged two years), most notably because of an association between radiation dose and mortality from chronic myeloid leukemia (excess relative risk per Gy 10.45, 90% CI 4.48–19.65). This study provided strong evidence of a causal association between protracted low-dose radiation exposure and leukemia.

4.3.2 Case–control study

As we saw in the previous section, a case–control design is simply an efficient sampling technique to measure exposure-outcome associations in a cohort. In theory, every case–control study takes place within a cohort although, in practice, it can be difficult or impossible to characterize the cohort. The cases are collected, for example, from a hospital, a neighborhood, or an insurance company's records. The risk factor status of these cases at a relevant time in the past then has to be ascertained. The identification of the appropriate source population from which to select controls is the primary challenge in the design of case–control studies (see ▢ Figure 4.9, Step 1). In essence, this source population is the collection of all individuals who would become the cases if they develop the outcome under study. Once the source population is identified, we have the ideal sampling framework for a suitable control group (see ▢ Figure 4.9, Step 2); in practice, this turns out to be quite complicated.

Once we have selected a case group and a suitable control group, we need to collect information on the past exposure to explanatory factors and confounders for all individuals in both groups (see ▢ Figure 4.9, Step 3). A case–control study does not follow the course of outcomes over time but looks back at the exposure history of the participants. This feature of case–control studies makes them quick to carry out, as all the relevant outcomes (and explanatory factors) have already taken place. Another important feature of case–control studies is that, by approximating an efficient sample of the source population, a small number of participants is usually needed. This advantage is lost, however, if we are dealing with a rare risk factor. Designing and carrying out a case–control study presents a substantial challenge in practice. Let us briefly discuss the main complications.

Selecting the cases

The participants that we find, for example, in a hospital only constitutes a selection of all individuals with the outcome or disease of interest. Milder cases do not generally end up in hospital and the worst cases may have already died. Some hospitals attract patients from outside their region because of their specialty. Furthermore, patients with the explanatory factor may be overrepresented because the presence of that

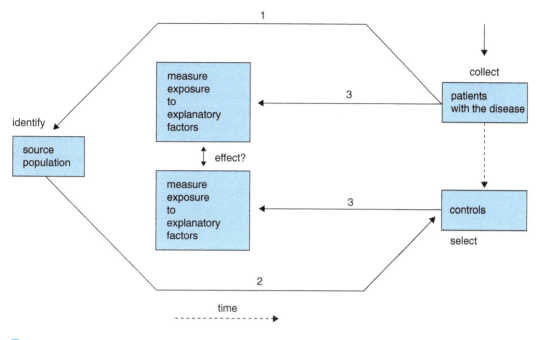

◻ Figure 4.9 Design of a case–control study.

factor has been used to diagnose them. These various selection mechanisms can potentially jeopardize the validity of the study. To avoid such problems, it is preferable to use incident (new) cases of the disease.

Selecting the controls

The purpose of having a control group is to show the frequency of the explanatory factor of interest and the confounders in the source population from which the cases are drawn. We then compare this distribution with those found among the cases. The controls should be taken from the population who have the potential to develop the outcome: in a study on the use of estrogen and endometrial cancer we would look for female controls with a uterus, for instance.

While there are often several options for the selection of a control group, we need to choose the option that maximizes validity and efficiency. Some commonly used options:

- *A population-based control group*. This is a sample from the general population (e.g. taken from the population register). We then assume that the population from which the controls have been selected is the same as the population from which all cases have been selected (the source population). The assumption is valid when incident cases

are recruited, for example, from a population cancer registry. Often, however, this is not the case because referral patterns may differ across geographical regions and depend on personal preferences.

- *A hospital-based control group*. This is made up of patients from the same hospital but with a different condition. Such controls are easier to find and contact, as they are usually more motivated to take part in a study than healthy controls. Another advantage is that the risk of recall bias is probably smaller, as the controls are themselves patients. It is important, however, to select for the control group only patients suffering from conditions not related to the explanatory factors being studied, otherwise we may be comparing two diseases related to the same explanatory factor, which will cause bias. This phenomenon is known as Berkson's fallacy. For example, if we were to examine the risk of smoking on heart attack and used lung cancer patients as the control group, the controls would not accurately reflect the source population.

- *A peer-based control group*. A quick, simple and inexpensive way of selecting controls is to ask cases to suggest friends or contacts from their social network. This provides a control group

4

◘ Table 4.1 Major differences between a case–control study and a cohort study.

Case–control study	Cohort study
Relatively inexpensive	Often expensive
Quick results	Often a long wait
Relatively small study population	Relatively large study population
Suitable for rare diseases	Suitable for common diseases
Unsuitable for rare exposure	Suitable for rare exposures
Complete information	Risk of loss follow-up, selective dropout
Susceptible to bias, especially selection bias, information bias (exposure measurement), confounding	Less susceptible to bias, but possible information bias (outcome measurement) Confounding, selective dropout, changes in measuring procedures
Only OR can be calculated (RR estimated), not incidences (risks)	Incidences (risks), AR and RR can be calculated directly

containing people who are comparable with the cases. The danger, however, is that the controls will also be comparable in terms of the exposures being studied. When the selection of controls is dependent on the explanatory factor of interest, selection bias can be introduced.

- A *family-based control group*. If we are prepared to ignore the effects of genetic factors, it may be useful to select family of the case as controls: in studies of twins, for example. There is family clustering of many environmental factors, however, so this method is not suitable for studying explanatory factors that correlate highly within families. The major differences between a case-control study and a cohort study is summarized in ◘ Table 4.1.

Measuring explanatory factors

In a case–control study, we usually have to rely on questionnaires to measure the explanatory factor of interest and the confounders in the time period relevant to the development of the outcome, which means relying on the respondents' memories. Some explanatory factors cannot be ascertained at all using this method

(e.g. concentrations of biomarkers in the blood sample), while others cannot be ascertained accurately (complex behaviors, e.g. diet during the teenage years). There is a real danger of explanatory factor measurement being affected by the fact that the researchers and the participants know what relationship the study is looking for. Blinding is by no means always feasible. When measuring the explanatory factor, it is also vital to ask the correct time period in the past. What we have said about measuring the explanatory factor of interest also applies to potential confounders and effect modifiers (see Chapter 5).

Matching

Matching is sometimes used in case–control studies. This involves selecting controls who are similar to the cases as much as possible with regard to important confounding factors. This strategy is more efficient than adjusting for confounding in a multivariable regression analysis within a non-matched case–control study. Matching can be done in two ways. Individual matching involves finding a suitable control for each case. Frequency matching involves selecting controls in such a way that the distribution of the matching variables among them is comparable to that among the cases.

Matching also has its disadvantages. Once matching has been done for a particular factor, the effect of that factor cannot be studied anymore. Matching in case–control studies introduces confounding and should always be followed by a stratified or multivariable analysis that adjusts for that confounding (see Chapter 5). Matching factors strongly associated with the primary explanatory factor would hide the relationship being studied (overmatching). When designing the study, we need to check whether the advantages of matching outweigh the additional time, money, and energy involved in finding suitable matched controls. Note that when calculating odds ratios from case–control data with individual matching, there is a special statistical method based on matched case–control pairs (see ◘ Table 4.2). If we calculated odds ratios using the standard method (see Chapter 3), we would underestimate the strength of the relationship. Matching is not only used in case–control studies. It can also take place in cohort studies (where exposed and non-exposed groups are matched to selected characteristics).

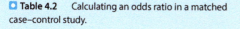 **Table 4.2**   Calculating an odds ratio in a matched case–control study.

Controls	Cases	
	Risk factor present	Risk factor absent
Risk factors present	a	b
Risk factors absent	c	d
OR = b/c		

Case 4.4 Traveler's Diarrhea, a Case–Control Study

Suppose we want to examine whether consumption of tequila, a local hard liquor, is the cause of traveler's diarrhea in German tourists on holiday in the city of Acapulco in Mexico. To answer this question, we collect all the German patients admitted to hospital in Acapulco with traveler's diarrhea. We then investigate their tequila consumption prior to the diarrhea episode. The next step is to find a suitable control group. A representative sample of the inhabitants of Mexico is not suitable, as their tequila consumption is different from that of the average tourist. A representative sample of Germans will not do either, as only Germans who travel to Mexico could drink tequila there or be admitted to hospital in Acapulco. The best control group is other Germans who traveled to Acapulco at the same time and did not have traveler's diarrhea during their stay there.

Case 4.5 Smoking and Lung Cancer, a Case–Control Study

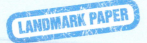

Richard Doll and Bradford Hill, two of the best-known epidemiologists of the twentieth century, were the first to track down the link between smoking and lung cancer using a case–control study – one of the most important epidemiological findings to date, which had a major impact on public health. In order to explain the high mortality from lung cancer in London, in 1950, Doll and Hill started questioning all patients with lung cancer in 20 London hospitals. When selecting a lung cancer patient, they looked for a control at the same hospital of the same gender and approximately the same age but without cancer. If they were unable to find suitable hospital controls at that hospital, they selected controls from other hospitals in the area. Each patient's diagnosis was checked using histopathology. In this way, Doll and Hill were able to include 709 lung cancer patients and an equal number of matched controls in their study. Although they initially hypothesized that lung cancer was related to car exhaust fumes, they found that the association with smoking was much stronger. Virtually all the lung cancer patients had smoked (99.7% of the men and 68.3% of the women), whereas the figures were far lower among the controls (95.8% of the men and 46.6% of the women). When they looked at the number of cigarettes smoked, they found the association was even stronger: the risk of developing lung cancer was 50 times greater in those who smoked 25 cigarettes a day than in non-smokers. Based on his findings, Bradford Hill stopped smoking himself.

4.3.3 Cross-sectional study

The study designs discussed earlier all have at least two different observation times for each individual, one for the explanatory factor under consideration and the confounders, and one for the outcome. In a cross-sectional study, the explanatory factor of interest, the outcome and all confounders are measured at the same time for each participant (see ◘ Figure 4.10), which will not necessarily be the same calendar time for all participants.

One problem of a cross-sectional study is that we are usually uncertain whether the risk factor was present before the occurrence of the outcome, one important criterion to establish a causal relationship. If we want to know whether stress is a cause of heart attacks, there is no point in measuring the current degree of stress in a group of patients recently admitted to hospital with an acute heart attack and a group of controls. Nor will a researcher find an answer to whether there is a causal relationship between regularly wearing a hat and baldness by comparing the degree of

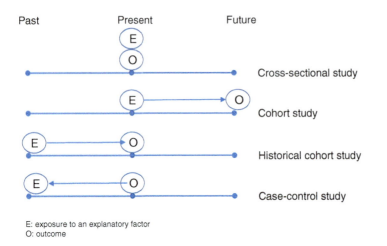

Past   Present   Future

E: exposure to an explanatory factor
O: outcome

Figure 4.10 The temporal relationship between observation times in various epidemiological study designs.

baldness in a sample of men with and without a hat. Only if we can satisfactorily demonstrate that the measured value of the explanatory factor under consideration remains stable over a long period (e.g. blood group, sex, personality, and other genetically determined characteristics) can we use a cross-sectional study for etiological research.

4.3.4 Ecological study

In the types of study described so far, the observations and measurements are always carried out on individuals and the comparison is between individuals. An eco-logical study does not have measurements on the individual level; instead, group characteristics are compared. Examples of groups include countries, regions, general practices, and schools. Outcome and explanatory factors are regarded as group characteristics, presented as population averages. These data are usually collected as a matter of routine, such as food consumption data and statistics on mortality or hospital admissions. To gain an understanding of the relationship between explanatory factors and outcomes, we can compare two or more populations – usually geographical units – at a particular point in time (geographical correlation studies), or we can examine the same population at two or more different times (time-trend studies). A hybrid approach can also be adopted. We could look, for example, at the differences in disease frequency between a region where a new medical facility has been introduced and a comparable region where

this has not been done (simultaneous comparison). Or, we could look for differences in outcome frequency in a region between the periods before and after the introduction of a new facility (pre-post comparison).

The fact that aggregate data are used to examine the relationship between the explanatory factor under consideration and the outcome is the Achilles heel of ecological studies. If we incorrectly translate associations at the population level to the individual level, we fall into the ecological fallacy, for example, because there is a systematic difference between the groups we are comparing. In nineteenth-century Europe, suicide rates were higher in countries that were more heavily Protestant than countries that were more heavily Catholic. The inference that suicide was promoted by the social conditions of Protestantism is incorrect because the Protestant countries were different from the Catholic countries in many ways besides religion (the problem of "confounding"). The association at the population level does not automatically characterize the relationship at the level of the individual.

In any epidemiological study, we need to check whether the research question is about individual risk or group risk. If it is about individual risk, the most that an ecological study can do is generate ideas about a possible relationship between exposures and outcomes. We then will need to select a study design that has the individual as the unit of observation and analysis, so as not to fall into the ecological fallacy.

The reporting of observational studies should follow the STROBE guideline and its extensions, available from the EQUATOR network's website.

Recommended reading

Gordis epidemiology Celentano, David D; Szklo, M (Moyses); Gordis, Leon, 1934–2015. Epidemiology, 6e. Philadelphia, PA: Elsevier, [2019]. (Chapters 7-11).

Szklo, M. and Nieto, F.J. (2019). *Epidemiology: Beyond the Basics*, 4e. Burlington, Massachusetts: Jones & Bartlett Learning. (Chapter 1).

Rothman, K.J., Lash, T.L., VanderWeele, T.J., and Haneuse, S. (2021). *Modern Eidemiology*, 4e. Philadelphia: Wolters Kluwer. (Chapters 8, 9 and 11).

Piantadosi, S. (2017). *Clinical Trials: A Methodologic Perspective*, 3e. New York: Wiley.

Source references (cases)

de Kieviet, J.F., Vuijk, P.J., van den Berg, A. et al. (2014). Elburg RM van. Glutamine effects on brain growth in very preterm children in the first year of life. *Clin. Nutr.* 33 (1): 69–74. (Case 4.1).

Biobank www.ukbiobank.ac.uk. (Case 4.2) (accessed 12 June 2022).

Leurand, K., Richardson, D.B., Cardis, E. et al. (2015). Ionising radiation and risk of death from leukaemia and lymphoma in radiation-monitored workers (INWORKS): an international cohort study. *Lancet Haematol.* 2: e276–e281. (Case 4.3).

Miettinen, O.S. (1985). The "case–control" study: valid selection of subjects. *J. Chronic Dis.* 38: 543–548. (Case 4.4).

Doll, R. and Hill, A.B. (1950). Smoking and carcinoma of the lung: preliminary report. *Br. Med. J.* 2 (4682): 739–748. (Case 4.5).

Source references (knowledge assessment questions)

Jensen, P., Ahlehoff, O., Egeberg, A. et al. (2016). Psoriasis and new-onset depression: a Danish Nationwide cohort study. *Acta Derm. Venereol.* 96 (1): 39–42. https://doi.org/10.2340/00015555-2183. PMID: 26086213. (Question 5).

Sardana, K., Gupta, T., Kumar, B. et al. (2016). Cross-sectional pilot study of antibiotic resistance in propionibacterium acnes strains in Indian acne patients using 16S-RNA polymerase chain reaction: a comparison among treatment modalities including antibiotics, benzoyl peroxide, and isotretinoin. *Indian J. Dermatol.* 61 (1): 45–52. https://doi.org/10.4103/0019-5154.174025. PMID: 26955094. (Question 6).

Teo, K.K., Ounpuu, S., Hawken, S. et al. (2006). Tobacco use and risk of myocardial infarction in 52 countries in the INTERHEART study: a case–control study. *Lancet* 368 (9536): 647–658. https://doi.org/10.1016/S0140-6736(06)69249-0. PMID: 16920470. (Question 7).

Knowledge assessment questions

1. The local department of public health in Mumbai has been alerted to a recent outbreak of Botulism. One hundred and forty-five people have been reported as cases in the last six days – the largest outbreak of the century. Researchers quickly mobilized to determine the source. Enrolling all cases and 145 controls without Botulism, researchers collect a detailed food intake history to try to determine the source of the outbreak. This study would best be described as: (select the one best answer)

   a. Analytical, observational, case–control study
   b. Descriptive, ecological, cross-sectional study
   c. Analytical, observational, cohort study
   d. Analytical, ecological, time trend study

2. You are designing a study you hope to generalize to the citizens of Lithuania. Which of the following would you deem to be a suitable study sample? (select all that apply)

   a. A cross-section of staff and students at Vilnius University in Lithuania
   b. All members of a random sample of 500 households from the last census
   c. A group of individuals who regularly participate in food-pantry distribution at a local elementary school
   d. A new mother's support group
   e. A random sample of phone numbers of residents throughout the country
   f. A cross section of the largest metropolitan hospital patients on a given day
   g. Respondents to a food-assistance government-offered program

3. Which of the following is NOT an advantage of a cohort study? (select the one best answer)

   a. Incidence and incidence rates can be calculated
   b. Information bias in the measurement and ascertainment of exposure is minimized compared with a case–control study
   c. Many health outcomes can be studied simultaneously
   d. Rare outcomes can be studied easily
   e. Clarity of temporal sequence

4. Which of the following is NOT an advantage of a case control study? (select the one best answer)

   a. Efficient for rare diseases or diseases with a long latency period between exposure and disease manifestation
   b. Less costly and less time-consuming compared with a cohort study
   c. Suitable when exposure data are expensive or hard to obtain
   d. Suitable when studying dynamic populations in which follow-up is difficult
   e. Exposures can be measured with little information bias

5. To study whether psoriasis is associated with an increased risk of depression, researchers in Denmark looked at all individuals aged ≥18 years from 2001 to 2011 from national registries. They excluded individuals with prevalent depression and/or psoriasis at baseline. The outcome of interest was the initiation of antidepressants or hospitalization for depression. The researchers compared the incidence rates of outcome in those with psoriasis and those without psoriasis. This study can be best described as a: (select the one best answer)

   a. Cross-sectional study
   b. Case–control study
   c. Cohort study
   d. Randomized controlled trial
   e. Time trend study

6. To study antibiotic resistance in isolates of *Propionibacterium acnes (P. acnes)*, researchers in India recruited 80 patients with acne vulgaris in a tertiary care hospital in India. They collected specimens from study participants. These specimens were then cultured, the growth identified, and antibiotic susceptibility and resistance were assessed. They isolated *P. acnes* in

52% of the cases. In these isolates, resistance for erythromycin, clindamycin, and azithromycin was observed in 98%, 90%, and 100% of the isolates, respectively. This study can be best described as a: (select the one best answer)

a. Cross-sectional study
b. Case–control study
c. Cohort study
d. Randomized controlled trial

7. To study tobacco use and risk of myocardial infarction, researchers identified 12,461 cases of first acute myocardial infarction and 14,820 age-matched and sex-matched controls from 52 countries. Trained staff administered a structured questionnaire and did physical examinations for all participants in the same manner. Participants were asked if they regularly used tobacco products. This study can best be described as a: (select the one best answer)

a. Cross-sectional study
b. Case–control study
c. Cohort study
d. Randomized controlled trial
e. Geographic correlation study

Precision and Validity

Textbook of Epidemiology, Second Edition. Lex Bouter, Maurice Zeegers and Tianjing Li.
© 2023 John Wiley & Sons Ltd. Published 2023 by John Wiley & Sons Ltd.
Companion website: www.wiley.com/go/Bouter/TextbookofEpidemiology

5.1 Introduction

You will undoubtedly have noticed that characterizing the epidemiological function is pivotal in epidemiological research. Here is that function once more:

$$P(O) = f(b_0 + b_1 F_1 + b_2 F_2 + \ldots + b_k F_k)$$

To put it in words: the probability of the occurrence of any health outcome ($P(O)$) is described as a mathematical function of a series of explanatory factors F_i (where i = 1, …, k, and k is the number of risk factors). The regression coefficients in the function indicate the slope of the association between those factors and the health outcome. In epidemiological research, we would like the estimated regression coefficient, and the epidemiological measure of association derived from it, to reflect the association between the explanatory factor and the outcome as accurately and validly as possible. Or, in other words, this should be as close as possible to the true association. For example, if a logistic regression equation in a sample yields a regression coefficient of 0.6 (corresponding to an odds ratio, or, of Exp(0.6) = 1.8), that number, in theory, should be a valid and precise representation of the association between that explanatory factor and the health outcome in the target population being studied. In an ideal world, we would not want any systematic or random error that could cause the observed odds ratio to be significantly higher or lower than the true value. A small discrepancy between the estimated parameter and the true strength of the link may not be disastrous (e.g. an odds ratio of 1.7 or 1.9 in this case), but a large discrepancy could lead to completely different conclusions about the strength of the association. As a rule of thumb, for binary risk factors (e.g. yes/no eating processed meat) an odds ratio that ranges between 0.80 and 1.20 is indicative of no association, while an OR <0.80 or >1.20 is indicative of an association. An odds ratio of <0.5 of >2.0 would be interpreted as substantial. This is because an odds ratio of >2.0 equates to an etiological fraction of >50% (see Chapter 3, Section 3.2.5). For continuous risk factors, the value of the OR depends on the measurement scale and no rule of thumb can be given.

5.2 Systematic and random errors

When estimating measures of frequency and measures of association (see Chapter 3) in epidemiological

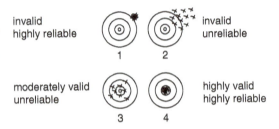

Figure 5.1 Validity and reliability expressed as throwing darts at a target.

research, just as when measuring just about anything, two types of errors can occur: systematic errors and random errors. Systematic errors occur when incorrect or inappropriate decisions are made during the design, execution of the study or the data analysis. These lead to a systematic over- or underestimation of the parameter. For this, epidemiologists use the term bias. If no bias exists, the study results are valid. Random errors, on the other hand, are non-systematic and can occur due to sampling error. The term precise refers to a lack of random sampling error, whereas the term reliable refers to the lack of random measurement error. This chapter mainly discusses validity and precision in study designs, moving on briefly to validity and reliability of instruments in Section 5.7.

The difference between validity and precision can easily be illustrated using a darts example: someone with a good (*read: valid*) but trembling (*read: unprecise*) arm may hit the bullseye on the dartboard by chance but will be more likely to hit randomly around it. A steady (*read: precise*) hand with a poor throwline (*read: invalid*), however, will consistently produce hits at the same, albeit wrong, spot. Only someone with both the correct throwline and a steady hand will always be able to hit the bullseye. The bullseye of a dartboard represents, in this metaphor, the true value of a frequency measure or measure of association in epidemiological research (see Figure 5.1).

5.3 Precision

A study design that repeatedly produces the same result (for example, an incidence, relative risk (RR) or difference of means) has high precision. In other words, when a study is precise, the study result should always be more or less the same if the study is repeated (with the same study design and analytical methods in a new sample from the source population).

5.3.1 Random error

Random errors can be due not only to random measurement errors in individual observations (see Section 5.7), but also to the fact that every epidemiological study is based on observations of random samples. The observed individuals (also called the study population or the sample) are a random representation of a larger source population from which the researchers want to draw inference to. Theoretically, all individuals who meet the study eligibility criteria could be included but, for practical reasons, almost always, only a much smaller number is recruited to participate in a study. The results of this sampling should be based purely on chance, so sampling error is a major factor in the precision of results from epidemiological research. The researchers could have recruited another randomly selected study population instead of the one with which they are now working. The larger a sample is, the smaller the effect of random errors on the precision of the results of a study.

Estimates of measures of frequency and association must be sufficiently precise, i.e. the magnitude of the random errors must be minimized in relation to the true value of the parameter. In statistics, sampling error is expressed as a standard error (SE), which can be interpreted as the standard deviation of the measured parameter, if the study was to be repeated many times using other samples from the same source population. The formulas for calculating the standard error of a proportion, the mean, the difference of means, the odds ratio and the RR are shown in ◻ Figure 5.2. We can see from these formulae that – as we would expect – the larger the sample, the smaller the standard error will be and thus, the greater precision is obtained.

Of course, not only the measures of frequency and association but any population parameter estimated from a sample has a standard error. Generally speaking, the standard error is determined by three factors:

- The measurement error of the separate observations in the sample.
- The distribution of the parameter in the population from which the sample has been taken.
- The size of the sample.

The standard deviation, then, should not be confused with the standard error. The standard error indicates the variation in a population parameter (mean, proportion, etc.) estimated from a sample.

SE of a proportion	$\sqrt{\dfrac{p(1-p)}{n}}$
SE of the mean	$\dfrac{s}{\sqrt{n}}$
SE of a difference of means	$\sqrt{\dfrac{s_1{}^2 + s_2{}^2}{n}}$
SE ln(OR)	$\sqrt{\dfrac{1}{a} + \dfrac{1}{b} + \dfrac{1}{c} + \dfrac{1}{d}}$
SE ln(RR)	$\sqrt{\dfrac{b}{a(a+b)} + \dfrac{d}{c(c+d)}}$

	Health Outcome	
Risk Factor	Present	Not Present
Present	a	b
Not Present	c	d

◻ **Figure 5.2** Calculation of the standard error (SE) for a proportion, a mean, the difference of means, the logarithm of the odds ratio (OR) and the logarithm of the relative risk (RR). P: proportion; s: standard deviation of the measurement in a sample; n: sample size.

It is the expected hypothetical standard deviation of population parameters between samples, if we were to repeat the study many times. The standard deviation indicates the spread of measurements within a specific sample. The latter is not dependent on sample size.

5.3.2 The confidence interval

The confidence interval (CI) indicates how precise the estimate of an epidemiological parameter is. A 95% CI is formally defined as the interval in which the population parameter would lie in 95% of cases if the study were to be repeated many times. Describing it more loosely, we could say that we are 95% confident that the CI covers the true value of the measure of association. Thus, the CI gives a good idea of how precise the results are. The smaller the interval, the more precise the estimate. For instance, an odds ratio of 2.0 of which we are 95% confident it lies between 1.5 and 2.7 has been estimated with greater precision compared to the same odds ratio but with a CI between 0.8 and 5.3. More (e.g. 99%) or less strict (e.g. 90%) CIs can also be calculated. From the same sample estimate, the higher the confidence required, the wider the interval will be. For example, we can say with 100% confidence that the actual RR lays between 0 and infinity (∞). Of course, this wouldn't be very informative. A CI only provides information on the precision (i.e. random error) of an epidemiological parameter, not on its validity (i.e. systematic error).

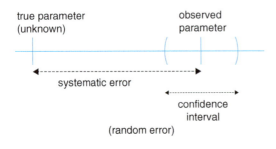

Figure 5.3 A confidence interval only provides information on the precision (random error) of an epidemiological parameter, not on its validity.

It is even possible that the true value of the estimated parameter lies outside the CI as is illustrated in Figure 5.3.

To calculate CIs we need an estimate of the standard error (SE_p) of the estimated parameter (P) (see Figure 5.2) and a translation of the confidence selected into a z-score on the standard normal distribution (e.g. 95% CI corresponds to a z-score of 1.96) (see Figure 5.4).

The 95% CI of an epidemiological parameter P in a sufficiently large sample which has an approximately normal distribution is thus:

$$95\% CI = P \pm 1.96 SE_p$$

In small samples (typically smaller than 30 observations), values from the t-distribution instead of the standard normal distribution are used. The t-distribution produces slightly wider CIs in small samples. Parameters such as RR and OR do not have a normal distribution as they can vary from 0 to ∞. But after log-transformation, these values can range from −∞ to +∞ and approximate a normal distribution. The 95% CI for ln(P) is thus:

$$95\% CI = \ln(P) \pm 1.96 SE_{\ln}(\ln(P))$$

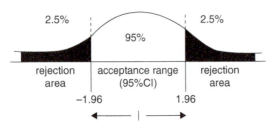

Figure 5.4 The standard normal distribution.

The result of these calculations can be interpreted as follows. Say an estimate of a cumulative incidence in a sample yields the following result: Cumulative Incidence = 5 per 10,000 = 0.0005. At a particular size of the sample, the 95% CI would then be:

$$95\% CI = 0.0005 \pm 0.0001 = (0.0004 - 0.0006)$$

This means that we are 95% confident that the actual cumulative incidence in the population from which the random sample has been selected lies between 4 and 6 per 10,000.

An estimate of the RR in a particular study, for example, yields the following result: RR = 1.52 (95% CI 1.27–1.81). This means that we can be fairly certain that there is a real, slightly increased risk. That would not have been the case if we had obtained a 95% CI of 0.82–2.33 for this RR of 1.52, as such a CI would imply, we are 95% confident the actual population RR indicates lower risk (RR between 0.82 and 1), no increased risk (RR = 1), a slightly increased risk (RR between 1 and 2), or a moderately increased risk (RR between 2 and 2.33).

A related, but usually misinterpreted, concept is the p-value. A p-value of 0.03, for instance, expresses that, if the null hypothesis is true (that a risk factor has no effect on the outcome), there is a 3% probability (p = probability) of obtaining results at least as extreme as those actually observed in the study. A very small p-value means that such an extreme observed result would be very unlikely under the null hypothesis. When the probability is regarded as low enough, for example, lower than a threshold of $\alpha = 5\%$, we conclude that the risk factor has a statistically significant effect on the outcome (see Figure 5.4). Note that there is a one-to-one relationship between α and CI. When testing with an α of 5%, it is accompanied by a 95% CI, whereas testing with an α of, e.g., 1%, a 99% CI would be calculated. This way, conclusions based on the p-value of the outcome of the statistical test and based on the CI would always be in agreement. Since the meaning of p-value is hard to grasp, misuse is widespread. The p-value does not measure the probability that the null hypothesis is true.

The use of statistical tests is based on the idea that we ultimately want to draw conclusions about whether the estimates can or cannot be explained by random variation with a degree of plausibility. A p-value of 0.03, then, indicates that the probability that this result is purely due to chance (or more precisely: sampling error) is so small that the null hypothesis could be rejected. Similarly, it is standard practice to interpret a p-value higher than 0.05 as indicating that the result obtained could have been caused by chance. Clearly, the p-value is not a gauge of the magnitude of an effect. Statistical tests can help answer the question of whether it is likely that there is an effect, not how large it is or could be. To estimate the magnitude of an effect, the p-value will not suffice; we are better off using a CI. Scientific conclusions should focus mainly on the size of the estimates of association, and the CI as a measure of precision.

5.3.3 Precision versus sample size

To calculate the number of participants needed to obtain results with a particular precision, we have a collection of sample size formulas to use. These are included in most statistical software packages.

To apply sample size formulas, we need – in the case of dichotomous outcomes – information on the following parameters:

1. The health outcome frequency in the reference group, if necessary, estimated based on the frequency in the source population.
2. The minimum size of the association that we would consider to be worthwhile to demonstrate. We would need to include fewer people in the study when the expected association is greater.
3. The probability that we mistakenly claim an association that is not actually there (type I error or α-error). For example, a type I error of 0.05 means a 5% chance of finding a statistically significant association that does not actually exist. The lower we want to make this probability, the more people we need to include in the study (see also 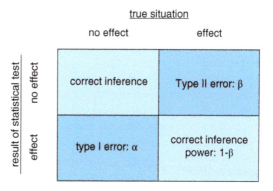 Figure 5.5).
4. The probability that we miss an association that actually exists (type II error or β-error). A type II error of 0.20, for instance, means a 20% chance of missing an association that actually exists. The lower we want to make this probability, the more people we need to include in the study (see also ▢ Figure 5.5). The complement of the type II error (1-β) is the power, i.e. the probability of detecting an association in the study that actually exists.
5. The desired ratio between the numbers of participants in each of the groups being compared, e.g. three times more controls than cases in a case-control study.

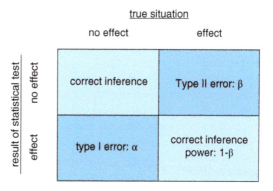

▢ Figure 5.5 The relationship between type I errors, type II errors and power.

6. The hypothesis we wish to test. In addition to the one described above, other options such as non-inferiority hypotheses and equivalence hypotheses can be chosen.

Precision in a study depends not only on the size of the study population but also on how that study population is assembled and divided into the various groups being compared. The efficiency of an epidemiological study is essentially related to the total amount of informative data available. The more participants and also the greater the amount of data per individual, the higher the statistical efficiency.

5.4 Validity

Although a result may be very precise as judged by a narrow CI (i.e. yielding similar estimates of effect on repetition – or in other words with limited random error), it may nevertheless be completely wrong because of the occurrence of systematic errors. We call this bias. Results from biased research present a distorted view of reality. This section discusses three types of bias in measures of association.

5.4.1 Selection bias, information bias and confounding

Bias occurs when associations systematically differ from reality (see ▢ Figure 5.1). A host of mistakes can be made that lead to invalid conclusions on the relationship between exploratory factors and health outcomes. Broadly speaking, these can be classified into three types of bias: selection bias, information bias, and confounding. Bias can cause the effect to be over-estimated, underestimated or even observed as going in the opposite direction to reality.

Suppose we want to examine the association between an explanatory factor and an outcome using a case-control design. The true association is OR = 2.5. Errors could result in the study producing an OR of 5.0: this is an overestimate of the association, also referred to as positive bias or bias away from the null value (no association, in the case of an OR this would be 1). The study could alternatively produce a result of OR = 1.5: this is an underestimate, also referred to as negative bias or bias toward the null value. Both over- and underestimations are considered quantitative bias (see also ◘ Figure 5.6). The study could even produce an OR of 0.7: here, the association changes into the opposite direction (switch-over bias). In this example, the risk factor was actually harmful, but as a result of errors in the design and execution, the study suggests that it is a protective factor, producing a qualitative bias in the association (see also ◘ Figure 5.7).

We need to anticipate potential bias during the design and execution of the study, since once the study has been initiated, there is not much that can be done about any remaining bias. Although the direction of the resulting systematic error might be predicted in most instances, it is not usually possible to ascertain the magnitude of the bias. Nevertheless, all information on the direction and potential size of bias, however limited and incomplete it may be, is vital to the interpretation of the results. For example, if a case-control study finds a fairly clear increased odds (OR = 3.0) and it can be argued that any bias must be toward the null hypothesis, the true OR would be greater than 3.0 and there is almost certainly a strong association in the target population. If only a slightly increased risk is found (e.g. OR = 1.1) and it can be argued that any bias is away from the null, the true OR is evidently less than 1.1, and what remains has little, if any, value. The true OR could even be less than 1.0, in which case, the true effect is in the opposite direction. And, if a substantially increased risk is found (e.g. OR = 8.0), there must be a very strong bias away from the null hypothesis if there is actually no effect.

Selection bias is a distortion of the estimate of effect due to errors in the selection or follow-up of the participants. Information bias is a distortion of the esti-mate of effect due to errors in measuring the variables in the study (risk factors, outcomes, confounders,

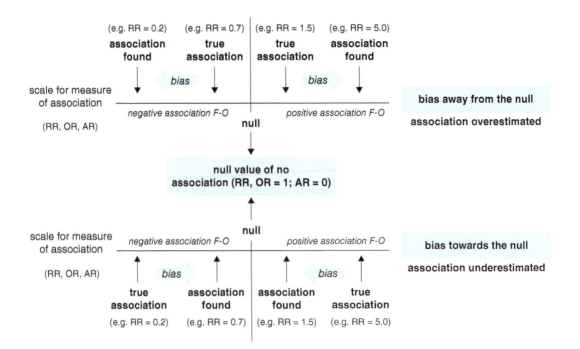

◘ **Figure 5.6** Quantitative bias in the association between explanatory factor (F) and disease outcome (O).

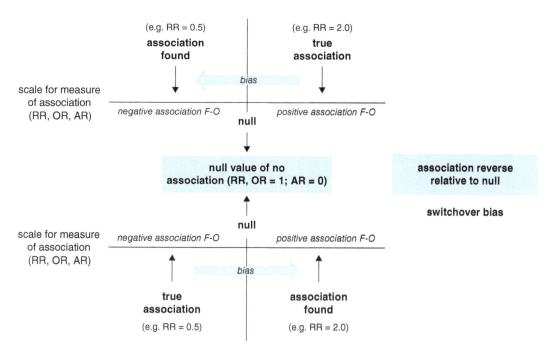

Figure 5.7 Qualitative bias in the association between explanatory factor (F) and disease outcome (O).

effect modifiers). Confounding results in a distorted estimate of effect because the groups being compared in the study have been exposed in non-comparable ways to other risk factors for the disease. This causes the effect of the primary factor to become mixed up, or confounded, with that of the other risk factors ("confounders" or "confounding variables") that we are not currently interested in.

These three categories of bias can overlap to some extent. Confounding can be introduced, for instance, by the selection of the participants. Nor is it always possible to make a clear distinction between confounding and information bias. The term "confounding" is usually reserved for known measurable risk factors for the health outcome in question that are unequally distributed among the groups being compared. If these variables have actually been measured, it is usually possible to adjust for them at the analysis stage of the study. Selection bias and information bias cannot be eradicated once the study data have been collected, unless the exact magnitude and direction of the selection and measurement errors are known, which is seldom the case in practice.

Sections "Selection bias", "Information bias", and "Confounding" look at the trio of selection bias, information bias, and confounding in more detail.

Selection bias

Selection bias occurs when the probability of people being included in the sample depends on the outcome being studied (in a cohort study) or on the explanatory factor being studied (in a case-control study). We will discuss this phenomenon separately for cohort studies and case-control studies.

As we have already seen in Chapter 4, in a cohort study, participants are recruited and classified on the basis of the status of the explanatory factor (e.g. being exposed or not exposed to a potential toxic). In this type of study, selection bias occurs if the probability of being included in the sample would somehow depend on the outcome measured at the end of the follow-up period. This is called differential selection. Non-differential selection can also occur in a study when the selection probability, although different for those with or without the exploratory factor, does not differ systematically for persons with or without the outcome at the end of the study. Only differential selection causes selection bias.

Selection bias, in theory, is of a lesser concern in the context of a cohort study, as in this type of study, the risk-factor status of potential participants in the study is established before the health outcome is present. However, selection bias cannot be ruled out in cohort studies. Take, for example, a cohort study into the association between physical activity and life expectancy in middle-aged people. Among the potential participants, there are people with a congenital heart defect or some other heart problem. These people will generally be at increased risk of mortality (from cardiovascular disease). Many of them could also conceivably have been advised to take it easy with regard to physical exercise, because of the increased risk of complications. This causes a problem: in the sub-cohort of people with little physical activity, the category with short life expectancy due to a congenital heart defect will be over-represented when compared with the general population. The association between physical activity and life expectancy will be distorted because of the over-representation of people with congenital heart defects in the less active group. To avoid this type of selection bias, everyone with a known heart problem could be kept out of the study sample by restriction. We need to be particularly wary of the possibility of selection bias in a cohort study if the preliminary stages or particular preclinical characteristics of the disease being studied are related to exposure to the explanatory factor.

Differential selection can also occur in a cohort study due to selective dropout of participants after the cohort has been assembled (attrition bias). Selective dropout occurs when some of the cohort members stop taking part in the follow-up measurements after a while, for reasons related to the outcome that we are interested in. This type of selection bias can also distort the results of a randomized trial. Take, for example, an experiment looking at the effects of a new weight-loss diet compared with a normal diet: it is quite conceivable that particularly those people who do not see any results will abandon the diet after a while. The remaining participants in the experimental group will be over-represented by people who have lost weight, resulting in an overestimation of the effect of the new diet.

The participants in a case-control study are selected on the basis of their outcome status (e.g. with or without the health outcome or disease). Unlike a cohort study, a case-control study is particularly susceptible to selection bias, as the participants are recruited after the relevant exposure to the risk factor being studied has taken place. Selection bias occurs when the probability of being included in the study sample as a case (with the disease) or control (without the disease) depends on exposure to the primary factor in the study.

Selection bias occurs when the researchers recruit the participants for the study, but the seed may already have been sown at an earlier stage. An example of this is the healthy worker effect: it has been found that morbidity and mortality rates among employees are usually lower than in the general

---

Case 5.1 Venous Thromboembolism and Use of the Oral Contraceptive Pill (Hypothetical Example)

A hypothetical study aims to examine the association between the use of the oral contraception pill (OCP) in adult women and the risk of venous thromboembolism (VTE), a vascular disorder. The study is carried out in a region where 100,000 women in the 25–45 age group (the inclusion criterion) live. Over a period of two years, 100 cases of VTE occur in this population. Half of all women take the OCP. In reality, use of the OCP is not related to the development of thromboembolism (see the left half of ▢ Figure 5.8). If all women were to be included in the study, it would find an OR RR of 1.0. However, the researchers opt for a case-control design to increase the efficiency, recruiting the patients from a hospital. At the time the study was initiated, the idea that use of the OCP could be a risk factor for VTE had already been put forward in the medical press. Women with symptoms suggestive of thromboembolism and who are also on the OCP are more likely to be referred to specialists than those who are not on the OCP (90% vs. 50%). As a result of this selective referral, of the aforementioned 100 women with symptoms of VTE, 70 are ultimately admitted to hospital, the majority of them OCP users. These women are included in the case-control study as cases. The control group is a random 0.2% sample from the general population (excluding the VTE patients). The analysis of the case-control study produces an estimated OR of 1.8, i.e. a substantial overestimate of the true association (positive selection bias). The cases in the study are not a representative sample of the source patient population about which the researchers wish to draw conclusions, as it contains an excessive proportion of exposed patients (OCP users).

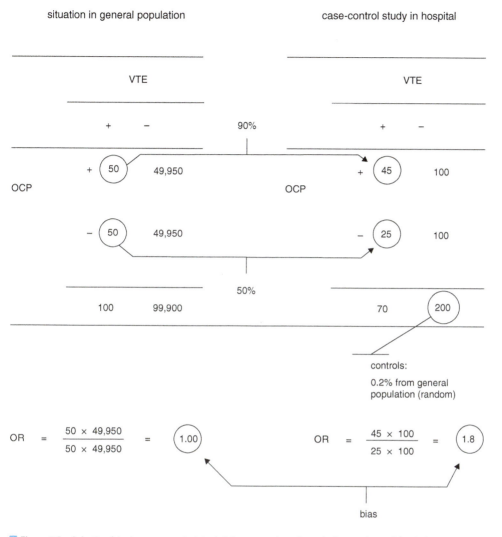

situation in general population

case-control study in hospital

Figure 5.8 Selection bias in a case-control study into venous thromboembolism and use of the Oral Contraceptive Pill.

population. This is related to the fact that people with serious illness or disabilities are less likely to participate in regular employment. For the same reasons, the general state of health of other groups too – e.g. vegetarians, physically active people, or migrants – may be better than that of the population as a whole (membership bias). The consequence of this differential selection is that certain health risks can escape attention. The incidence of non-specific respiratory tract disorders among upholsterers, for instance, will be lower than that in the population as a whole, although their working conditions are actually presumed to be associated with an increased risk of respiratory tract disorders.

Selective survival or selective mortality of the population being studied before the participants are recruited can also result in selection bias. In case-control studies in particular, there is a danger that patients whose disease lasts only a short time (they die soon or get better quickly) and patients with a mild form of the disease will be underrepresented in the study sample. Take, for example, a case-control study that examines risk factors for acute myocardial infarction based on patients admitted to hospital after an infarction. The risk profile of those who survive an infarction can potentially be very different from that of those who die from it immediately.

Case 5.2 *Cervical Cancer and Pap Smear Frequency (Hypothetical Example)*

Suppose there is a case-control study that examines whether regular pap smear tests can prevent cervical cancer. In other words: the risk factor studied is not having had a pap smear test plus missing the diagnostic and therapeutic actions that a positive pap smear test may have led to. The study is carried out on women in the 35–65 year age group in a region. Pap smear frequency is divided into two categories: pap smears or no pap smears during the previous five years. A total of over 10,000 women are potentially eligible for the study. In this population, 200 women die of cervical cancer within a few years. In the total population from which both cases and controls are sampled, 80% of these 200 women had a pap smear (PAP) while 90% of the surviving women had as is shown in the top part of ▢ Figure 5.9. Suppose a case-control study is conducted that takes as cases all 200 deaths from cervical cancer during this period. The control group is a 10% sample from the general population. These women are contacted for a telephone survey, in which they are asked, among other things, about the frequency of pap smears in the past. The response is poor, only 20%. A non-selective response would lead to the results shown at the bottom left of the diagram (no bias). In practice, however, it is mainly women in the lower socioeconomic group, who often do not have pap smears done, who are contactable by telephone. As a result of this selective non-response, the control group contains 18% of the invited women who did have pap smears done and 40% of those who did not. The result, as the right-hand side of the diagram shows, is a substantial underestimate of the protective effect of pap smears (negative selection bias).

Case 5.1 also illustrates the fact that hospitalized patients are generally different from those who are not hospitalized. If this selection is related to the exposure that we are interested in, the effect is biased (admission rate bias). This is also known as Berkson's fallacy. This bias is sometimes due to a particular referral policy (referral bias), for example, because complicated patients (with a non-standard risk profile) are referred to an academic medical center and uncomplicated patients to a general hospital.

Selection bias can also occur after the study sample has been selected, because the people who have been selected and agree to take part in the study differ systematically from those who decline to take part (non-respondent bias), or the other way round (volunteer bias). We have already mentioned the danger of selective dropout during the follow-up period (withdrawal bias).

Information bias

Information bias is caused by measurement errors, which can relate to the explanatory factors, the health outcome, or both. When these factors are binary or categorical, participants can be classified into the wrong risk factor and/or health outcome category (misclassification). The misclassification can differ from one group to another. This is referred to as differential misclassification (systematic measurement error): the error frequency in recording the outcome depends on the explanatory factor level measured, or conversely the error frequency in measuring the explanatory factor depends on the outcome recorded. In a cohort study, for example, the disease we are interested in may be diagnosed more accurately in participants who have been exposed to the risk factor than those participants not exposed to it. And, in a case-control study, more effort may be put into finding out about prior exposure to a risk factor with regard to cases than with controls. Differential misclassification of the risk factor and/or outcome can result in an underestimate, overestimate or even reversal of the true association between the risk factor and the outcome.

The term non-differential misclassification (random measurement error) is used when the errors in measuring one variable are independent of the measured values of the other variable. Also, non-differential misclassification usually distorts the association, but the direction is generally clear: non-differential misclassification biases the results toward the null. In the case of random measurement errors on a continuous variable, there can also be exceptional cases where there is no distortion.

Misclassification not only affects explanatory factors and outcomes but also confounders (see Section 5.4.4). When such errors in measurements of the confounder occur, adjustment for confounding

situation in general population

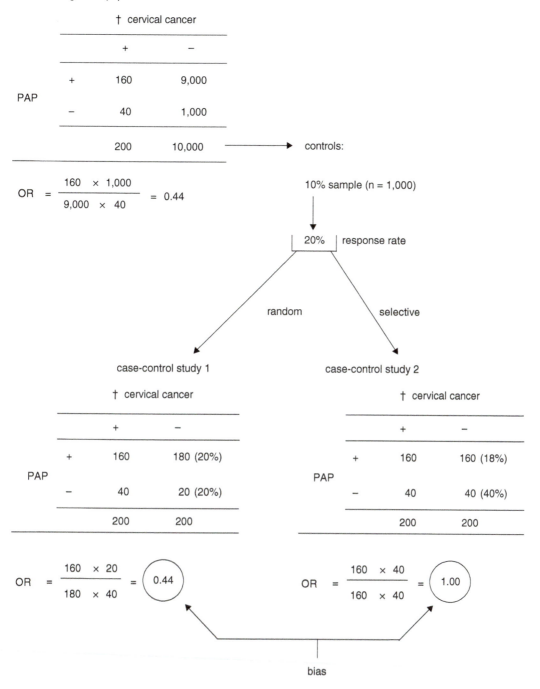

Figure 5.9   Selection bias in a case-control study into cervical cancer and pap smear frequency.

during analysis can only be partially implemented. For strong confounders in particular, misclassification will lead to substantial residual confounding.

In principle, information bias can affect all types of study. The danger is particularly great, however, when collecting information on the past, based on self-reporting (in case-control studies). Knowing the outcome status can, for instance, lead the researchers to search fanatically for the suspected risk factor among the cases, especially if there is already a strong suspicion that that factor is harmful. For instance, in a case-control study looking for teratogenic risks, women who have a baby with a congenital abnormality (cases) will search their memories more thoroughly for potentially hazardous substances than women with a normal pregnancy outcome, resulting in systematic differences in the amount and quality of the information (recall bias). Information bias occurs in a cohort study when prior knowledge about the harmful nature of a particular explanatory factor affects the intensity and outcome of the diagnostic process. The source of information bias, then, can be the researcher, the participant with their limited or biased memory, or the instrument used.

Confounding

Confounding is caused by mixing up the association with the primary explanatory factor with that of one or more other explanatory factors.

For example, a study finds that open surgery has the probability of success of 75% in removing kidney stones, and a percutaneous nephrolithotripsy (an endoscopic procedure) has a probability of success of 82% in removing kidney stones. Based on the study, we would conclude that an endoscopic procedure is to be preferred. If the size of the kidney stone is included in the analysis, however, the effect is very different. In the case of small stones (under 2 cm), the success probability is 93% for open surgery and 83% for an endoscopic procedure; in the case of larger stones the success probability is also higher for open surgery (73% as against 69%). As endoscopic procedures are performed mainly on small kidney stones, they appear to have a higher success probability than open surgery (◘ Figure 5.10). If the confounder (size of the stones) are not accounted for in the analysis, preference would be given to the wrong treatment. We call this reversal of association due to confounding Simpson's paradox. Reversal of an association is an extreme example; confounding can also cause overestimation or underestimation of the true effect.

Another example is a case-control study into whether alcohol consumption is a cause of laryngeal cancer. Cigarette smoking is also associated with an increased risk of laryngeal cancer, and people who drink a lot of alcohol are also more likely to be smokers, therefore, the effect of alcohol consumption will be overestimated if the smoking is not included in the analysis, since part of the effect is due to the drinkers' smoking behavior.

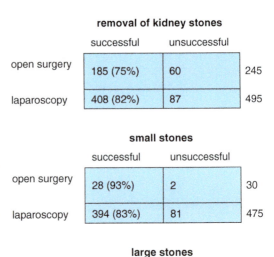

◘ **Figure 5.10** Simpson's paradox.

A confounder must meet the following criteria:

1. The factor is itself an independent risk factor of the disease or health outcome being studied.
2. The factor must be associated with the exposure (or the primary explanatory factor) under study in the source population. This association need not be causal; a marker of a causal factor (age, socioeconomic status, etc.) can also act as a confounder. Prior knowledge (from the literature) is needed to determine what the suspected risk factors for the particular disease are.
3. The factor must not be affected by the exposure (or the primary explanatory factor) or the disease. In particular, it cannot be an intermediate step in the causal path between the exposure and the disease. If the potential confounder is part of the mechanism linking the primary explanatory factor to the disease (an intermediary factor), this is not confounding but a chain of successive effects referred to as mediation. Although an association may then be found between the potential confounder and the primary explanatory factor, this is due to the relationship between the primary explanatory factor and the disease itself. In such cases, we must not adjust for confounding; we can carry out a mediation analysis instead. The situation is similar if the

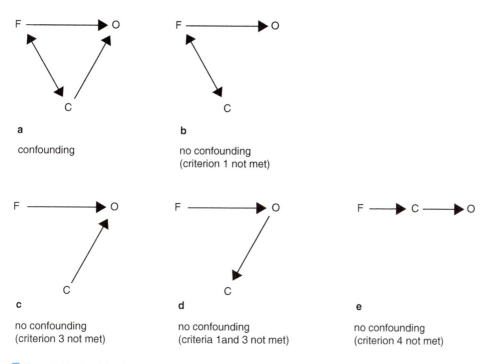

a

confounding

b

no confounding
(criterion 1 not met)

c

no confounding
(criterion 3 not met)

d

no confounding
(criteria 1and 3 not met)

e

no confounding
(criterion 4 not met)

Figure 5.11 Possible relationships between primary risk factor, potential confounder and disease.
F: risk factor
O: health outcome;
C: potential confounding factor;
↔: association;
→: causal relationship

potential confounder is due to the disease (e.g. a symptom): here again, there is a secondary association between the primary explanatory factor and the disease that is not due to confounding.

Figure 5.11 outlines a number of situations where confounding is or is not present.

Examples of potential confounders (situation a):

- Smoking in a study into the relationship between alcohol consumption and laryngeal cancer (see above).
- Physical exercise in a study into the relationship between fat consumption and being overweight
- Driver's age in a study into the relationship between wearing seat belts and the risk of a fatal road accident.

Examples of situations where a risk factor could wrongly be regarded as a confounder:

- Alcohol consumption in a study into the relationship between cigarette smoking and pulmonary emphysema (situation b in Figure 5.11).

- Chronic cough in a study into the relationship between smoking and lung cancer (situation b in Figure 5.11).
- Dietary habits in a study into the relationship between blood group and the risk of an infectious disease (situation c in Figure 5.11).
- Consumption of tissues in a study into the relationship between dietary vitamin C intake and the common cold (situation d in Figure 5.11).
- Birth weight of the baby in a study into the relationship between malnutrition in pregnant women and infant mortality (situation e in Figure 5.11).

If a variable is wrongly treated as a confounder – i.e. if criteria one to two above are not met – this generally has adverse effects only on the efficiency of the study. However, intermediary factors (situation e) must never be adjusted for, as that would "adjust away" the true relationship between the exposure and the health outcome.

Confounding can cause positive bias (overestimation), negative bias (underestimation), or even reversal of the direction of the effect (Simpson's paradox). What effect confounding has in a specific study will depend on the direction and strength of the associations between the variables concerned: the stronger the associations, the greater the bias in the estimation of effect. Confounding presents a real danger in all types of research.

To assess whether there actually is confounding in a study, a stratified analysis can be carried out. The following steps are involved:

1. Calculate the association between the primary explanatory factor (F) and the health outcome (O) for the sample as a whole (crude association).
2. Calculate the association between the explanatory factor and the outcome for each category (stratum) of the suspected confounder (C) (stratum-specific association).
3. Compare the crude association with the stratum-specific associations: there is confounding only if the crude association significantly differs from the stratum-specific associations.

Stratified analysis is also a way to adjust for confounding (Section "Selection bias"). Cases 5.3 and 5.4 further illustrate the evaluation of confounding. These are based on the simplest possible situation: the explanatory factor, the health outcome, and the potential confounder are all binary and only one confounder is considered at a time.

Case 5.3 *Physiotherapy or General Practitioner (GP) Treatment for Back Problems (Hypothetical Example)*

Suppose a cohort study is conducted among patients with back problems to find out if patients who opt for treatment by a physiotherapist (F) are more likely to be symptom-free (O) one year after therapy, compared to people who opt for treatment by their GP (F̄). At the start of the treatment, the researchers ascertain, among other things, whether the participants engage in regular sporting activities (C1) and for how long they have had the back problems (C2). ▢ Figure 5.12 shows the results of the analysis.

Case 5.4 *Smoking and Risk of a Second Heart Attack (Hypothetical Example)*

Assume a case-control study into the association between second heart attacks (O) within five years of the first attack and continued smoking of cigarettes (F). The severity of the first attack (C1) and the age of the patients (C2) are regarded as potential confounders. The results of the analysis are summarized in ▢ Figure 5.13.

Substantial differences between stratum-specific associations are called effect modification, a concept discussed in Section 5.5. Chapter 6 returns to the subject of confounding in detail in relation to causality.

5.4.2 Bias and study design

A number of measures to deal with bias were discussed in Chapter 4. Randomization, restriction, and matching are examples of strategies to minimize selection bias and confounding during the design and execution stages. Information bias can be minimized in various ways. The blinding of researchers, participants, and outcome assessors can reduce information bias. To avoid differential misclassification, objective outcomes (e.g. death, lab measurements) that leave little room for interpretation by the researcher or the participant should be used wherever possible. We introduce randomization, restriction, and matching below as measures taken at the design stage to improve internal validity. Other measures that can be used at the analysis stage to control for confounding in the collected data are stratification, standardization, and multivariable regression analysis.

Randomization

An experimental study in which the researchers can manipulate the allocation of the intervention being studied offers the possibility of randomization (random allocation). In principle, random allocation results in the intervention group and the comparison group (or groups) being equal in all respects at

Assessing confounding in a cohort study into the effectiveness of treatment for back problems

F = treatment by physiotherapist

$\bar{F}$ = treatment by GP

O = treatment unsuccessful: still symptoms after 1 year

$\bar{O}$ = treatment successful: no more symptoms after 1 year

C_1 = regular sports

$\bar{C}_1$ = no regular sports

C_2 = duration of symptoms > 1 month

$\bar{C}_2$ = duration of symptoms < 1 month

1

	O	$\bar{O}$	
F	160	240	400
$\bar{F}$	480	720	1,200
			1,600

$$RR_{FO} = CRR = \text{crude RR} = \frac{160/400}{480/1,200} = 1.0$$

a. Is regular sports a confounder? (details: 2a–5a)

b. Is duration of symptoms a confounder? (details: 2b–5b)

2a

C_1			
	O	$\bar{O}$	
F	20	100	120
$\bar{F}$	60	300	360
			480

$\bar{C}_1$			
	O	$\bar{O}$	
F	140	140	280
$\bar{F}$	420	420	840
			1,120

$$RR_{FO|C_1} = RR_1 = \frac{20/120}{60/360} = 1.0 \qquad RR_{FO|\bar{C}_1} = RR_2 = \frac{140/280}{420/840} = 1.0$$

3a $RR_{FO} = 1.0$: physiotherapy is no more successful than treatment by a GP.
$RR_{FO|C_1} = RR_{FO|\bar{C}_1} = 1.0$: GPs and physiotherapists achieve the same results in both people who play sports regularly and people who do not play sport regularly; there is no confounding and no effect modification.

4a

	C_1	$\bar{C}_1$	
F	120	280	400
$\bar{F}$	360	840	1,200
	480	1,120	1,600

$$\frac{P(C_1|F)}{P(C_1|\bar{F})} = \frac{120/400}{360/1,200} = 1.0$$

no link between intensity of sports and nature of treatment.

5a

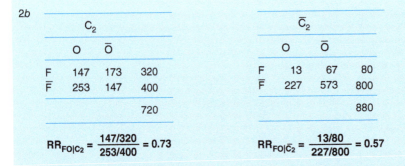

	O_1	$\bar{O}$	
	$\bar{F}$		
C_1	60	300	360
$\bar{C}_1$	420	420	840
			1,200

$$RR_{C_1|\bar{F}} = \frac{60/360}{420/840} = 0.33 \ (\neq 1.0)$$

back pain patients treated by a GP who play sports regularly are more likely to get better than patients who do not play sports regularly.

in summary:
no confounding (see Fig. 5.12a)

2b

	O	$\bar{O}$	
	C_2		
F	147	173	320
$\bar{F}$	253	147	400
			720

$$RR_{FO|C_2} = \frac{147/320}{253/400} = 0.73$$

	O	$\bar{O}$	
	$\bar{C}_2$		
F	13	67	80
$\bar{F}$	227	573	800
			880

$$RR_{FO|\bar{C}_2} = \frac{13/80}{227/800} = 0.57$$

3b RR_{FO} = 1.0: physiotherapy is no more successful than treatment by a GP if the duration of the symptoms is ignored.

$RR_{FO|C_2}$ = 0.73; $RR_{FO|\bar{C}_2}$ = 0.57: physiotherapists achieve better results than GPs in both patients with long-standing symptoms and patients with recent symptoms; the efficacy of physiotherapy was initially underestimated (bias towards the null); there is also some effect modification.

4b

	C_2	$\bar{C}_2$	
F	320	80	400
$\bar{F}$	400	800	1,200
	720	880	1,600

$$\frac{P(C_2|F)}{P(C_2|\bar{F})} = \frac{320/400}{400/1,200} = 2.4 \ (\neq 1.0)$$

patients treated by a physiotherapist are more likely to have long-standing symptoms than patients treated by a GP.

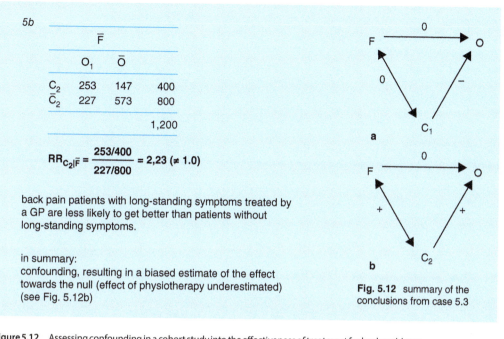

Figure 5.12   Assessing confounding in a cohort study into the effectiveness of treatment for back problems.

the start of the experiment, including the distribution of potential confounders. Randomization does away with both the known and unknown, as well as difficult-to-measure confounders. It does not guarantee that the various treatment groups will be completely equal, however; when the sample size is small, random differences in the distribution of confounders due to chance can happen. Pre-stratification can improve comparability in such instances. This involves classifying members of the sample into strata based on their values for the main confounders, and subsequently carrying out randomization within each stratum. This will substantially increase the likelihood that each group has the same distribution of these important confounders. Note that the stratification variables need to be adjusted for in the analysis.

A random sequence itself does not prevent selection bias. Importantly, the random sequence must be concealed such that, at the time of randomization, the intervention being assigned to the next eligible participant is unknown and cannot be changed. Concealed randomization is critical to the validity of a randomized trial, as without allocation concealment, the person giving the intervention will be likely to allocate the experimental intervention to those patients expected to benefit most from it (e.g. those with a favorable – or unfavorable – prognosis). This causes serious bias in the results, confounding by indication, since differences in effect are no longer related solely to the intervention chosen but also to differences in prognosis between the patients to whom the various interventions are allocated.

Randomization is the crucial element in an intervention study but, as we have seen, it does not always guarantee that the various confounding factors will actually be distributed equally between groups. Should an unequal distribution of confounders occur, a stratified analysis can adjust for the resulting distortion. A stratified analysis can only be used, however, if the confounder in question is known and has been measured, which is not always the case. Unknown and unmeasurable confounders are, in fact, the main reason for randomizing.

Assessing confounding in a case-control study into smoking and risk of heart attack

F = smoking after first heart attack
$\bar{F}$ = no smoking after first attack
O = second attack
$\bar{O}$ = no second attack
C_1 = severe first attack
$\bar{C}_1$ = minor first attack
C_2 = age $\geq$ 55
$\bar{C}_2$ = age < 55

1

	O	$\bar{O}$	
F	100	200	
$\bar{F}$	100	600	
	200	800	1,000

$$OR_{FO} = cOR = \text{crude OR} = \frac{100 \times 600}{200 \times 100} = 3.00$$

a. is the severity of the first attack a confounder? (details: 2a–5a)
b. is age a confounder? (details: 2b–5b)

2a

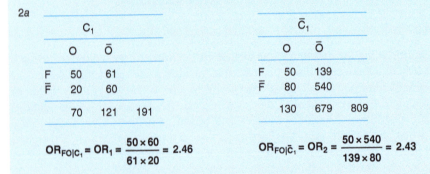

	C_1		
	O	$\bar{O}$	
F	50	61	
$\bar{F}$	20	60	
	70	121	191

$$OR_{FO|C_1} = OR_1 = \frac{50 \times 60}{61 \times 20} = 2.46$$

	$\bar{C}_1$		
	O	$\bar{O}$	
F	50	139	
$\bar{F}$	80	540	
	130	679	809

$$OR_{FO|\bar{C}_1} = OR_2 = \frac{50 \times 540}{139 \times 80} = 2.43$$

3a OR_{FO} = 3.00 : patients with a second heart attack are more likely to have continued smoking after the first attack.

$OR_{FO|C1} = OR_{FO|\bar{C}1} = 2.44$: smoking is a prognostic factor for a second attack in both patients with a severe first attack and patients with a minor first attack; the effect is not as strong as in the group as a whole.

4a

	C_1	$\bar{C}_1$	
F	111	189	300
$\bar{F}$	80	620	700
	191	809	1,000

$$\frac{P(C_1|F)}{P(C_1|\bar{F})} = \frac{111/300}{80/700} = 3.24 \ (\neq 1.0)$$

O			
	C_1	$\bar{C}_1$	
F	50	50	100
$\bar{F}$	20	80	100
	70	130	200

$\bar{O}$			
	C_1	$\bar{C}_1$	
F	61	139	200
$\bar{F}$	60	540	600
	121	679	800

$$\frac{P(C_1|FO)}{P(C_1|\bar{F}O)} = \frac{50/100}{20/100} = 2.50 \ (\neq 1.0)$$

$$\frac{P(C_1|F\bar{O})}{P(C_1|\bar{F}\bar{O})} = \frac{61/200}{60/600} = 3.05 \ (\neq 1.0)$$

patients with a severe first heart attack are more likely to smoke, both in the group with a second attack and in the control group.

5a

$\bar{F}$			
	O	$\bar{O}$	
C_1	20	60	
$\bar{C}_1$	80	540	
	100	600	700

$$OR_{C_1O|\bar{F}} = 2.25 \ (\neq 1.0)$$

non-smoking patients with a second heart attack are more likely to have had a severe first attack than patients without a second attack.

in summary:
confounding, resulting in a biased estimate of the effect away from the null (effect of smoking overestimated) (see Fig. 5.13a).

5

2b

	C_2		
	O	Ō	
F	85	115	
F̄	65	235	
	150	350	500

$OR_{FO|C_2} = 2.67$

	$\bar{C}_2$		
	O	Ō	
F	15	85	
F̄	35	365	
	50	450	500

$OR_{FO|\bar{C}_2} = 1.84$

3b $OR_{FO} = 3.00$

$OR_{FO|C_2} = 2.67$; $OR_{FO|\bar{C}_2} = 1.84$: smoking after the first heart attack is a prognostic factor for a second attack in both older and younger patients; the effect is not as strong as in the group as a whole, however: age is a confounder; the magnitude of the effect also differs between the two age groups: age is also an effect modifier.

4b

	C_2	$\bar{C}_2$	
F	200	100	300
F̄	300	400	700
	500	500	1,000

$$\frac{P(C_2|F)}{P(C_2|\bar{F})} = \frac{200/300}{300/700} = 1.56 \, (\neq 1.0)$$

	O		
	C_2	$\bar{C}_2$	
F	85	15	100
F̄	65	35	100
	150	50	200

$$\frac{P(C_2|FO)}{P(C_2|\bar{F}O)} = \frac{85/100}{65/100} = 1.3 \, (\neq 1.0)$$

	Ō		
	C_2	$\bar{C}_2$	
F	115	85	200
F̄	235	365	600
	350	450	800

$$\frac{P(C_2|F\bar{O})}{P(C_2|\bar{F}\bar{O})} = \frac{115/200}{235/600} = 1.47 \, (\neq 1.0)$$

older patients who have had a first heart attack are more likely to smoke than younger patients, both in the group with a second attack and in the control group.

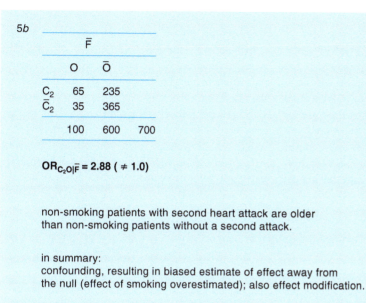

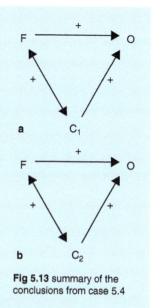

$$OR_{C_2O|\bar{F}} = 2.88\ (\neq 1.0)$$

non-smoking patients with second heart attack are older than non-smoking patients without a second attack.

in summary:
confounding, resulting in biased estimate of effect away from the null (effect of smoking overestimated); also effect modification.

Fig 5.13 summary of the conclusions from case 5.4

Figure 5.13 Assessing confounding in a case-control study into smoking and risk of heart attack.

Restriction

The most rigorous method to avoid confounding in a study design is restriction, ensuring that these variables no longer vary. As the entire study sample will then have the same value for the confounder in question, it cannot cause bias. Examples of restrictions are allowing only men to take part in the study, or only non-smokers. We can then be certain that gender or smoking cannot act as confounders, thus increasing the internal validity of the study. On the other hand, restriction of a variable to a single category will often affect the generalizability of the study finding (see Section 5.6). If a study involving only men does find an effect, it will not be possible to generalize this to women without qualification. In addition to avoiding confounding, restriction of the study sample can also be used to obtain an optimal (efficient) distribution among the categories of the explanatory factors, so as to guarantee sufficient contrast in the distribution of the explanatory factor status (see Chapter 4). In a randomized trial, restriction is used to reduce the source population to a more or less homogeneous group (e.g. people in the same age group, of the same gender, with the same disease, at the same stage of the disease). This involves setting inclusion and exclusion criteria that the people must meet before enrolment into a study.

Matching

Matching refers to the selection of a comparison group – persons not exposed to the explanatory factor in a cohort study, or controls in a case-control study – who are identical (as much as possible) to the index group – in terms of the distribution of one or more potential confounders. Intuitively, matching would seem to be a very attractive and obvious measure to improve the quality of a study design. As we shall see below, intuition is deceptive sometimes, notably in case-control studies where matching is quite popular.

Matching in a cohort study involves selecting the members of the subcohorts to be compared (exposed/nonexposed to the primary explanatory factor) in such a way that there is an equal distribution of one or more potential confounders between the exposed and nonexposed. This eliminates the matching factors as confounders. On the other hand, matching in a cohort study is often resource-intensive and therefore expensive, as many prospective participants have to be assessed, measured – and often rejected from participation – in order to achieve the matching. The validity of a study can be attained just as well by measuring confounders in all participants followed by adjustment procedures at the data analysis stage. In most cohort studies, adjustment in the analysis is more efficient than matching in advance. Case 5.5 gives an example of the use of matching in a cohort study.

Matching in a case-control study involves selecting controls from the population from which the cases originate in such a way that both the cases and controls have an equal distribution of one or more potential confounders. As the second part of Case 5.5 shows, matching in a case-control study does not always increase validity and sometimes even reduces it by introducing confounding. Matching can improve the efficiency of a case-control study, but this benefit is soon lost if a lot of resources have to be invested in the matching process itself. When matching is used in a case-control study, it is important to take into account matching in the analysis, as that eliminates the problem of any confounding introduced by the matching.

As Case 5.5 clearly shows, matching is not usually warranted. The advantages of matching will only outweigh the drawbacks when confounders are very strong and very unequally distributed among the primary risk factor categories.

Case 5.5 Alcohol and Road Traffic Accidents (Hypothetical Example)

Suppose we have a source population comprising 500,000 men and 500,000 women. A study is initiated in this region to assess the influence of alcohol consumption on the risk of becoming a road accident victim. Alcohol consumption is self-reported and expressed as the average number of alcoholic drinks per day (for the sake of simplicity we assume that there is no information bias). Participants are classified into "high alcohol consumption" (two or more glasses of alcohol per day, A in Figure 5.14) and "low alcohol consumption" (less than two glasses of alcohol per day, Ā). Records are then kept over a period of one year of who has fallen victim to a road traffic accident ("accident injury" = I) and who has not ("no accident injury" = Ī). Now let us look at what consequences matching in the study design would have produced, given the events outlined for the source population.

Figure 5.14 shows what the results of the study would be if the entire source population were to be followed over the period of one year.

Clearly, there is confounding in the population in question. The RR for injury due to accident for "high alcohol consumption" is 3.38, compared to a risk ratio of 2.00 for men and women when analyzed separately. Gender is a confounder because (i) there is a link in the population between gender and the amount of alcohol consumption (80% of the people with high alcohol consumption and only 20% of those with low alcohol consumption are male) and (ii) the risk of accident injury is higher for men than for women, regardless of their level of alcohol consumption. If a cohort study were to be carried out to examine the association between alcohol consumption and the risk of accident injury, and the cohort – e.g. comprising 100,000 people

(10%) – were to be selected at random from the source population, the confounding present in the source population would manifest itself in the same way in the study sample.

Now, suppose we decide to carry out a cohort study on 100,000 people in which we match individually for the gender variable. This means recruiting a subcohort of 50,000 people with "high alcohol consumption" and an equally large subcohort of people with "low alcohol consumption" from the source population in such a way that each "exposed" male is matched with a "nonexposed" male and each "exposed" female is matched with a "nonexposed" female. This strategy would produce a study sample comprising 80% men and 20% women, i.e. a completely different gender distribution than in a cohort study based on a random sample. The expected results of a matched cohort study of this kind are shown in Figure 5.15.

These calculations show that matching has eliminated confounding due to gender. The RR is no longer being overestimated. This non-confounded estimate of the effect of alcohol consumption on the accident risk could also have been achieved, however, by analyzing the data from a sufficiently large random sample using stratified analysis. Another point is that the matched cohort study includes a larger number of accident injuries (330) than the non-matched version (285). This shows the higher statistical efficiency of a matched approach.

Now, suppose the population described above is used as the basis for a case-control study into the relationship between alcohol consumption and accident risk. The cases in the study are the 2,850 people from the source population identified as having an accident injury during a period of one year. They

			I	Ī	total	risk of I in 1 year
males (500,000)		A	2,000	398,000	400,000	0.0050
		Ā	250	99,750	100,000	0.0025
females (500,000)		A	200	99,800	100,000	0.0020
		Ā	400	399,600	400,000	0.0010
total (1,000,000)		A	2,200	497,800	500,000	0.0044
		Ā	650	499,350	500,000	0.0013

$RR_{A/\bar{A}} = RR_{crude} = 0.0044 / 0.0013 = 3.38$

$RR_{A/\bar{A}|male} = 0.0050 / 0.0025 = 2.00$

$RR_{A/\bar{A}|female} = 0.0020 / 0.0010 = 2.00$

$RR_{m/f} = \dfrac{2.250 / 500,000}{600 / 500,000} = 3.75$

Figure 5.14 Alcohol consumption and accident injuries in a hypothetical source population.

		I	Ī	total	risk of I in 1 year
A (50,000)	M	200	39,800	40,000	0.0050
	F	20	9,980	10,000	0.0020
Ā (50,000)	M	100	39,900	40,000	0.0025
	F	10	9,990	10,000	0.0010
total (100,000)	M	300	79,700	80,000	0.0037
	F	30	19,070	20,000	0.0015

$RR_{A/\bar{A}} = RR_{crude} = \dfrac{220 / 50,000}{110 / 50,000} = 2.00$

$RR_{A/\bar{A}|male} = \dfrac{200 / 40,000}{100 / 40,000} = 2.00$

$RR_{A/\bar{A}|female} = \dfrac{20 / 10,000}{10 / 10,000} = 2.00$

Figure 5.15 Cohort study into alcohol consumption and accident injuries in 1,00,000 people (matched for gender).

comprise 2,250 (79%) males and 600 females, of which 2,200 (77%) have high alcohol consumption and 650 have low alcohol consumption. In a non-matched case-control study with an equal number of controls from the general population, the controls are randomly selected from the source population from which the patients are taken, resulting in a control group of 2,850 people containing 50% men and 50% people with high alcohol consumption. The crude OR is (2,200×1,425)/(1,425×650) = 3.38. The confounding present in the source population is thus "copied" to the study sample, resulting in a substantial overestimate of the odds ratio.

In a matched case-control study, for the 2,250 male cases, 2,250 male controls are recruited from the source population. The expectation is that 1,800 (80%) of them

		I	$\bar{\text{I}}$	
males	A	2,000	1,800	
	$\bar{\text{A}}$	250	450	
	total	2,250	2,250	
females	A	200	120	
	$\bar{\text{A}}$	400	480	
	total	600	600	
total		2,850	2,850	

$$OR_{A/\bar{A}} = RR_{crude} = \frac{(2{,}000 + 200) \times (450 + 480)}{(1{,}800 + 120) \times (250 + 400)} = \frac{2{,}200 \times 930}{1{,}920 \times 650} = 1.64$$

$$OR_{A/\bar{A}|male} = RR_{A/\bar{A}|male} = \frac{2{,}000 \times 450}{1{,}800 \times 250} = 2.00$$

$$OR_{A/\bar{A}|female} = RR_{A/\bar{A}|female} = \frac{200 \times 480}{120 \times 400} = 2.00$$

Figure 5.16 Case-control study into alcohol consumption and accident injuries in 2,850 people with accident injuries and 2,850 controls from the general population (matched for gender).

will have a high level of alcohol consumption. Similarly, for the 600 female cases, 600 female controls are recruited, of whom 120 (20%) are expected to have a high level of alcohol consumption. As Figure 5.16 shows, the matching results in an OR of 1.64, which is an underestimate of the true RR of 2.00.

Evidently, matching introduces confounding that does not reflect the confounding initially present in the source population, causing bias in the opposite direction. The explanation for this phenomenon is as follows: the purpose of a control group in a case-control study is to estimate the distribution of exposure levels in the population from which the cases are taken. However, if the controls are matched with the cases for a factor related to the primary explanatory factor, this will make the distribution of the primary explanatory factor in the control group similar to that in the case group. The result is an underestimate of the true association between the explanatory factor and the disease. If the correlation between the matching factor and the explanatory factor is very strong, the effect of the explanatory factor on the outcome could even be canceled out entirely. In this example, if all the

men in the population have high and all the women have low alcohol consumption (a perfect correlation), matching for gender in a case-control study into the association between alcohol consumption and accident risk would result in an OR of 1. In a case-control study, then, matching can introduce new confounding. This can even happen if we match for a factor that is not a confounder but is merely associated with the health outcome, as shown in Figures 5.17 and 5.18.

Confounding introduced by matching in a case-control study can be eliminated at the analysis stage by carrying out a stratified analysis to control for the same matching variables (see later in this chapter). As Figures 5.14–5.18 show, the stratum-specific odds ratios give a correct indication of the effect being studied. Indeed, we could have carried out a stratified analysis even if we had not matched for the confounders in question. It should be noted that a stratified analysis to control for the matching variables is not needed in a matched cohort study. Finally, it is often difficult to find matches. It may be necessary to screen a large number of potential candidates for the comparison group to find one single person who is suitable.

		I	Ī	total	risk of I in 1 year
males (500,000)	A	2,000	398,000	400,000	0.0050
	Ā	250	99,750	100,000	0.0025
females (500,000)	A	500	99,500	100,000	0.0050
	Ā	1,000	399,000	400,000	0.0025
total (1,000,000)	A	2,500	497,500	500,000	0.0050
	Ā	1,250	498,750	500,000	0.0025

$RR_{A/\bar{A}} = RR_{crude} = 0.0050 / 0.0025 = 2.00$

$RR_{A/\bar{A} \mid male} = 0.0050 / 0.0025 = 2.00$

$RR_{A/\bar{A} \mid female} = 0.0050 / 0.0025 = 2.00$

$RR_{M/F} = \dfrac{2,250 / 500,000}{1,500 / 500,000} = 1.50$

$RR_{M/F \mid A} = \dfrac{2,000 / 400,000}{500 / 100,000} = 1.00$

$RR_{M/F \mid \bar{A}} = \dfrac{250 / 100,000}{1,000 / 400,000} = 1.00$

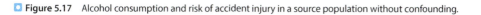

Figure 5.17 Alcohol consumption and risk of accident injury in a source population without confounding.

		I		Ī	
males	A	2,000		1,800	
	Ā	250		450	
	total		2,250		2,250
females	A	500		300	
	Ā	1,000		1,200	
	total		1,500		1,500
total		3,750		3,750	

$OR_{A/\bar{A}} \approx RR_{crude} = \dfrac{(2,000 + 500)\,(450 + 1,200)}{(1,800 + 300)\,(250 + 1,000)} = \dfrac{2,500 \times 1,650}{2,100 \times 1,250} = 1.57$

$OR_{A/\bar{A} \mid male} \approx RR_{A/\bar{A} \mid male} = \dfrac{2,000 \times 450}{1,800 \times 250} = 2.00$

$OR_{A/\bar{A} \mid female} \approx RR_{A/\bar{A} \mid female} = \dfrac{500 \times 1,200}{300 \times 1,000} = 2.00$

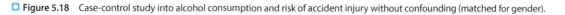

Figure 5.18 Case-control study into alcohol consumption and risk of accident injury without confounding (matched for gender).

Stratification and standardization

In epidemiological research, stratified analysis is one way of dealing with confounding once it is detected. The steps involved are as follows:

1. Calculate the association between the explanatory factor under consideration and the effect being studied in the total population (the crude effect).
2. Create strata based on the potential confounder categories.
3. Calculate the effect for each stratum and assess whether there is any substantial difference in the stratum-specific effects (to rule out effect modification: see Section 5.5).
4. Calculate the weighted average of the stratum-specific effects. This is the overall effect adjusted for confounding.

There are various ways of averaging out stratum-specific effects to obtain an effect adjusted for confounding, with differences in the weighting factor used. A method commonly used in epidemiology is the Mantel-Haenszel estimate, which can be used to pool stratum-specific odds ratios, RRs, or risk differences. The Epidemiology Calculator iPhone app, for example, provides a convenient way of doing this.

Here, we show how a Mantel-Haenszel odds ratio can be calculated manually:

$$OR_{MH} = \frac{\Sigma\left(\dfrac{a_i d_i}{N_i}\right)}{\Sigma\left(\dfrac{b_i c_i}{N_i}\right)}$$

where a_i, b_i, c_i, d_i and N_i represent the figures in cells a, b, c, and d and the total number of participants in the stratum respectively. Applying this to the data from Case 5.4 we obtain the following result:

$$OR_{MH} = \frac{\left[(50\times60)/191\right]+\left[(50\times540)/809\right]}{\left[(61\times20)/191\right]+\left[(139\times80)/809\right]}$$

The crude OR is 3.00 and the OR_{MH} adjusted for confounding is 2.44.

Another way of obtaining a weighted average of stratum-specific effects is to use the standardization technique for RRs or RDs.

Standardization is not traditionally used for odds ratios. Although the procedure is very different, the effect is the same: it eliminates confounding by the factor for which standardization is carried out. From the statistical point of view, the Mantel-Haenszel method is preferable to standardization, as it lends the greatest weight to the strata containing the most information, and therefore the smallest sampling error. This is not the case with standardization, where the weighting is based on the distribution in an arbitrarily selected standard population. Therefore, standardization is nowadays used as a technique to adjust for confounding only when analyzing and interpreting health statistics.

Multivariable modeling

If many confounders or several categories exist for each confounder, the information available on each stratum will be too limited for stratified analysis. We can then use multivariable analysis techniques based on statistical models. This is, in fact, a very logical choice, which links up directly with the epidemiological function that lies at the heart of this book: a mathematical description of a model that describes the interrelationships between the health outcome (O), the primary explanatory factor (F) and the other factors (confounders, C) as completely and accurately as possible.

Of all the statistical analysis models available, the various types of multivariable regression analysis have become the standard for confounder adjustment in epidemiology. The starting point is the linear model, which describes e.g. the relationship between the dependent variable (health outcome) and the exploratory factors such as a straight line (see ◻ Figure 5.19).

Here, the distribution of the outcome variable is regressed to the values of the explanatory factor. The straight line that shows the relationship between F and O is therefore referred to as the "regression line." This line can also be used to estimate the outcome for a given risk factor. Linking the outcome variable to a single risk factor is done in univariate regression analysis.

Analyzing more than one risk factor at the same time is referred to as "multiple" or "multivariable" regression. Thus, multivariable linear regression describes the occurrence of the outcome using a linear combination of explanatory factors (primary risk factor, confounders):

$$O = b_0 + b_1 F + b_2 C_1 + b_3 C_2 + \ldots$$

To describe a relationship of this kind, we need a multidimensional instead of a two-dimensional space (see e.g. ◻ Figure 3.5).

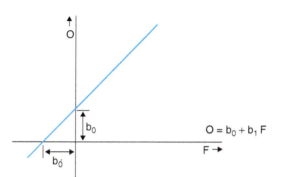

O = frequency of health outcome

F = level of exposure to risk factor

b_0 = value of O if F = 0; the intercept of the regression line

b_1 = regression coefficient = tangent of the slope of the regression line with the O = 0; $b_1 = b_0 / b_0'$

◘ Figure 5.19 Linear regression model describing the relationship between explanatory factor and outcome.

In epidemiology, we generally study disease frequencies, i.e. probabilities with a value between zero and 1. Because probabilities do not produce straight lines, a transformation is necessary to obtain a linear model. A model commonly used in epidemiology, especially in case-control studies, is multivariable logistic regression, represented by the following general formula:

$$P[O] = 1 / \left[1 + e^{-(b_0 + b_1 + F + b_2 C_1 + b_3 C_2 + ...)}\right]$$

Logit transformation of this function describes the outcome variable based on a linear combination of explanatory factors:

$$ln\left[O / (1 - O)\right] = b_0 + b_1 F + b_2 C_1 + b_3 C_2 + ...$$

This model is particularly suitable when analyzing dichotomous outcomes (e.g. diseased/not diseased). Other examples of multivariable models that can be used for different types of outcomes are the proportional hazards model and the log-linear models. All these models are derived from this basic linear model and are closely related to the multivariable logistic regression model. Of course, non-linear models could also be used. Any statistical modeling, linear or any other model, has limitations: in particular, the difficulty of ascertaining the biological plausibility of the underlying assumptions, and the problem of interpreting the results correctly. Ideally, statistical models should be based on prior knowledge of the underlying biological or pathophysiological mechanisms. There are various ways of ascertaining which model is best suited to a particular data set. Without careful checks, these analyses may produce misleading results.

Causal diagrams

The definitions of confounding can easily be applied in the case of a single outcome variable O, a single risk factor D, and a single potential confounder C. Things might become complex, however, when several interdependent variables are involved. Take the case of four variables in ◘ Figure 5.20a. Do we need to adjust for both C1 and C2 in order to study the relationship between F and O? And in the case shown in ◘ Figure 5.20b, with five variables, do we need to adjust for C if there are two – latent, unmeasured – variables L1 and L2?

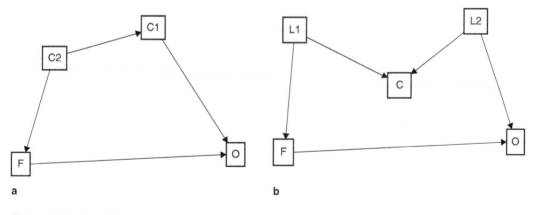

a   b

◘ Figure 5.20 Causal diagrams.

If we adjust for too many confounders, we run the risk of overcorrection (resulting in unnecessarily wide confidence intervals). If we adjust for too few confounders, there is a risk of undercorrection (resulting in residual confounding). It is important, therefore, to look at all the characteristics of participants relevant to the study – including those not being measured – and determine what set of variables needs to be considered to minimize confounding (the adjustment set). These variables are best set out in a causal diagram as shown in ■ Figure 5.20. Please keep in mind that covariates in a statistical model are, by definition, measured variables, and thus exclude the unmeasured variables.

These diagrams are referred to as Directed Acyclic Graphs (DAGs) in the literature. A DAG contains all the variables relevant to the research question and the causal relationships between them. If the DAG rules are applied strictly, the DAGs will help to identify the adjustment sets. These rules are as follows:

1. Include all the variables, including the unmeasured ones.
2. Show only direct causal relationships between variables using an arrow (an arrow A → B in a DAG means that A has a direct causal influence on B).
3. Successive arrows are referred to as a "path"; more than one variable may lie on a path.
4. Only paths that connect F and O and start with an arrow pointing in the direction of F can yield an adjustment set.

Adjusting for one of the variables in an adjustment set adjusts for the confounding effect of all variables on that path because it blocks the path. In ■ Figure 5.20a, for example, variables C1 and C2 both meet the criteria for confounding (risk factor of the health outcome and associated with F), but there is only one adjustment set because both variables lie on the same path F ← C2 → C1 → O, so it is enough to adjust for C1 or C2. Once we have controlled for one confounder on this path, we no longer need to adjust for the other one.

A variable on a path with two arrows pointing to that variable is referred to as a collider. In ■ Figure 5.20b, for example, the variable C is a collider on the path F ← L1 → C ← L2 → O. C is not a confounder, even although it is independently associated with F (via L1) and O (via L2), as the diagram does not show any correlation between L1 and L2. This path does not therefore meet the criterion for an adjustment set. If "just to be on the safe side" we were to

control for C, we would in fact create a link between L1 and L2, thus introducing bias that was not there before. This is referred to as collider bias. As this example also shows, it is not a good idea to control for all sorts of "pre-treatment" variables, as is often recommended, unless a properly described DAG indicates that there is an adjustment set.

For a full description of the rules for determining adjustment sets we refer to the literature listed at the end of this chapter. In practice it is often better – especially in the case of large DAGs – to carry out software analyses. A useful free software program is DAGitty.[1] Causal diagrams can also be used to examine effect modification, which is discussed in Section 5.5.

5.5 Effect modification

We present effect modification in this chapter to show how it differs from confounding, although effect modification is not really a topic that should be discussed in a chapter about the validity and precision of study designs. The term effect modification is used when the effect of an explanatory factor on the health outcome frequency differs for the various categories of another variable (often another explanatory factor of the health outcome).

Effect modification occurs in the language of stratified analysis, as described in Section "Selection bias", when the stratum-specific effects are substantially different (see ■ Figure 5.21).

If we use a multivariable regression model to analyze the data from an epidemiological study, we can examine effect modification by including interaction terms in the model. An interaction term in a model is the multiplication of the two variables that interact.

One obvious example of effect modification is the combined effect of alcohol and car-driving on the risk of having a road traffic accident. Both factors are risk factors for having an accident, but the combination of the two is a far stronger risk factor of accidents than each one separately. We find similar phenomena if we include skin color when investigating whether exposure to sunlight causes skin cancer: in this example, the effect of sunlight on skin cancer is modified by skin color. The paler the skin color, the higher the risk of skin cancer due to sunlight. ■ Figure 5.22 describes an arrow diagram representing effect modification. Compare this with the arrow diagram for confounding (■ Figure 5.11).

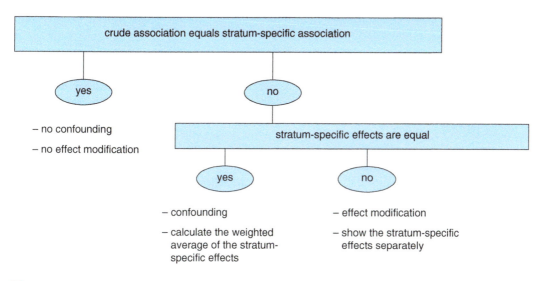

Figure 5.21 Rules for decision making on effect modification and confounding in stratified analysis.

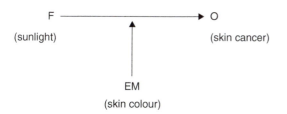

Figure 5.22 Effect modification represented as an arrow diagram.

Effect modification is of scientific interest that should be examined in epidemiological research; whereas confounding causes a spurious association and therefore should be avoided or controlled. Effect modification is based on two biological concepts: synergism, i.e. interaction between two or more factors in bringing about a biological effect, and antagonism, i.e. opposition between two or more factors in bringing about a biological effect. In other words, synergism and antagonism act at the biological level. The extent to which synergism and antagonism are expressed as effect modifiers in an epidemiological study will depend on whether the study is capable of uncovering these more complex types of causal relationships. It will need a sufficient sample size to distinguish effect modification from random variation, for instance. Case 5.6 describes a hypothetical example of effect modification by smoking on the relationship between exposure to asbestos and lung cancer.

Various combinations of confounding and effect modification due to an external factor can occur.

Sometimes, there will be no confounding and no effect modification. In other cases, there will only be confounding, no effect modification. In yet other cases, there will be both confounding and effect modification. Lastly, the effect modification can be so strong that confounding is a "non-issue": if the effect under consideration varies widely for the various strata of a variable, there may be confounding due to that variable but there is no point in calculating an overall effect measure adjusted for confounding. Evidently there is not a single effect, but different effects for different subgroups in the study sample, which need to be reported separately. See the decision tree in Figure 5.21.

Confounding is a nuisance, a smokescreen within the data set that obscures the view of the true relationships between the variables. We can gain an impression of the magnitude of the distortion by making an estimate of the parameter adjusted for the influence of a potential confounder. Effect modification reflects the true situation in the population, showing the natural variability of the extent to which people react to specific risk factors.

When investigators are interested in studying effect modification, they need to inspect the data and examine the differences between the stratum-specific effects, taking precision into account. The number of participants in each stratum must be large enough to enable a sufficiently precise estimate of the stratum-specific effect. But even if researchers are not particularly interested in effect modification, they will still need to ascertain whether there are

Case 5.6 Asbestos, Lung Cancer, and Smoking (Hypothetical Example)

Suppose we are conducting a cohort study into the relationship between exposure to asbestos and lung cancer in an industrial population that has been exposed to asbestos (A_1) and a control group of employees who have not been exposed to asbestos (A_0). Both groups include cigarette smokers (S_1) and non-smokers (S_0).

Based on exposure to these two risk factors of lung cancer, we can identify four different risk-factor groups, A_0S_0, A_1S_0, A_0S_1, and A_1S_1. Let us assume that the study finds the following risks of lung cancer for these subpopulations:

- $R_{A0S0} = R_{00} = 23/100{,}000$ per year
- $R_{A1S0} = R_{10} = 117/100{,}000$ per year
- $R_{A0S1} = R_{01} = 244/100{,}000$ per year
- $R_{A1S1} = R_{11} = 1{,}244/100{,}000$ per year

For these subpopulations, comprising people with different combinations of smoking behavior and exposure to asbestos, we can calculate ARs and RRs of lung cancer compared with the subpopulation with the lowest lung cancer incidence, whose members do not smoke cigarettes and have not been exposed to asbestos (background risk):

- $RR_{00} = R_{00}/R_{00} = 1.0$
- $RR_{10} = R_{10}/R_{00} = 5.1$
- $RR_{01} = R_{01}/R_{00} = 10.6$
- $RR_{11} = R_{11}/R_{00} = 54.1$
- $AR_{00} = R_{00} - R_{00} = 0$
- $AR_{10} = R_{10} - R_{00} = 94/100{,}000$ per year
- $AR_{01} = R_{01} - R_{00} = 221/100{,}000$ per year
- $AR_{11} = R_{11} - R_{00} = 1{,}221/100{,}000$ per year

Clearly, the combination of asbestos and cigarettes presents a far higher risk than each of these risk factors separately. So, does that mean there is effect modification? If we look at the RRs and multiply the effect of asbestos (RR = 5.1) with that of smoking (RR = 10.6), the result is close to the increased risk that we find in the group with combined exposure (RR = 54.1). In other words, there does not appear to be any interaction on the scale of RRs. If we look at the attributable risks, on the other hand, there is clearly interaction, since the additional risk in the group with combined exposure (AR = 1,221/100,000 per year) is far higher than the sum of the separate effects (AR = 94 + 221 = 315/100,000 per year). So, it depends on the model being used: the RR model (also referred to as the multiplicative model) or the attributable risk model (also referred to as the additive model).

From the perspectives of the participants in the study, we find that there are a whole lot of people (12 44−224−117+23 = 926/100,000 per year) who would not have developed the disease without the combined exposure. For interpretation at the individual level, then, the additive model is generally more informative. The absence of effect modification on the multiplicative scale provides information on the causal effects of smoking: the risk is increased more than tenfold, regardless of the presence of asbestos as an additional important risk factor. Note, however, that this is a special case, and there will usually be some effect modification on both the additive and the multiplicative scale.

large differences between the strata, since there is no point in calculating the weighted average of two totally different effects.

▢ Figure 5.23 shows the principle of effect modification in diagrammatic form. Panel A shows that the effect of salt consumption on the incidence of high blood pressure affects the various age groups. in line with a multiplicative model. As the effect at each age expressed in terms of RR ([a + b]/b) is the same, this suggests that the multiplicative model fits the data well. In other words, there is no effect modification on the multiplicative scale in panel A. But when looking

at panel A in terms of an additive model which is considering the difference between risks, the effect of salt consumption on the incidence of hypertension does depend on age (the difference increases with age). To put it another way, on the additive scale in panel A, age is an effect modifier of the relationship between salt consumption and the incidence of hypertension. The reverse is true in panel B, where the difference in the incidence of hypertension between high and low salt consumption is the same for each body weight category. On the additive scale, then, body weight is not an effect modifier, but on the multiplicative scale, the

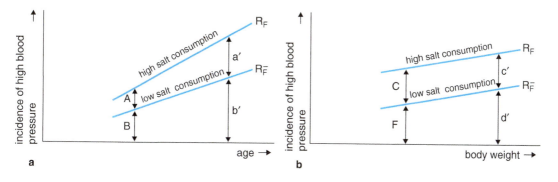

Figure 5.23 Illustration of effect modification on an additive scale (a) and a multiplicative scale (b).

effect of salt consumption on the incidence of high blood pressure does depend on body weight. In fact, the RR reduces at higher level of body weight. This is why there is effect modification on the multiplicative scale in panel B.

5.6 External validity

Internal validity of a study refers to the extent to which the results obtained represent the truth in the population we are studying. The external validity of a study, on the other hand, refers to the generalizability of the results – the extent to which results from a study can be applied to other situations or populations.

5.6.1 Study sample

Both the internal and external validity are strongly influenced by the choice of study sample. As we saw earlier, the aim of epidemiological research is to answer an epidemiological question on, for example, the occurrence of a health outcome or the relationship between an outcome and one or more explanatory factors. This relationship can be represented in the form of an epidemiological function (see Section 1.1.4) showing how the health outcome in question relates to a series of explanatory factors

When selecting the study population for a scientific study, the first step is to define the domain (see ◻ Figure 4.1). The domain is an abstract concept referring to the type of person to be studied. The domain is defined by individual characteristics such as gender, race and age. The domain needs to be

narrowed down particularly if we expect the effect of the exposure on the outcome to be substantially different in one subdomain than in the other: in other words, an effect modifier is present (see Section 5.5). For example, if it is clear that the effect or association will be different between men and women, baseline disease severity, people with and without an accompanying chronic condition, etc. we will want to express this in the definition of the domain, either by limiting it to a single category (only women, only people without a chronic condition), or by explicitly having two subdomains on which to collect separate and sufficiently precise estimates.

Once the domain has been defined, the next step is to find a suitable source for identifying people of the kind required for the study. Sources (sampling frameworks) could be a voting registry, the patient population of a hospital, people registered with one or more general practices, or members of a student association, for example. The source needs to contain a sufficient number of representatives of the domain. The people in the source who fall into the domain constitute the source population for the study. Within that population, we will want to examine events relevant to the study (exposure to risk factors, development of the outcome), as these are the people who can provide information for the epidemiological function. The ultimate study population is that part of the source population from which we actually collect data for the study.

Errors can easily be made when translating the domain or target population into a study sample. If these errors are systematic, they can affect generalizability. Systematic differences between the study population and the domain or target population can creep in at various levels and stages of the recruitment process:

- Authorities may refuse to grant researchers access to their population register.
- People in the source population may have to be excluded from the study because they are unable to take part (due to comorbidity, comedication, temporary absence, visual, hearing, speech or motor disorders, etc.).
- Other people, who are qualified to take part, may decide not to do so for personal reasons.
- The people finally included in the study may ultimately not all be included in the analysis and counted in the final results (due to dropout or poor patient compliance).

5.6.2 Extrapolation

High internal validity can be guaranteed by ensuring that the study meets certain methodological standards. The level of external validity, on the other hand, is far more difficult to assess. Generalization of research findings must involve a careful consideration and judgment as to whether relevant aspects of the population and condition are actually comparable.

In order to generalize the frequency of a health outcome, we will need a study sample that is representative with respect to all risk factors of the health outcome in question. It will not be possible to generalize from a study into the frequency of HIV among drug users in Barcelona to all drug users in Europe. A study of nursing home residents in Vienna will not suffice to understand the frequency of falls among the elderly in general.

The situation is different when it comes to generalizing causal relationships. Here again, the study sample needs to be representative of the domain, but it does not need to be representative of all the risk factors of the health outcome in question, only of the relationship under consideration. It could be argued, for instance, that an effect of smoking on the development of lung cancer found in a study of men will also apply to women (although more men are smokers), as women's lungs will display the same reaction to the chemical stimulus of cigarette smoke as men's. We would be less inclined, on the other hand, to extrapolate a relationship between physical activity and osteoporosis (bone decalcification) found in a study of women to the male population, as we know that the hormonal status of women may affect the effect of physical activity on osteoporosis. In other words, in the case of the smoking and lung cancer example, gender is probably not an effect modifier, but it is likely to modify the effect of physical exertion on osteoporosis (see Section 5.5).

The example in the previous paragraph, where we suggested that the effect of smoking on lung cancer among men could also be applied to women, can be contested in the sense that the strength of the effect could well differ somewhat between men and women. Quantitatively speaking ("how strong is the effect?"), the result obtained among men can perhaps not be generalized to women exactly, but this does not affect the conclusion in practice: smoking is such a strong risk factor of the risk of lung cancer in both men and women that everyone should be discouraged from it. So, qualitatively speaking ("is or isn't there an effect?") it is perfectly acceptable to generalize the results in this case.

A study that sets out to answer a clear quantitative question ("how large, how strong, how many?") requires a sample that is representative of all the factors that can influence the strength of the association. Many studies, however, are designed to find qualitative links between risk factors and health outcomes, in which case, a sample that is representative of only the parameters under investigation may suffice. Thanks to this phenomenon, it is possible to use research carried out in the United States or Europe, and the results of research conducted 50 years ago are still useful. And also, thanks to this phenomenon, it can even be justified to use only animal experiments to answer certain medical questions: in those cases, the laboratory animals can serve as a model for the relationship that we would really like to examine in humans.

5.6.3 Selection

One of the threats to the internal validity of an epidemiological study is selection bias (see Section 5.4.1). Having read the example in Case 5.5, however, readers might conclude that selection is unavoidable. In fact, we saw in Chapter 4 that selection can actually be used as a way of improving the validity and efficiency of a study. This apparent contradiction is easy to resolve. Selection is a tool for researchers that enables them to design a good study and achieve maximum internal validity with minimum effort. They must however ensure that the selection is carried out equally in the groups being compared: in other words, it must be non-differential (see Section 5.4.1). Differential selection, i.e. different degrees of selection between the groups being compared, causes bias and adversely affects the internal validity of the study.

For example, in a cohort study into the association of using a computer mouse on the development of arm, neck, and shoulder problems, it is a good idea to carry out the study on 30–50-year-old, full-time office workers at a large insurance company who use a mouse for more than five hours a day, provided that the comparison group (with low mouse usage) also comprises 30–50-year-old full-time office workers at the same company. This selection will increase the chance of obtaining a valid answer to the research question with relatively low effort compared with taking a random sample of all adult residents of a particular country and classifying them into mouse users and non-mouse users. The results will, however, probably be generalizable to the whole working population of that country.

A case-control study into the effect of folic acid on the occurrence of congenital heart defects could be carried out among children with such defects operated on at St George's Hospital in the UK, provided that the control group accurately reflects the population from which the patients are taken – for example, a control group of children with another severe congenital abnormality assumed not to be related to folic acid intake. The results of such a study could be useful internationally, in spite of the selection.

5.7 Validity, reliability, and responsiveness of instruments

To minimize information bias, instruments used in epidemiological studies to measure exposures and outcomes must be suitable for the purpose. In particular, epidemiologists will want to test whether newly developed instruments or modifications to existing instruments produce reproducible and valid data. Reproducibility means being able to achieve more or less the same results on repeated measurement. Validity of an instrument means that it measures what it is intended to measure. Sometimes researchers want answers to other questions: for example, whether the

instrument is sufficiently responsive (i.e. sensitive enough to detect relevant changes over time). When we talk about random variation due to measurement error, we use the word reliability instead of precision (see Section 5.2).

5.7.1 From concept to instrument

Variables that need to be measured in an epidemiological study correspond to theoretical constructs (concepts). Everyone will have some idea of what is meant by concepts such as "heart attack," "hearing loss," "alcohol consumption," "age," and so on, but this will not suffice if we want to measure these concepts. The theoretical constructs need to be defined precisely if they are to be measured. In an epidemiological study, it is important to assign a value to each unit of observation – usually an individual person – for each outcome, risk factor, confounder, or effect modifier. Both a good theoretical definition of the parameter (the concept) and a satisfactory operational definition (that can be used in practice) are required in an instrument.

The following steps need to be taken to make a parameter specific and measurable:
1. Decide what you want to measure: a conceptual definition of the variable (e.g. blood pressure, headache, heroin use).
2. Decide what possible values you wish to identify with this concept. This is referred to as the conceptual scale (e.g. high, normal, or low blood pressure; presence or absence of headache; presence or absence of heroin use).
3. Translate the conceptual definition into an operational definition of the variable. This essentially boils down to choosing or developing an instrument that can provide valid, precise information on the parameter of interest (e.g. systolic and diastolic blood pressure measured using a sphygmomanometer after five minutes in a recumbent position; use of a headache powder; visible signs of use of an intravenous needle on the forearm).
4. Choose the empirical scale on which you will actually measure the participants, i.e. the possible values that you wish to identify when measuring in practice (e.g. diastolic and systolic blood pressure in mmHg measured using a sphygmomanometer after five minutes in a recumbent position; the number of times that headache medication has

been used during the past year; presence or absence of intravenous needle scars on the forearm). The empirical scale, then, refers to the instrument ultimately used, including the response options, assessment criteria and scoring rules.

It is important to ensure that the theoretical concept, conceptual scale, and empirical (or operational) scale are linked as closely as possible. For example, in a study on alcohol and accident risk, we would like to have information on the amount of ethanol in the brain tissue during the last few minutes before the accident (the theoretical concept). This is translated into the number of glasses of alcohol individuals have had during the hours preceding the accident (the operational definition). We could measure this by asking "How many glasses of alcohol did you drink during the past six hours?" If we were interested in alcohol consumption as part of a study into the development of cirrhosis of the liver, the theoretical concept would be completely different (the lifetime cumulative amount of alcohol that the liver has had to process). In operational terms, this could be translated into total alcohol consumption over the previous 20 years. The instrument ultimately used, however, is likely to ask about the number of years that the person has been drinking alcohol and the average alcohol consumption per week. The product of these two numbers (multiplied by 52) yields the value of the variable.

A whole range of instruments are used in epidemiological research, for example:

- Observations of signs and symptoms of a disease.
- Questionnaires or interviews (self-reported behavior or symptoms, as entered by the respondents themselves or recorded by an interviewer).
- Examination based on direct sensory observation (looking, listening, feeling, smelling, tasting).
- Physical measurements (body weight, blood pressure, muscle strength, etc.).
- Biochemical and other laboratory tests (serum, urine, hair, tissue biopsies, etc.).
- Imaging (X-rays, CT scans, angiograms, MRIs, PET scans, etc.).

5.7.2 Reliability of an instrument

Testing for the reproducibility of the results produced by an instrument involves examining the extent to which the results are consistent when obtained on the

same individual from repetitive tests. It goes without saying that such testing will be carried out on people who are representative of the people we ultimately want to include in the epidemiological study and on whom we shall carry out the measurement. Provided the measuring conditions remain constant, and assuming the parameter being measured does not change, we can expect repeated tests to produce the same results when the test is reliable.

Various terms are used to indicate the degree of similarity between repeated measurements and the absence of random measurement errors, e.g. reproducibility, repeatability, reliability, agreement, consistency, and precision.

There are many ways to assess the reliability of an instrument. First, we can check whether a particular assessor who repeats the test on the same individual comes up with the same findings (low intra-observer variability). This entails at least carrying out the test a few times. Successive tests should be independent of each other and not too close together, to avoid knowledge of the first observation influencing the second one. They should not be too far apart either, as the underlying condition or parameters could change over time biologically. Secondly, we can check whether two or more assessors who carry out the test on the same people simultaneously reach the same results (low inter-observer variability).

Various measures can be used to quantify reproducibility. Intra-observer and inter-observer reproducibility or agreement of continuous measures are often expressed as intraclass correlation. A commonly used measure for categorical test results is the agreement rate (between the first and second rating or between the first and second rater). Cohen's kappa is a measure of inter-rater and intra-rater agreement that indicates actual agreement as a proportion of agreement after adjusting for random agreement. This topic is discussed in more detail in Chapter 9.

5.7.3 Validity of an instrument

To test the validity of an instrument, we need to compare the test results obtained in a series of individuals with results in the same individuals obtained using a reference instrument. An instrument with 100% validity is termed the gold standard. In reality, no instrument is 100% valid, and therefore we use the term reference standard instead. In contrast to testing for reproducibility, testing for validity has a clear dependent variable (the result from the reference standard, Y) and a clear independent variable (the result from the instrument being tested, X). The question of validity can therefore be simply translated into an epidemiological function ($Y = b_o + b_1 X$), where the distribution (SD) in the regression coefficient b_1 is a measure of the instrument's validity. This distribution should ideally be zero, as we can then perfectly predict what the true value will be once we have carried out the measurement. Note that when the regression line does not pass through the zero point at an angle of precisely 45°, we can use transformation to arrive at the values of the reference standard. The true value could be deduced from each measurement using a calibration line obtained from the above test. Calibration is not even needed for an etiological study comparing the average measurements between groups. Systematic measurement errors will be eliminated when the groups are compared. The validity of instruments is discussed in more detail in Chapter 9.

Recommended reading

Altman, D.G. (2010). *Practical Statistics for Medical Research*, 2e. London: Chapman & Hall.

Carneiro, I. and Howard, N. (2011). *Introduction to Epidemiology*, 2e. Maidenhead: Open University Press.

Elwood, J.M. (2017). *Critical Appraisal of Epidemiological Studies and Clinical Trials*, 4e. New York: Oxford University Press.

Gordis, L. (2014). *Epidemiology*, 5e. Philadelphia: Elsevier Saunders.

Grobbee, D.E. and Hoes, A.W. (2015). *Clinical Epidemiology: Principles, Methods, and Applications for Clinical Research*, 2e. Burlington: Jones and Bartlett Learning.

Harrell, F.E. (2015). *Regression Modeling Strategies: With Applications to Linear Models, Logistic Regression, and Survival Analysis*, 2e. New York: Springer International Publishing Ag.

Haynes, R.B., Sackett, D.L., Guyatt, G.H., and Tugwell, P. (2006). *Clinical Epidemiology: How to Do Clinical Practice Research*, 3e. Philadelphia: Lippincott, Williams & Wilkins.

Morgan, S.L. (2013). *Handbook of Causal Analysis for Social Research*. Dordrecht: Springer.

Pearl, J. (2009). *Causality: Models, Reasoning and Inference*. New York: Cambridge University Press.

Rosner, B. (2015). *Fundamentals of Biostatistics*, 8e. Boston: Cengage Learning.

Rothman, K.J., Greenland, S., and Lash, T.L. (2012). *Modern Epidemiology*, 3e. Philadelphia: Lippincott, Williams & Wilkins.

de Vet, H.C.W., Terwee, C.B., Mokkink, L.B., and Knol, D.L. (2011). *Measurement in Medicine*. Cambridge: Cambridge University Press.

Webb, P. and Bain, C. (2017). *Essential Epidemiology: An Introduction for Students and Health Professionals*, 3e. Cam-bridge: Cambridge University Press.

Weiss, N.S. (2006). *Clinical Epidemiology: The Study of The Outcome of Illness*, 3e. New York: Oxford University Press.

White, E., Armstrong, B.K., and Saracci, R. (2008). *Principles of Exposure Measurement in Epidemiology*. Oxford: Oxford University Press.

Knowledge assessment questions

1. Researchers are three weeks into their study when they realize that their scale has been wrongly calibrated and adds an extra 5 lb to every participant's weight. Explain whether this would lead to differential or non-differential misclassification and how you reached that conclusion.

2. In each example, determine which of the following sources of error could cause the point estimate to differ from the population parameter: selection bias, information bias, confounding, sampling error.
   a. An uncalibrated heart monitor consistently measures all participants with a heartbeat 10 beats per minute too fast
   b. In an Argentinian study, researchers prefer to speak English over Spanish, and opt to only thoroughly interview those participants who are English-speaking
   c. In an exercise study, a miscommunication among team members results in all children who are positive for thyroid disease being excluded from a study that did not exclude them from being eligible for participation
   d. Researchers struggle to recruit participants and their resulting sample has confidence intervals that are too wide to draw meaningful conclusions from their data

3. Selecting the controls is an important part of a patient-control examination. Name three differences between a so-called "hospital-based-case control study" and a "population-based-case control study." Briefly explain your answers and explain whether the difference you describe has to do with validity or reliability.

4. In a cohort study, the association was studied between frequent music festival attendance and the occurrence of hearing damage. The frequency of festival visits was divided into three categories. The results are shown below.

	Hearing damage (+)	Hearing damage (−)	
>6 times per year	80	20	100
1–6 times per year	60	50	110
Never	60	40	100
	200	110	310

   a. Calculate the relative risk of visiting a music festival > 6 times a month compared to "never" of developing hearing damage. In the next step of the analysis, the researcher wants to examine whether there is effect modification or confounding by gender when comparing visiting a music festival > 6 times a year compared to never. To this end, he performs a stratified analysis. Out of a total of 100, 40 men visit a festival > 6 times a year and have suffered hearing damage. In total, there were 70 men with hearing damage at the follow-up measurement. Fifty men never attended a festival. Of the 50 women who attended a festival > 6 times a year, 10 did not suffer any hearing damage. Even although they never attended a festival, 30 women still suffered hearing damage.

b. Construct the corresponding 2×2 tables and calculate the RRs for both men and women

c. According to these results, is gender an effect modifier or a confounder? Briefly explain your answer.

Notes

1. The free software package DAGitty, for drawing and analysing causal diagrams (Textor et al.) (application). http://bit.ly/1FjBVdu

Etiology and Causality

Textbook of Epidemiology, Second Edition. Lex Bouter, Maurice Zeegers and Tianjing Li.
© 2023 John Wiley & Sons Ltd. Published 2023 by John Wiley & Sons Ltd.
Companion website: www.wiley.com/go/Bouter/TextbookofEpidemiology

6.1 Introduction

Etiology is the study of possible causal factors for a specific health outcome. But what does it mean if we say that a factor is the *cause* of an outcome? Causality implies that the outcome *always* follows the presence of the factor. This is not necessarily correct. First, a causal relationship need not be completely deterministic (in fact, it most often isn't!): smoking is an important cause of lung cancer, but not all smokers get lung cancer; and not all lung cancer patients smoke or have smoked in the past. Second, even if the outcome would seemingly always follow the factor, that alone would not suffice as proof for causation: every time the rooster crows the sun rises, but this does not mean that the rooster's crowing causes the sun to rise, or that if the rooster would stop crowing in the morning, the sun would not rise. The latter is an example of the well-known fallacy *Post hoc ergo propter hoc,* Latin for *after this therefore because of this.*

Causality has something to do with what would have happened in case the presumed cause were not present. If the rooster had not crowed, the sun would still have risen, but many lung cancer patients would not have developed lung cancer if they had not smoked. Smoking is not the only cause of lung cancer and, by itself, is not a sufficient cause in the sense that it doesn't lead to lung cancer in all smokers. That is why we do speak of causality in the case of smoking but not in the case of the crow: smoking may be the main cause of lung cancer in most patients, a rooster's crowing is never the cause of the sun rising.

Often, whether an association is causal or not is less clear-cut as in these examples. Epidemiologists are interested in differentiating between causal and non-causal associations, and in quantifying to what extent different causes contribute to the occurrence of a health outcome or its course over time. For example, knowledge of disease etiology is of great value in trying to prevent or delay this disease from occurring or recurring, or for intervention allowing for the best possible course. By encouraging smoking cessation, we can prevent or delay the occurrence of lung cancer; lobectomy or resection of the affected lobe of the lung, may result in curation. So causal relationships are quintessential in many epidemiological studies.

Often, the purpose epidemiological research is to establish whether there is an association between the presumed cause, or causes, and the health outcome under consideration. The association is usually estimated using statistical models and quantified as OR, HR, RR, or AR, and are all too often dichotomized into being present or absent using statistical tests. Identifying an association through statistical modeling is not enough to prove causality, as we have seen. We will likely find a rather strong association (e.g. an OR much higher than "1") between carrying a lighter and the occurrence of lung cancer, but that doesn't imply that possessing that lighter is a cause of developing lung cancer. In this example, smoking is the actual cause, and carrying a lighter is merely associated with smoking and hence, associated with the occurrence of lung cancer. The situation is less obvious in reality, and it may remain uncertain whether we have tracked down the "real" cause or just a correlate. We epidemiologists need to be particularly careful here, as associations in epidemiological research are often reported as news, even when no causal relationship has been established (see ◘ Figure 6.1). Higher socioeconomic status is associated with longer life expectancy, for example, but in etiological epidemiology, we need to know whether the explanation for this association truly lies in the components used to quantify it (i.e. education level, having a paid job, or household income) or that the association can be explained by other factors, factors associated with socioeconomic status such as lifestyle factors (smoking, physical exercise, particular dietary factors) and/or particular living conditions (air pollution, hygiene, occupational exposure). Once we have identified the main causal factors, preventive measures can be taken: a vaccine against the virus that causes a disease, education to change lifestyle, statutory measures to ensure that environmental pollution is reduced, and so on.

Preventive interventions are not always possible for all etiological factors (for example, genetic variation, age and gender). It is nevertheless useful to know about these non-modifiable causal factors as these help us understand why, under apparently similar circumstances, some people develop a certain health outcome and others do not.

6.1.1 Etiologic, prognostic and predictive factors

In addition to studying factors that cause the development of a disease, etiology is also concerned with prognostic factors that determine the course after disease onset. Again, etiological research in epidemiology aims to determine what factors actually cause

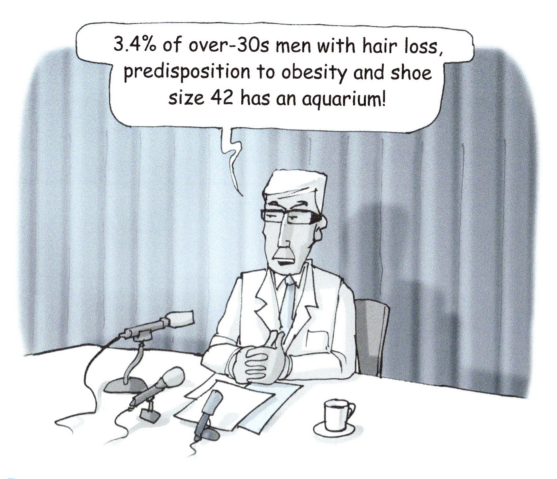

the course to go in certain directions (progression, the occurrence of comorbidities, etc.). This should not be confused with prediction research, yet another branch of epidemiological research, that is primarily interested in providing accurate predictions, regardless of whether those predictors are causal or not. These predictors can either be diagnostic factors that predict disease status or prognostic factors that predict disease course.

Sometimes prognostic factors that are causally associated with the course of a disease will be the same as those that caused its occurrence. We know, for example, that smoking plays a role not only in the development of coronary heart disease but also in the course of the disease after the first myocardial infarction, but this is by no means always the case. As Case 6.1 shows, some causal factors for breast cancer also play a role in the prognosis for the disease, whereas others do not.

Case 6.1 Etiologic Factors and Prognostic Factors for Breast Cancer in Women

Being overweight is a risk factor for the development of breast cancer in postmenopausal women. It is also associated with poorer breast cancer survival, partly because overweight women have other comorbidities. Even if we adjust for these comorbidities, however, being overweight remains a prognostic factor for the survival of breast cancer patients.

Age, on the other hand, is a factor that has different effects on the development and course of breast cancer respectively. Older age is associated with a higher risk of breast cancer, whereas young age is associated with higher mortality from it, probably because women who develop it at a young age may have a more aggressive type of tumor.

We know that various hereditary variants play a role in the development and/or survivability of breast cancer. Variant *1100delC* in the *CHEK2* gene is a fairly rare variant, occurring in up to 1.5% of individuals in North-West Europe.

Women with this variant in their DNA have more than double the risk of developing breast cancer, both the primary tumor and contralateral tumor in the other breast (◯ Figure 6.2). Results show that *CHEK2*1100delC* is also associated with a poorer prognosis: women with a hormone receptor-positive breast tumor and the *CHEK2*1100delC* variant in particular were at increased risk of dying from breast cancer, compared with breast cancer patients who did not have the *CHEK2*1100delC* variant; the multivariate corrected hazard ratio was 1.63 (95%–CI 1.24–2.15).

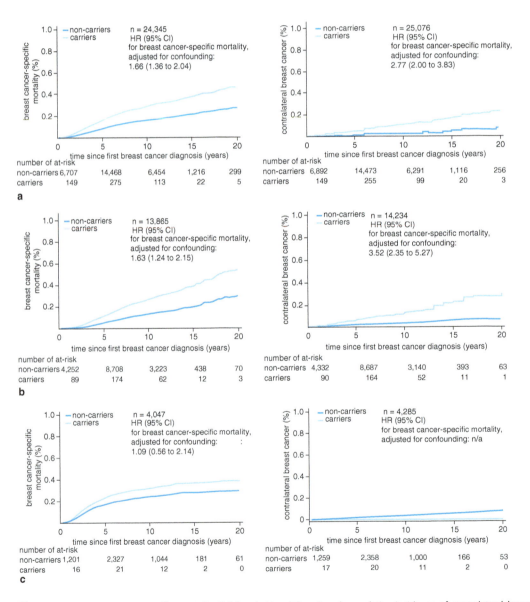

◯ **Figure 6.2** Breast cancer-specific mortality (*left*-hand side of figure) and cumulative incidence of contralateral breast cancer (*right*-hand side of figure) in carriers and non-carriers of the *CHEK2*1100delC* genetic variant, stratified for estrogen receptor status. (a) all participants, (b) receptor-positive patients, (c) receptor-negative patients.

In some cases, factors that cause a disease to occur may simultaneously be protective for its course. For instance, evidence suggests that an excess amount of exercise causes wear of the knee and ankle joints, and thereby contributes to the occurrence of arthrosis. Despite that, arthrosis patients are recommended to exercise, albeit in a way that doesn't harm the joints that much, to delay arthrosis progression.

Seemingly paradoxical findings may also be caused by what is called index-event bias or collider bias. Smoking is a known cause of stroke, but many studies have suggested that continuing to smoke after an initial stroke does not increase mortality. Restricting analyses on those who have already experienced a stroke (the collider in this case), can result in an association between smoking status and other risk factors, even if smoking and these other risk factors are completely independent. If not analyzed properly, this can result in bias *to* the null (i.e. the estimated association between smoking status and mortality is smaller than in reality), or bias *through* the null (i.e. in the opposite direction), causing such a paradox. To minimize such errors in etiological research, causal diagrams are used to visualize causal associations before analyses.

6.1.2 Causal diagrams

Typically, multiple factors are involved in the causal chain leading to the occurrence of a disease, or any health outcome for that matter. This is called multicausality. For example, mere exposure to a virus is not a sufficient cause of clinical manifestation of an infection: a previous infection or vaccination may decrease someone's susceptibility dramatically. Various factors in a causal chain may affect one another, and each factor in turn has its own causes. These causal chains can be very complex and, in most cases, only partly known. To aid interpretation of the causal chain and to detect potential biases due to confounding, concepts explained in the previous chapter, we often draw

a causal diagram. A causal diagram is a simplified theoretical representation of how the health outcome develops due to the interplay of various factors. A causal diagram takes the form of a Directed Acyclic Graph (DAG), which was introduced in the previous chapter.

Case 6.2 presents a simplified causal chain of the development of tuberculosis. We can deduct from the causal diagram that although exposure to the tuberculosis bacterium (*Mycobacterium tuberculosis*) is an essential factor, there are other factors that determine whether an individual will actually develop tuberculosis. As the causal diagram clearly shows, socioeconomic factors are important when combating tuberculosis in the population. This contention is supported by the observation that deaths from tuberculosis fell sharply between the nineteenth and twentieth centuries, whereas the tuberculosis bacterium was not discovered until 1885, and antibiotic therapy did not become available until 1948.

A causal diagram can be drawn for any outcome, whether it describes its occurrence or its course. Our understanding of the causal chain is constantly improved and refined due to findings from epidemiological and pathophysiological research. With sufficient empirical support, causal diagrams can be used as a basis for preventive or therapeutic interventions, even if the etiology has not been completely unraveled. For instance, the complex pathophysiology of preeclampsia, a hypertensive disease during pregnancy, is not yet fully understood. Nonetheless, research has provided obstetricians with a number of treatments that help delay or completely prevent preeclampsia from occurring, such as calcium supplementation and aspirin intake during pregnancy, thereby improving health outcomes for both mother and child. In addition, the availability of an etiological model, as shown in a causal diagram, will help epidemiological researchers to better formulate the research question (usually a single relationship in this model) and design the study required to answer that question and minimize the likelihood of introducing bias.

Case 6.2 The Etiology of Tuberculosis

Tuberculosis is caused by a type of bacterium called M. tuberculosis. The bacterium invades and grows in the host tissue (lungs, bones and brain), eventually causing the disease. From the pathogenic point of view, combating the disease is a question of eliminating the bacterium with an effective antibiotic or vaccine.

These drugs have been developed successfully through biomedical research, but the causal chain leading to tuberculosis is far more complex (see 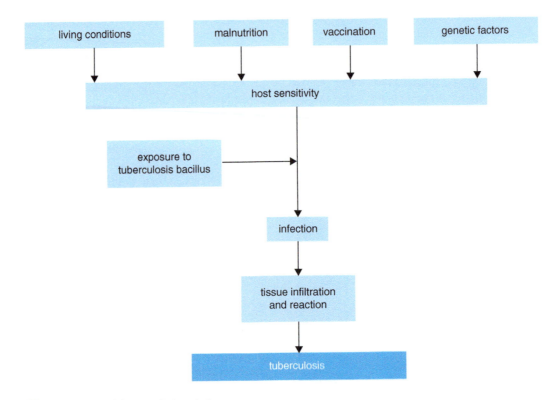 Figure 6.3). Whether it actually develops in an individual depends on how susceptible the host is and the degree of exposure to the bacterium. Whether individual susceptibility is a "cause" of tuberculosis is a matter for debate, but it is certainly an important factor when it comes to prevention and treatment. Indeed, improved diet and living conditions – and preventing HIV infection – have proved more important worldwide in combating tuberculosis epidemics than antibiotics and vaccines.

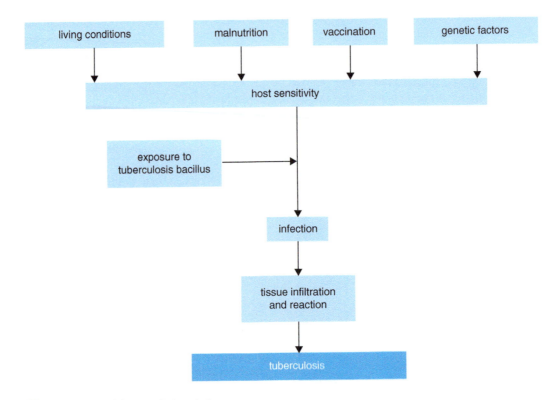

Figure 6.3 Causal diagram of tuberculosis.

6.2 Causality

6.2.1 Definition

Our understanding of causality is based first and foremost on simple, everyday observations: when we flip the light switch on the wall, we see straight away that the light goes on or off. If the bulb is faulty or there is a power failure, however, we realize that it takes more than just flipping the switch to turn the light on. There would be no electric light if the home did not have the correct wiring. Clearly, the position of the light switch is not the sole cause; it forms part of a multitude of factors (electricity in the grid, correct wiring, a working bulb, etc.). The tendency to regard the switch as the unique cause of the light coming on is understandable in that it is the last factor in the causal chain that eventually produces the result, light.

Etiological epidemiology involves searching for the multiple causes of a health outcome. Research often focuses on the factors that we can modify to alter the process that results in disease, such as smoking cessation to prevent lung cancer from occurring. We must not forget that all sorts of other factors contribute to that process. Many of these factors are not modifiable (e.g. genetic predisposition), but this does not make them any less important in understanding causality.

Ideally, we would want to investigate whether a particular modifiable factor makes a causal contribution to the development or course of a particular health outcome by manipulating the presumed cause and seeing whether the effect under consideration (the health outcome) actually occurs or in fact disappears. This is what we emulate in a randomized controlled trial (RCT). Obtaining empirical evidence of causality from RCTs is not always a practically or ethically tenable proposition in epidemiology. In that case, we aim to emulate the design and analysis of an RCT as closely as possible using observational data.

6.2.2 Sufficient and necessary causes

We refer to a set of factors that together will inevitably result in the health outcome under consideration as a sufficient cause. If one of these causal factors is missing from the set – e.g. the light switch in our example above is not switched on – the outcome will not occur.

Figure 6.4 shows a model of three such sufficient causes, all three of which would result in the same hypothetical outcome. In other words, there are three ways in which the outcome can develop. Each of the three sufficient causes is made up of eight causal factors that together – provided they are all present – result in the outcome. Some of these factors (C, E, and

H) occur in all three of the sufficient causes, and these are referred to as the necessary causes. Without these factors, the outcome cannot develop. Exposure to a virus may not be sufficient for developing subsequent viral infection, it is a necessary cause in the sense that the infection will not occur in absence of the virus.

Sufficient causes, then, are in fact always combinations of component causes, necessary or otherwise. An example of a necessary cause is deep vein thrombosis (DVT) in the case of pulmonary embolism: an embolism will not develop without thrombosis in the leg or pelvis. Clearly, once we have discovered a necessary cause, in principle we hold the key to the effective prevention of the condition in question. We have succeeded, for example, in eliminating malaria in large parts of the world by killing the mosquito that transfers the pathogen (a microorganism) from the infected to healthy people, since the malaria mosquito is a necessary cause for the development of malaria (as is the microorganism itself, of course). Similarly, vaccination has been successful because inadequate immune response is a necessary cause for the development of infectious diseases.

We will use smoking to illustrate the difference between a necessary cause and a sufficient cause. Smoking is a major risk factor for lung cancer, but it is certainly not a sufficient cause, as over 90% of smokers will not develop lung cancer. Nor is smoking a necessary cause of lung cancer, as lung cancer also occurs in non-smokers. This is relatively rare, however, and lung cancer is usually the result of a sufficient cause that includes smoking, so abstaining from smoking could prevent over 90% of lung cancer cases. The causal model outlined in Figure 6.4 is mainly illustrative, as

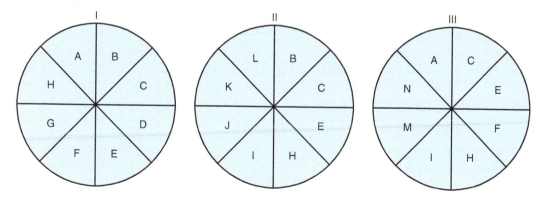

Figure 6.4   Causal model of the development of a disease with three sufficient causes.

in reality, it is extremely difficult to identify all the components of the various sufficient causes, and in many cases, causes can be more than just present or absent. As a rule, all we can estimate from epidemiological studies are the associations (usually expressed as OR, HR, RR, or AR) between particular factors and the development of a disease or an outcome. The known causal factors will generally only be part of a much larger set of factors that influence the development of the disease or outcome, many of which we do not know or may not be able to measure.

6.2.3 Causal interpretation

Etiological research can be compared to a court case, with the epidemiologist playing the role of the prosecutor. Just as it is the job of the prosecutor to prove (beyond reasonable doubt) that the defendant, not someone else, is guilty (alone or with others) of the criminal offense, an epidemiologist needs to convince the readers of their study that the factor is causally co-responsible for the development of the health outcome of interest. Nowadays, epidemiologists are indeed consulted in court cases involving damage to health (smoking, side effects of medical drugs, medical errors, food contamination, exposure to pesticide, occupational health). For more information see Section 6.3.1.

The causal model discussed in Section 6.2.2 also illustrates scenarios when there is confounding and/or effect modification. A confounder is not part of the set of factors that, together with the factor of interest for a study, constitute sufficient cause; on the contrary, confounders are found in the other mechanisms (sufficient causes) that can result in the disease. In □ Figure 6.4, for example, the risk factors I, J, K, L, M, and N are potential confounders of the relationship between risk factor G and the development of the outcome. Whether these risk factors actually act as confounders will depend on whether they are associated with the presence of G in the population. If there is an association of this kind between the factor of interest (G) and the confounders (I, J, K, L, M, and N), the difference between the incidences of the outcome when G is present and when it is absent will be due not only to factor G (and sufficient cause I) but also to the other sufficient causes (II and III in □ Figure 6.4) that do not include G but do include the confounders.

Causal factors that together constitute a sufficient cause are dependent on the presence of the other factors to achieve their effect. If there is a relationship of this kind between risk factors, this is referred to as effect modification (see Section 5.5). This does not mean that the two factors cannot separately form part of other sufficient causes, but there is evidently at least one mechanism (sufficient cause) where it is necessary for both factors to be present. In Figure 6.4, for example, it is possible for causal factor A to result in the health outcome without B (via mechanism III); conversely, causal factor B could contribute to the health outcome via mechanism II without A being present. But there is another mechanism (I) which only results in the health outcome if both A and B are present: this is referred to as modification of the effect of factor A by factor B (and vice versa). Thus, A has a greater effect on the development of the health outcome if factor B is also present (and vice versa). A familiar example of effect modification is the way smoking and asbestos influence the development of lung cancer (see Case 5.6). Both smoking and exposure to asbestos each increase that risk substantially, but smokers who are also exposed to asbestos run a far greater risk of lung cancer than we would expect from simply adding the separate risks due to smoking and asbestos.

In the example shown in □ Figure 6.4 the factors K and J, and also M and N, display effect modification but, here, the effect of one factor is entirely dependent on the presence of the other factor: J has no effect without K (and vice versa), and N has no effect without M (and vice versa).

The situation where a factor acts as both a confounder and an effect modifier corresponds to risk factors B and E, I and J, and H and I in □ Figure 6.4 which have some sufficient causes in common but not all. Age is an example of a risk factor that is both a confounder and an effect modifier in the case of the association between total serum cholesterol and coronary heart disease in women. Age is an effect modifier because the association between total serum cholesterol and coronary heart disease in women is much stronger after the menopause than before it. But age is also a confounder, because it is a determinant of coronary heart disease in both premenopausal and postmenopausal women and is also associated with total serum cholesterol.

To establish whether an association found in an observational study can be interpreted causally, so as to draw conclusions on the strength of the effect and any effect modification, we try to rule out other possible explanations step by step. Specifically, the alternative explanations are as follows:

1. The association found can be explained (at least partly) by selection bias or information bias (see Section 5.4.1). To find out whether this alternative is likely, we need to discuss the design and procedures of the study in detail. Even if no association is found, it is important to look at bias, as this can make a real relationship invisible in a study.

2. The association found can be attributed wholly or partly to confounding (see Section 5.4.1). We can use stratified analysis of the data to see whether this is a likely explanation of the association found, provided that information on these confounders is available on all participants in the data set. If the crude association does not differ substantially from the association within the strata of the confounders, confounding is probably not the explanation.

3. The association found may be due to chance. We can use statistical techniques (such as constructing confidence intervals) to determine whether this is likely. A narrow confidence interval that does not include the value of 1 (for OR, HR, and RR) or zero (for AR) provides support for an association.

If all three of these explanations are unlikely, a causal relationship becomes more likely, but this does not give us absolute certainty regarding the presence of a causal relationship. It could be said, following the philosopher of science Karl Popper, that researchers are constantly trying to reject (i.e. falsify) the hypothesis of causality based on the results of research (see Section 1.1.5). The credibility of the hypothesis that there is a causal relationship increases the more rigorous and varied the researchers' attempts to test and rule out alternative explanations.

To support the discussion of causality, sensitivity analyses are often used to explore the influence of bias and random errors on the estimation of association. To identify selection bias, information bias, and confounding we examine what values could be realistic and use these to simulate the resulting distribution of possible outcomes. If this range of alternative values does not lead to substantially different conclusions, causality is more likely. It will not be possible to interpret a weak association between alcohol consumption and lung cancer correctly if we have not carefully controlled for the influence of smoking. Conversely, a strong association between smoking and lung cancer will not be greatly affected if we add realistic assumptions about bias due to the absence of good data on alcohol consumption. Sensitivity analysis is commonly used in situations where there are uncertainties in the design and execution of the study, for example, in comparative research into the cost-effectiveness of two or more treatments. A conclusion as to the superiority of one treatment over another, based on research of this type, will be strengthened if we can show by a sensitivity analysis that this conclusion does not change substantially if we use other plausible values for uncertain factors that have a substantial influence on the results.

Section 3.2.6 introduced the concept of population attributable risk (PAR). This is a measure of the contribution made by a particular factor to the occurrence of the health outcome in a particular population. The model of causality described in ▢ Figure 6.4 shows that the PAR depends on the frequency with which the other factors in the same sufficient cause occur in the population. Suppose the three sufficient causes in ▢ Figure 6.4 are responsible for 80%, 15%, and 5% respectively of the cases of the condition under consideration. The population attributable proportion for risk factor K, for instance, is thus 15%, since eliminating cause K in the population eliminates sufficient cause II (which accounts for 15% of the disease cases). For a necessary cause (e.g. C, E, and H in ▢ Figure 6.4) the PAR is always 100%. As these examples show, there is no point in adding up PARs, as the sum will soon exceed 100%. This is because – despite the fact that a combination of various factors is needed for a disease to develop – eliminating just one of those factors can prevent cases of the disease.

The same principle is illustrated by the following example. Suppose the incidence density (ID) of head and neck cancer per 100,000 person-years among smokers and drinkers is distributed as shown in ▢ Table 6.1.

▢ **Table 6.1** Hypothetical incidence density of head and neck cancer per 100,000 person-years.

	Non-smokers	Smokers
Non-drinkers	1	4
Drinkers	3	12

We can calculate from the table that, in the group of smoking drinkers, $12 - 3 = 9$ of the 12 incident cases of head and neck cancer per 100,000 persons can be attributed to smoking and $12 - 4 = 8$ of the 12 to drinking. The etiological fraction among the exposed (EFe) is thus 75% for smoking and 67% for drinking. The sum is significantly more than 100%, because effect modification (see Section 5.5) is taking place: without smoking and without drinking there would have been one case of cancer per 100,000 person-years. With smoking alone, there would have been three additional cases, and with drinking alone, two additional cases. This means that the combination of smoking and drinking has caused $12 - 1 - 2 - 3 = 6$ cancer cases per 100,000 person-years. Without this effect modification, the attributable proportions for the group of smoking drinkers would have been $(6 - 3)/6 = 50\%$ for drinking and $(6 - 4)/6 = 33\%$ for smoking respectively.

We can also infer from the model in 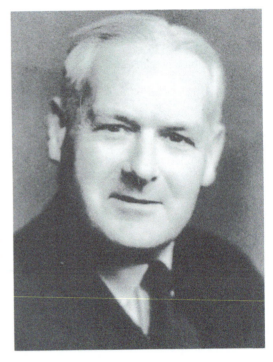 Figure 6.4 that the attributable risk (AR) for a necessary cause is equal to the incidence of the health outcome in question. In the absence of a necessary cause, the incidence is zero by definition, so the relative risk (RR) will then be infinitely large. In the case of non-necessary factors, the magnitudes of AR and RR depend on the relative contributions made by each of the sufficient causes, with and without the factor, to the total incidence. This means, then, that the strength of association (expressed in terms of AR or RR) depends on the population under consideration.

Figure 6.5 Biostatistician Austin Bradford Hill formulated criteria for arguing the likelihood of causation in the 1960s. Source: Bradford Hill.

6.2.4 Hill criteria

Observational epidemiological research cannot prove causality. Over the years, guidance has been developed on how to argue the likelihood of causality. The best-known example are the Hill criteria for causation of Austin Bradford Hill (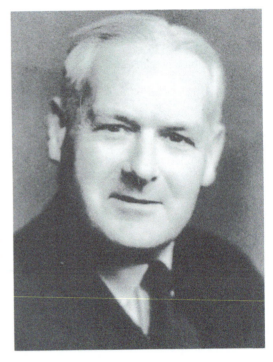 Figure 6.5).

Experimentation

A hierarchy of study designs that provide ascending levels of evidence was presented in Chapter 4 (see Figure 4.4). The Bradford Hill criteria also use a hierarchy of this kind, as some study designs provide more ways of controlling bias and confounding than others (Chapters 4 and 5). The hierarchy, from low to high, is as follows: case report, case series, case control study, cohort study, and RCT. RCTs are rare in etiological research as it is often impractical or unethical to randomize participants into exposure groups. Therefore, most etiological research is observational in nature. It is debatable as to the relative merits of case control studies and cohort studies, as the power of these two designs for exploring causal relationship is potentially the same. In practice, it is often easier to avoid bias (including confounding) in cohort studies than in case control studies.

Over the years, variations of levels of evidence have been published, often in the form of a pyramid, with systematic review or RCT at the top and case reports or expert opinion at the bottom. Levels of evidence are used routinely nowadays when devising practice guidelines. The Grading of Recommendations Assessment, Development and Evaluation (GRADE) system provides a further refinement.[1]

Coherence

Coherence of findings – preferably based on the presumed biological mechanism of action – refers to the fact that a causal relationship found for one population is also likely to apply to other populations. The more coherent an association is, the more likely it is to reflect a causal effect.

Plausibility

The question of theoretical or biological plausibility is whether a causal relationship is likely, given our current knowledge of human biology. For example, the idea that there is a causal association between smoking and lung cancer makes sense to everyone, but a suggested association between smoking and cervical cancer is less self-evident. No one will be surprised to be told that there is a relationship between aircraft noise and sleep disorders, but it makes less sense to attribute the occurrence of cleft lip to aircraft noise. Biological plausibility is not a hard and fast criterion: what seems like a reasonable biological explanation to one researcher may be rejected by another. The history of medicine is riddled with examples of hypothetical descriptions of biological mechanisms that eventually turned out to be incorrect. Relevant findings from basic biomedical research, especially research on animals, are very important when assessing this criterion. A proven causal relationship in laboratory animals does not of course automatically mean that the relationship also exists in humans, but it often provides a suggestion in that direction.

Temporality

A cause must precede its effect: this is a necessary precondition, and in fact the only absolute criterion of causality. If it can be shown that the presumed effect preceded the cause, there cannot be causality. Unfortunately, the converse of this rule is not true: the correct time sequence does not at all guarantee a causal relationship. For this reason, cross-sectional study designs, i.e. designs that use data from only a single point in time, can provide only limited evidence of causal associations. Longitudinal designs, such as cohort studies can be employed to measure exposure and health outcome over the course of follow-up.

Strength

A strong association tends to suggest a causal relationship more than a weak one, as a strong association is not very likely to be explained by bias and confounding. As we saw in Section 6.2.3, the strength of an association is determined to a large extent by the frequency of the other factors in the complex of suf-

ficient causes. Also, a weak association does not rule out causality.

Biological gradient

A biological gradient or dose–response relationship provides further support for causality. Researchers investigate whether a higher dose or longer exposure coincides with a higher frequency of the response. A dose–response relationship can also be due to a confounder, however. Moreover, the absence of a dose–response relationship cannot generally be interpreted as an argument against causality in and of itself. There could be a threshold below which there is no response, for instance. Or there could be a threshold for the risk factor above which the response is always maximized. Another possibility is that the causal relationship between dose and response is U-shaped.

Consistency

If the same association has been shown by different researchers, at different times and places, in different populations and using different study designs, that is an argument in favor of causality. However, this criterion – consistency – is not absolute either. If different subgroups in the study population (both men and women, both older and younger people, both rural and urban areas, etc.) demonstrate a similar association, it is an argument in favor of causality. A lack of consistency can be due to effect modification, as particular causal relationships could conceivably manifest themselves only in special circumstances. If different studies or subgroups show opposite effects (increased risk in one subgroup and reduced risk in another), causality is less likely.

6.2.5 Individual versus population level

When interpreting associations, it can be useful to argue separately what would have happened in the population if the factor was not present for each element in the causal chain. Would the health outcome have occurred with the same frequency if the situation were completely identical except for the absence of that one factor? In this type of thought experiment then, the argument is based on the converse situation (counterfactual). If the health outcome only occurs if the factor is present, and not if it is absent (as in the light switch example in Section 6.2.1), the factor is a necessary cause. If the health outcome still occurs, but to a lesser extent, the factor is evidently one of the set of factors that, together, constitute a sufficient cause for the condition in question, but it is not a necessary factor. If the health outcome occurs with the same frequency with or without the presence of the factor (all other factors remaining equal), that factor evidently does not influence the development of the heath outcome and is not part of the causal chain. In this case, we need to find some other explanations for the association found – by chance, for example, or by showing that the factor in question often coincides with another factor that is causally related to the health outcome (take for instance, carrying a cigarette lighter in relation to the development of lung cancer as described in Section 6.1).

At the individual level, it is very difficult to show what the causal factor is. For example, did grandfather get lung cancer because he smoked a lot of cigarettes during his lifetime? Or did he get lung cancer earlier than he would have because he smoked? Smoking is not a necessary cause of lung cancer, so we do not know what would have happened if he had not smoked. Only if we are dealing with a necessary cause can we say with certainty that the individual would not have developed the health outcome if he had not been exposed to the factor.

Causality is easier to establish at the population level. "Was the lung cancer epidemic caused by large numbers of people that had started to smoking cigarettes?" Yes, because we know for sure that the incidence of lung cancer in the population would have been much lower if – in the converse situation, but in otherwise similar circumstances – everyone refrained from smoking cigarettes. It is precisely these population-based conclusions, founded on sound epidemiological research that have shown that the incidence of lung cancer increased sharply when the number of smokers in the population had increased, that can be applied to individuals: smokers are at much greater risk of developing lung cancer and dying from it than if he or she did not smoke. But, just as the population would not be immune from lung cancer if nobody smoked, there is no guarantee that a non-smoking individual will be immune from lung cancer. The converse is also true: smokers do not always develop lung cancer, and the incidence of lung cancer in a population of hardened smokers is far below 100%. Smoking is undoubtedly a cause of the disease, but it is neither a necessary cause nor a sufficient one. Population data can be translated into disease risks, but not into conclusions on individual causality.

Case Study 6.3 Caffeine Intake and Risk of Melanoma

Ultraviolet (UV) radiation is the major environmental cause of cutaneous malignant melanoma, a common type of skin cancer. Caffeine, a central nervous stimulant that is present in coffee and tea, had previously been shown to inhibit UV-induced thymine dimers and sunburn lesions in the epidermis of mice, acting as a sunscreen. Also, earlier studies had concluded that caffeine enhances UV-induced cell apoptosis and had shown that caffeine inhibits growth of melanoma cells both *in vivo* and *in vitro*. This led to the hypothesis that caffeine intake could reduce the risk of melanoma on locations that are most exposed to sunlight.

To test this hypothesis, data from three large cohorts were combined. The Health Professionals Follow-Up Study (HPFS) was established in 1986 and provided data on 39,424 male health professionals aged 40–75 years. The purpose of the HPFS study was to evaluate a series of hypotheses about men's health relating nutritional factors to the incidence of serious diseases such as cancer, heart disease and other vascu-

lar diseases. This all-male study was designed to complement the all-female Nurses' Health Study that began in 1976. The Nurses' Health Study and the Nurses' Health Study 2 (1989) contributed data on 74,666 and 89,220 female nurses aged 30–55 and 25–42 respectively. Participants were selected based on the availability of a completed dietary questionnaire and had to have no history of any cancer at baseline. Participants in all three cohorts received biannual questionnaires on disease outcomes.

Caffeine intake was categorized as quintiles. The lowest quintile (<60 mg) amounts to less than half a cup of coffee per day; the highest quintile (≥393 mg) amounts to drinking at least three cups of coffee each day. In total, 2,254 new cases of melanomas were observed in over four million person-years of follow-up. Cox proportional hazards regression was used to compute hazard ratios (HRs), which were adjusted for known melanoma risk factors and potential confounders.

⬜ Table 6.2 shows that people consuming ≥393 mg of caffeine per day as compared to <60 mg/day were less likely to report incident melanomas (HR = 0.71). However, this inverse association was more pronounced in women (HR = 0.66) than in men (HR = 0.82). The difference between men and women could be due to differing sun exposure patterns because of different dress styles, but it might also be due to effect modification by gender. This was also suggested by the finding that women reported more melanomas on extremities (53.5% of all melanomas) compared to men (29% of all melanomas). The generalizability of the results may be limited, since both cohorts comprise mostly white, well-educated health professionals. Skin color is a major risk factor of melanoma risk, making these results difficult to apply to people of different ethnicities. In terms of the Hill criteria for causality, this example is based on a strong study design, and argues that a protective effect of caffeine is plausible and provides some evidence of a dose-response relationship. Furthermore, the temporal sequence is probably correct, unless preclinical melanomas were already present at the baseline measurement.

⬜ **Table 6.2** Relative risk of cutaneous malignant melanoma for quintiles of caffeine intake.

	Q1 (<60 mg/day)	Q2 (60–140 mg/day)	Q3 (141–246 mg/day)	Q4 (247–392 mg/day)	Q5 (≥393 mg/day)
Pooled for women and men	1.0	0.83 (0.70, 0.99)	0.79 (0.67, 0.95)	0.87 (0.66, 0.93)	0.71 (0.59, 0.86)
Women	1.0	0.79 (0.63, 0.99)	0.82 (0.66, 1.0)	0.73 (0.59, 0.91)	0.66 (0.53, 0.83)
Men	1.0	0.91 (0.68, 1.2)	0.74 (0.54, 1.0)	0.89 (0.66, 1.2)	0.82 (0.59, 1.1)

RRs are adjusted for family history of melanoma, personal history of non-skin cancer, natural hair color, number of moles on legs or arms, sunburn reaction as a child/adolescent number of blistering sunburns, time spent in direct sunlight since high school, cumulative ultraviolet flux since high school, body mass index, smoking status, physical activity, total energy intake and alcohol intake. HRs are computed including 95% confidence intervals. Q1 served as the reference quintile.

6.3 Applications

6.3.1 Forensic epidemiology

Questions of causality in epidemiological research are increasingly being used in court cases, recently resulting in a new spin-off from the discipline: forensic epidemiology. This subdiscipline uses epidemiological and statistical methods to assess and quantify causal relationships in court cases with a medical connection. It is applied in both criminal and civil law, although the majority of cases involve civil law (in particular liability law), for example, with respect to medical negligence, occupational safety negligence, side effects of pharmaceutical products, faults in medical devices, and serious road accidents.

In liability cases, the plaintiff has to prove that the medical condition was likely caused by the factor in question (e.g. a drug, medical device, food product, or working condition) and not by something else.

Conversely, the defendant will do everything in their power to prove that the research leaves a lot of doubt (potential bias) as to the alleged causality of the relationship. The result of forensic epidemiological research is a well-founded quantitative estimate of the likelihood that the observed association is based on a causal effect.

Forensic epidemiologists generally follow these four steps:

1. Assess all the elements relevant to the case, including conflicting theories concerning causality and liability.
2. Carry out a quantitative analysis of the theories put forward by both parties. Are the estimations of likelihood correct and properly substantiated? Can they be quantified and compared?
3. Carry out an additional examination of the medical literature and/or other data.
4. Make a quantitative, substantiated estimate of the likelihood that the association is causal, based on all the available evidence.

6.3.2 Prevention

Etiological research produces scientific knowledge of the causes of diseases and factors that influence their course. This knowledge is used to devise preventive and therapeutic strategies. After all, if one of the causal factors can be eliminated from the complex of sufficient causes, the disease will no longer be able to develop through that mechanism or, if the disease is already present, run a different course. It is not necessarily true, however, that removing a cause of a disease will eliminate that disease in patients who already have it: sometimes this will be the case (e.g. antibiotics kill the bacterium responsible for the persistence of the infection), but often it will not (e.g. noise-induced hearing loss will not be reversed by starting to wear hearing protectors). Eliminating the cause may well have an effect on disease progression, as wearing hearing protection may prevent further deterioration of hearing.

Knowledge of the causes of a disease does not automatically lead to effective preventive measures; conversely, full knowledge of the causes is not always needed for prevention to be effective. Take safe sex and AIDS prevention, for example: this effective measure was advocated before the main cause of the disease (the HIV virus) was known. Generally speaking, prevention and knowledge of the etiological factors go hand in hand. Examples of preventive interventions include changing the physical environment (sewers, crash barriers), laying down statutory rules (food safety, speed restrictions), prescribing prophylactic medication (folic acid, fluoride), carrying out preventive surgery (circumcision, angioplasty), and health education.

There are three levels of prevention: primary, secondary and tertiary. The purpose of primary prevention is to prevent the health outcome from developing. The focus here is on etiological factors for occurrence. Quitting smoking – or better still, not starting – so as to prevent such things as asthma, coronary heart disease, and lung cancer is an example. The aim of secondary prevention is to detect a condition early once it has developed, so as to increase the likelihood of cure. An example is advocating breast self-examination so as to detect breast cancer at an early stage. Screening programs are also examples of secondary prevention. Tertiary prevention is carried out on patients who

have the condition and can be used to minimize its effects, reducing the likelihood of relapse, or to improve quality of life, among other examples. Health education provided to diabetes patients is an example. In essence, all forms of treatment could be regarded as tertiary prevention, whether curative or palliative in nature.

Recommended reading

Bonita, R., Beaglehole, R., and Kjellstrom, T. (2006). *Basic Epidemiology*, 2e. Geneva: World Health Organization.

Fletcher, G. (2020). *Clinical Epidemiology: The Essentials*, 6e. Baltimore: Wolters Kluwer.

Freeman, M. and Zeegers, M. (2016). *Forensic Epidemiology: Principles and Practice*. San Diego: Elsevier.

Grobbee, D.E. and Hoes, A.W. (2015). *Clinical Epidemiology: Principles, Methods, and Applications for Clinical Research*, 2e. Burlington: Jones and Bartlett Learning.

Hernán, M.A. and Robins, J.M. *Causal Inference: What if*, 1e. Boca Raton: Chapman & Hall/CRC.

Hill, A.B. (1965). The environment and disease: association or causation? *Proceedings of the Royal Society of Medicine* 58: 295–300.

Rothman, K.J., Greenland, S., and Lash, T.L. (2020). *Modern Epidemiology*, 4e. Philadelphia: Lippincott, Williams & Wilkins.

Szklo, M. and Nieto, F.J. (2019). *Epidemiology: Beyond the Basics*, 4e. Burlington: Jones and Bartlett Learning.

Source references (case and figure)

Weischer, M., Nordestgaard, B.G., Pharoah, P. et al. (2012). CHEK2*1100delC heterozygosity in women with breast cancer associated with early death, breast cancer-specific death, and increased risk of a second breast cancer. *Journal of Clinical Oncology* 30 (35): 4308–4316. (Case 6.1).

Fletcher, R.H., Fletcher, S.W., and Fletcher, G.S. (2012). *Clinical Epidemiology: The Essentials*, 5e. Baltimore: Lippincott, Williams & Wilkins (Case 6.2).

Wu, S., Han, J., Song, F. et al. (2015). Caffeine intake, coffee consumption, and risk of cutaneous malignant melanoma. *Epidemiology* 26 (6): 898–908. (Case 6.3).

Knowledge assessment questions

1. Which of the following best describes the main difference between association and causation?
   A. Association is a relationship while causation is a model
   B. Association reflects an underlying relationship while causation reflects an outcome
   C. Association quantifies the relationship between an explanatory variable and an outcome, while causation concludes that this relationship is causal
   D. Association can only be determined by determining temporality of the underlying relationship

2. Researchers at Edinburgh University are conducting a study on respiratory disease and air pollution exposure. In a sample of 547 hospitalized individuals, they find a relationship between exposure to high levels of air pollution and incidence of respiratory disease in the previous year (odds ratio 9.61). This association makes sense – exposure to high levels of pollution may irritate the lining of the lungs and increase susceptibility to respiratory disease. However, when researchers repeat their analysis in the general population with a sample of 5,000 individuals, the association is not detected (odds ratio 1.07). Upon conducting a stratified analysis, researchers conclude that both respiratory disease and exposure to high levels of pollutants caused individuals to be hospitalized.

Draw and label the variables and relationships in the study described using a directed acyclic graph. Describe what type of bias explains the different findings in the hospital and the general population samples. Which of these two provides the more valid odds ratio?

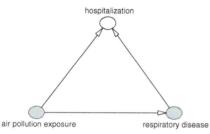

3. Match these Hill criteria for causation with their description. The names of the criteria are strength, consistency, temporality, biological gradient, plausibility, coherence, experimentation

Criterion	Description
	This criterion requires that exposure precedes the onset of disease by a reasonable amount of time.
	This criterion suggests evidence from clinical trials, *in vitro* experiments, animal models, and so on support the theory.
	This criterion says increase in the level, intensity, duration, or total level of exposure to the factor leads to progressive increases in risk. This is in keeping with the general dose–response relationship seen with many biological phenomena.
	This criterion holds that large associations provide firmer evidence of causality than do small ones, and that the most direct measure of association is found in the form of ratio measures of association such as the risk ratio.
	This criterion holds that diverse methods of study carried out in different populations under a variety of circumstances by different investigators provide non-contradictory results.
	This criterion suggests that all available evidence concerning the natural history and biology of the disease "sticks together" as a whole. By that, the proposed causal relationship should not conflict or contradict information from experimental, laboratory, epidemiological, theory, or other knowledge sources.
	This criterion suggests that it is helpful for an association to be based on known biological fact. This, of course, is contingent on the state of the biological knowledge of the day.

Notes

1. The Grading of Recommendations Assessment, Development and Evaluation (GRADE) system (website). http:// http://bit.ly/1IQ69Ub.

Genetic Epidemiology

Textbook of Epidemiology, Second Edition. Lex Bouter, Maurice Zeegers and Tianjing Li.
© 2023 John Wiley & Sons Ltd. Published 2023 by John Wiley & Sons Ltd.
Companion website: www.wiley.com/go/Bouter/TextbookofEpidemiology

7.1   Introduction

Risk factors for disease can, broadly speaking, be divided into three categories: biology, behavior, and environment (see Chapter 3). Genetic epidemiology studies primarily fall in the first category, and also concern the complex interactions between genetic markers or with environmental or behavioral factors. It is thus closely related to molecular epidemiology, which is concerned with the role of biological or molecular markers of exposure to risk factors and susceptibility to disease. Once the human genome had been mapped, interest in genetic factors of any health outcome – and hence in genetic epidemiological research – increased enormously. The reason we devote a separate chapter to genetic epidemiology is the existence of specific biological mechanisms that transfer genetic traits from one generation to the next. These enable researchers to tackle questions regarding the genetic factors of disease occurrence differently and more efficiently than for other categories of risk factors. Consequently, genetic epidemiology uses some substantially different study designs and analytical methods, in addition to general epidemiological methods.

7.1.1   Terminology

Genetic epidemiology is the study of how hereditary variations in the human genome influence the risk of diseases in human populations, either in interaction with behavioral and environmental factors, or on their own. There are many concepts from the field of genetics that need to be introduced. Below, you will find a summary. The Recommended Reading list of this chapter provides more in-depth reading.

Hereditary information is stored in chromosomes, which are composed of deoxyribonucleic acid molecules (DNA). Everyone has two copies of each chromosome – and therefore of each gene: one from the father and one from the mother. The exceptions to this are the X and Y chromosomes that define sex: females have XX and males XY. Each person has 22 pairs of homologous (meaning the same) chromosomes and two sex chromosomes. One chromosome of these pairs comes from the father and the other from the mother. Any two individuals' genomes will be 99.9% identical, but there are millions of sections in the DNA string where people can differ from one another. An

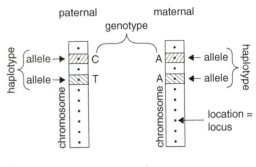

Figure 7.1   Genetic terminology.

allele is a DNA variation (or variant) at the same location (or locus) on a chromosome. Alleles come in one, two or more variants. If a specific allele variant has a frequency of less than 1% in the population it is referred to as a mutation. If the frequency of an allele variant is greater than 1%, it is referred to as a polymorphism. The most common allele variant is also called the wild type and the least common the mutant form of that allele. Sometimes we don't make this distinction and just call them all genetic variants. A pair of alleles on the same locus of the maternal and paternal chromosome is called a genotype. Depending on the number of allele variants available, many pairs, thus many different genotypes can be formed. Because of the different genotypes in a population, people differ in eye color, hair color and many other physical characteristics including their susceptibility to diseases. ◘ Figure 7.1 also shows two homologous copies of a chromosome (one paternal, one maternal) with groups of alleles. If alleles are near enough to each other, they usually get inherited together as a one "block" of alleles (also called haplotypes or haplotype block).

Genetic variants can be associated with the risk of contracting certain disorders. In monogenetic disorders, a structural defect in a chromosome or a mutation in a gene is a necessary and sufficient cause of developing the disorder. Familiar examples of this are Down syndrome (trisomy 21) and Huntington's disease (caused by an abnormal gene on chromosome 4). Without the genetic defect, the disease cannot develop. These monogenic defects may be caused by a chance mutation with no prior history in the family, as in the case of Down syndrome (a "de novo" mutation). In other cases, a disease develops due to heredity, as is almost always the case with Huntington's disease. Where there is a strong association between a genotype and a phenotype (a measurable trait, disorder, or disease as the result of a genotype) there is said to be high penetrance. Penetrance is a term used by geneticists that is identical to the term etiological fraction that epidemiologists use (see Section 3.2.5). If highly penetrant variants are passed on from one generation to the next, we will see an increased incidence of the phenotype within families. If these variants lower the number of offspring due to poor survival rate or low fertility, we say that these variants have low fitness. Variants with high penetrance and low fitness are less common in the population because of their difficulty to inherit from one generation to the next. It can also happen that a single gene mutation can cause multiple distinguishable phenotypes. This is called pleiotropy.

Far more common than monogenic phenotypes are multifactorial or complex phenotypes where multiple genetic variants, combined with environmental and behavioral factors, determine the risk in a more complex pattern. The number of genetic factors involved, their penetrance, and the frequency can vary substantially from one multifactorial phenotype to another. Until recently, it was thought that only a few underlying genetic factors were involved in these multifactorial phenotypes, namely common factors (with an allele frequency of over 5%) with only mild effects (the "common disease-common variant" hypothesis). In recent years, however, it has become clear that it is more likely that rare, relatively low-penetrance genetic factors are important in the development of multifactorial phenotypes (the "common disease-rare variant" hypothesis). In some cases, different genetic profiles can cause identical phenotypes (genetic heterogeneity), or a phenotype can be due to effect modification between genes and environmental factors. Multifactorial phenotypes don't cluster in patients' families due to their complex etiology. Nowadays, most genetic epidemiologists study multifactorial phenotypes. Hence, the greater emphasis in this chapter on the genetic epidemiology is on the methodology to study these genetic variants.

7.1.2 Research questions

This chapter looks at various methods and techniques used in genetic epidemiological research and provides examples of how they are used. The questions that can be posed in genetic epidemiology follow a certain natural order, gradually zooming in on the genetic factor.

The first research question is whether genetic variation is suspected to be relevant to a health outcome. If there is familial aggregation, i.e. the health outcome is more common among family members than would be expected based on the frequency of the health outcome in the general population, there is a high likelihood that factors shared by family members – environmental, behavioral or genetic – are involved. The use of case-control studies, family-based cohort studies and twin studies to explore familial aggregation is discussed in section 7.2. If we suspect that genetic variation may be of relevance to the occurrence of the health outcome, the next question is which loci are involved. If we do not wish to make assumptions about the location, we carry out a genome-wide linkage analysis (GWLA). This is a family-based study, in which the segregation of large numbers of DNA variants in the genomes of family members is observed and compared with the occurence of the health outcome in the different family members. A GWLA is an efficient way of tracking down monogenic disorders that are strongly aggregated within families. These linkage analyses are often supplemented with, or replaced by, techniques that identify all the variants in the genomes or exomes (the coding part of the genome) of family members. In practice, these analyses tend to fall in the domain of genetics rather than that of epidemiology, and they are therefore described only briefly (in Section 7.3).

Population-based studies are generally used to localize low-penetrance variations for multi-factorial phenotypes. The classic case-control study is often used in the design of genome-wide population or association studies (GWAS): this is described in detail in Section 7.3.4. If the approximate location is known, we can zoom in using more markers that are increasingly close together. Specific bioinformatic methods can be used to track down the possible genes involved, but these last methods fall outside the domain of epidemiology. Once these questions have been answered, further bioinformatic analysis is carried out into the possible biological pathways by which the variant influences the development of the phenotype, the underlying inheritance model, the prevalence of the variant in highly predisposed families, and in sporadic cases (where the patient has no affected family members). That information is used to decide whether it would be worthwhile to screen families and/or specific populations for the DNA variant.

It should be noted that the scope for genetic epidemiological research has been and still is highly dependent on advances in technology for measuring genetic variation in the human genome.

7.2 Family-based studies

Familial aggregation of a health outcome can be indicative of genetic variation playing a major role. Classic case-control studies (see Chapter 4) can identify familial predisposition by asking whether patients and controls have a negative or positive family history. The odds ratio (OR) (see Chapter 3) is then computed as a measure of association between having a positive family history and the health outcome. In the case of relatively rare health outcomes, the OR can be interpreted as the relative risk (RR) associated with a positive family history. This approach, however, can give a distorted picture of the degree of familial aggregation of a disease, as the likelihood of it occurring in the family will depend on the size of the family, the ages and gender distribution of the members, the genetic relationships of the participants and each family member's risk factor pattern due to other factors.

Familial aggregation of health outcomes is therefore ideally studied in family-based cohorts of patients and controls. The incidence of the health outcomes in the two cohorts is calculated. The ratio between these incidences – the RR – indicates the additional risk for patients' family members compared with the controls' family members (the base risk). The RR may then also be referred to as the familial relative risk. As the occurrence of the health outcome among family members may of course also depend on age (there is more competition from other causes of death in later life), suitable measures of frequency and analytical strategies need to be used (incidence densities [IDs], survival rates: see Chapter 2), just as in classic cohort studies. The central factor in these family-based cohort studies is therefore the familial relationship with the patients or the controls. The analysis can be stratified by degree of kinship if necessary: the risk of the disease among a patient's first-degree relatives can be compared with that of a control's first-degree relative. Information on potential confounders or effect modifiers can also be collected for each family member and included in the analysis: regression models can then be used to estimate IDs or hazard ratios (HRs), adjusted for confounders, enabling an initial impression of the relative contribution of the genetic component to the causation of the disorder. However, these analyses need to take the statistical dependence of family members into account. To achieve this, regression models can be expanded to take clustering into account, e.g. by using multilevel models. Case 7.1 gives an example of a family-based cohort study.

> ### Case 7.1 Clustering of Breast Cancer in Families
>
> Various case-control studies and family-based cohort studies in the closing decades of the twentieth century showed that a positive family history is a risk factor for breast cancer and that the risk is greater the earlier the age at which the family member was diagnosed with it. One of these was a family-based cohort study from 1990, which included 4,730 breast cancer patients and 4,688 controls in the 20–54 age range. The patients had been recorded in the cancer registries of the National Cancer Institute in the United States between 1 December 1980 and 31 December 1982. Information on the incidence of breast cancer in female family members (first-degree relatives and paternal and maternal grandmothers and aunts) was obtained from interviews with the patients and controls within 6 months of the first primary breast cancer diagnosis in the patient. To study the family clustering, the incidence of breast cancer among the patients' family members was compared with that among the controls' family members. The study showed that in all the age groups, the risk of breast cancer for patients' mothers was approximately twice as high as that for controls' mothers. It also showed that the risk was highest among women whose family members had been diagnosed at an early age. The familial relative risk (in this case, the cumulative incidence ratio [CIR]) of breast cancer in mothers of patients who had been diagnosed before the age of 30, 40, or 50 was 4.3, 2.7, and 1.7 respectively.

To study the contribution of genetic variation to continuous traits such as blood pressure or cholesterol level, the correlations of such traits between family members with various types of kinship, are often compared. If there is a strong correlation among relatives who share a lot of their genetic material (e.g. monozygotic twin pairs) and a weak correlation in pairs who share little genetic variation (e.g. second cousins), it is indicative of a strong genetic component for the trait. Most traits are affected by a combination of genetic and environmental or behavioral factors. To study the relative contributions of these factors based on correlations between family members with different degrees of kinship, we ideally need families that vary with respect to genetic, behavioral and environmental factors. In these genetic epidemiological study designs, the classic Mendelian laws are taken as a reference. A parent-child pair share half of their genetic material, a grandparent-child pair one quarter. At the same time, brothers and sisters in a family are often more alike in behavioral and environmental factors in childhood than second cousins. Combining these data on kinship and shared behavioral and environmental factors with measurements of continuous traits provide information on the relative contributions of heredity (nature) and behavior/environment (nurture). Studies of twins provide an efficient way of studying the genetic component of continuous traits, for one thing because they enable monozygotic and dizygotic twin pairs to be compared. Case 7.2 gives an example.

Case 7.2 All Human Traits are Heritable

Scientists have always been interested in the causes of individual differences in human traits. This has led to a lively "nature versus nurture" debate going back to the eighteenth century, but adequate methods to study the etiology of human trait variation only became available in the last few decades. The foundation of this type of research has been twins, as they enable high-quality natural experiments to disentangle the effects of nature (heritability), and nurture (environmental influences). Monozygotic (MZ) twins are genetically identical, while dizygotic (DZ) twins share 50% of their genes on average.

Usually, the environment that twins have in common (i.e. "the shared environment," such as the home environment) is 100% for MZ as well as DZ twins, at least during childhood. Comparison of the within-pair resemblance for a given trait in MZ twins versus DZ twins – usually presented as MZ and DZ twin correlations – indicates to what extent genes or the environment contribute to trait variation. Higher within-pair MZ correlations in comparison to DZ correlations suggest the presence of genetic influences, as the only difference between MZ and DZ twin pairs is the within-pair genetic similarity.

A large meta-analysis of all twin correlations and heritability estimates of the past 50 years was published in 2015 and is still the most comprehensive overview to date. This was based on 2,748 twin studies that reported on 17,804 traits of a total of 14.5 million twin pairs. One of the main findings was that all the traits investigated were heritable: not one trait had a heritability estimate of zero. The results of the meta-analysis, across all traits regardless of age and gender, showed that the contribution of genetic and environmental influences was equal. Thus, genetic and environmental influences each contribute about 50% to overall human variation. When zooming in on different traits it became clear that heritability estimates differ across traits. High heritability estimates were reported for "diseases of the skin" (69%), while one of the lowest heritability estimates was noted for voice and speech functions (15%). Heritability estimates may also be dynamic over time. For instance, intelligence is highly heritable in adulthood, while in childhood environmental influences are equally important. Heritability estimates for same sex pairs (SS), males (M) and females (F) were very similar across traits, indicating no gender differences in the contribution of genetic and environmental effects to trait variation. ◻ Figure 7.2 shows an example of results obtained from the website.

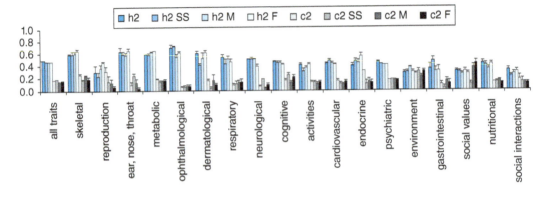

Figure 7.2 Shows the heritability estimates (h2) for "all traits" and other investigated trait domains from the MATCH web tool. The h2 estimates are shown in shades of blue and shared environmental influences (c2) in shades of grey. The remainder of the variation is due to the contribution of unique environmental influences.

7.2.1 Linkage analysis

As already noted, finding highly penetrant mutations for monogenic disorders is primarily the domain of genetics. GWLA of selected families with several affected members have resulted in various highly penetrant disease genes being localized. The principle of linkage analysis is simple. When the causal DNA variant is unknown, a multitude of DNA markers across the genome are used to find the location of the causal variant. This can be done by assessing the inheritance of the alleles of each of these DNA markers and the target phenotype in the families. Target genes and their DNA markers are more strongly associated when they are situated nearer to each other on the chromosome. When the target gene is indeed causal, we also expect to see a high correlation between the nearby DNA marker and the health outcome itself. In genetic terms this is referred to as linkage. If the DNA marker is not in linkage with the outcome, it is evidently far enough apart from the health outcome variant for recombination to have broken the link between the alleles of the two variants.

The concept of recombination is illustrated by an example in Section 7.3.3. The strength of the linkage between the marker and the health outcome variant can be quantified using the log-odds score (LOD score). As family members share long segments of their genome, only a few thousand markers need to be measured for a GWLA. Figure 7.3 shows a family for which the genotype of a single DNA marker with two

alleles (1 and 2) has been determined for a grandparent pair, the parents and four children. The squares represent males, the circles females. A hatched symbol for a family member means that the person has the disease. Where this is the case, it is assumed that the person carries the D allele (in other words, has the genotype DD), so there is full penetrance and dominant inheritance.

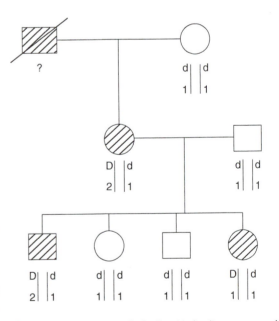

Figure 7.3 Family tree of a family with the disease gene and the marker on the same chromosome.

The affected mother is found to have received a 1-allele from the healthy grandmother and therefore both the health outcome and a 2-allele from the grandfather. This means that the mutated D allele of the gene associated with the health outcome has to be inherited along with the 2-allele of the marker in this family. The father has both two 1 alleles and two d-alleles and therefore does not provide any information on recombination during meiosis. A recombination event during meiosis must have occurred. The children have all received a chromosome with a 1-allele and a d-allele from the father. The leftmost child has the health outcome and has received a 2-allele from the mother, which means that there was no recombination between D and 2 during this child's maternal meiosis. The second child from the left is healthy and has received a 1-allele from the mother, so this is also a non-recombinant. Only the rightmost child deviates from this pattern: she has received the 1-allele from the mother but nevertheless has the health outcome, which means that a recombination during meiosis must have occurred. The likelihood of linkage in this family (with r = 1 recombinant from n = 4 informative meioses), assuming for example that the recombination fraction (θ) between the gene and the marker is 0.05, can be calculated as follows:

$$L(\theta) = (\theta/2)^r \times \left[(1-\theta)/2\right]^{n-r}$$
$$= (0.05/2)^1 \times \left[(1-0.05)/2\right]^{4-1} = 0.0027$$

The likelihood of the alternative hypothesis of no linkage is:

$$L(\theta = 0.5) = (0.50/2)^4 = 0.0039$$

The LOD score is the 10 log of the likelihood ratio, in this case:

$$LOD = \log\left[L(\theta = 0.05)/L(\theta = 0.50)\right] = 0.69$$

Of course, we do not know whether the recombination fraction is 0.05, so we calculate the LOD score for several recombination fractions between 0.005 and 0.25 (higher fractions would provide little evidence

that there is a marker near the gene). The recombination fraction for the highest LOD score indicates the distance between the marker and the gene. If more families have been described, each with a particular LOD score for a specific recombination fraction, the LOD scores for different families can be added up. Fewer recombinations will lead to higher LOD scores for low recombination fractions, and hence to more evidence that the marker is linked to the health outcome. An LOD score higher than zero suggests that the marker is linked to the unknown health outcome gene, but because of random variation we can only assume linkage if the LOD score is high (say 3 or higher).

It is important to realize that it is only the relationship between the location of the marker and that of the unknown gene that is relevant in link-age analyses; an allele variant of the marker does not relate to any pathophysiological function (they do not cause the health outcome to occur). So, it can be the case that in one family allele 2 of a particular marker is co-inherited with the phenotype and in another family allele.

The marker is merely a coordinate on the genomic map, as it were; whether that coordinate has been marked on the map in red, blue or black is not important in linkage analysis. This is very different from genetic association studies, which are discussed later on: they examine the association between a phenotype and a specific allele. It is also important to realize that this technique only provides a rough indication of the location of the gene concerned: the region that displays linkage is likely to contain dozens of genes. Further research will be needed to zoom in on the region (fine mapping) and ultimately lead to the identification of the gene. Case 7.4 describes a classic study of the localization of the *BRCA1* gene using linkage analyses before it was possible to clone this gene. When searching for highly penetrant mutations for monogenetic disorders, modern sequencing techniques that map all the variants in the human genome are often used. Here again, the search is for the one causal, highly penetrant mutation that explains the presence of the disease or phenotype in the family. One of the advantages of this technique is that it enables the causal variant to be identified directly.

Case 7.3 Localization of the Highly Penetrant Breast Cancer Gene

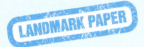

Family-based studies have shown that a genetic component is important in the development of breast cancer. Segregation analyses carried out by the group of the American researcher Marie-Claire King pointed to a rare, highly penetrant variant in combination with an autosomal dominant inheritance model as the best explanation for concentration of breast cancer in a large selection of high-risk families and families of young breast cancer patients. Blood was collected from 329 people in 23 families with a large number of breast cancer cases (a total of 146 patients) from North America, Puerto Rico, the United Kingdom and Colombia. The genotypes of 183 markers in each person were identified. It was found that a marker called D17S74, on chromosome 17q21, was inherited along with the breast cancer in the families, especially in those where the patients were diagnosed at a very early age. The linkage with the marker was not found in the families of older patients. The LOD score was just under 6, which is a very strong indication of a gene with the causal mutation (or mutations) near the marker. In the race to find the gene, King's group was beaten by Mark Skolnick's, which first identified it in 1994. This gene, now known as *BRCA1*, turned out to be a tumor suppressor gene that is important in repairing DNA damage. A host of different mutations were found in it, and women with such mutations were at high risk not only of breast cancer but also of cancer of the ovaries, where the gene is also expressed. Nowadays, women with a positive family history can be tested for mutations in the gene at clinical genetics centers. Women found to have a relevant *BRCA1* mutation are monitored closely for breast cancer and ovarian cancer. Some women who tested positive have their breasts or ovaries removed as a preventive measure.

7.3 Association studies

The linkage studies described above are a very powerful method for localizing unknown genetic variants on the genome for rare disorders that are highly clustered in families. Because of the complexity of the underlying genetic etiology, however, variants generally have small effects. Without high-risk families to study, linkage analysis is inefficient for studying multifactorial disorders. Multifactorial disorders are generally identified using population or association studies in which the classic case-control design is used. DNA is collected from patients and controls and the prevalence of variant alleles in the two groups is compared. The rationale behind an association study is that those with the phenotype of interest (i.e. the cases) are descendants of one and the same distant ancestor, who developed the causal allele(s) in the past, and that the controls are less closely related to that ancestor. This design of genetic association studies is discussed in Section 7.3.4. In essence, the starting point for an association study is that patients with the phenotype are descendants of one and the same distant ancestor, who was the first to receive the allele through a mutation (see Section 7.3.3). Among the controls who do not have the phenotype, we would expect fewer people to be descendants of that ancestor.

These association studies require genetic variants to be measured. Unlike those in a linkage study, however, these variants can be functional (i.e. affect the functionality of a protein) and be located in genes already suspected to influence the risk of the disease or phenotype. This is referred to as a direct association study and a candidate gene approach. In an indirect association study, the genetic variant merely serves as a coordinate in the genome and, if an association is found, it is indicative of linkage disequilibrium between the measured variant and the non-measured causal variant. This is explained in more detail in Section 7.3.3. An association between a genetic variant and a health outcome found in a case-control study can hence be indicative of causality or linkage disequilibrium with the causal variant, but also of two other phenomena, namely population stratification or chance (in small-scale studies). The phenomenon of population stratification is explained in Section 7.3.5.

7.3.1   Case-control design

Although any type of observational study design can be used for genetic epidemiological research, case-control design is used predominantly because many of the biases that normally apply to case-control studies are irrelevant in the genetic context. For example, genetic case-control studies do not suffer from differential misclassification (via information bias or recall bias), as the genetic information stored in the DNA is stable. Also, the risk of selection bias in genetic research is very low, as the likelihood of selection as a control or a patient in the study is unlikely to depend on the presence of an underlying – as yet unobserved – genetic variant. Lastly, disorders whose genetic factors we wish to study will generally have low prevalence, which makes case-control studies more efficient than cohort studies (see Chapter 4). Case 7.4 gives an example of a case-control study of a variant in a biologically plausible gene (candidate gene). Although case-control studies are very efficient when searching for genetic factors alone, cohort studies are also recommended, especially when studying gene-environment interactions.

Case 7.4 *APOE* and The Risk of Diabetic Nephropathy

Apolipoprotein E (*APOE*) plays a major role in the metabolism of lipids in the blood. There are three different functional alleles of the *APOE* gene that commonly occur: ε2, ε3, and ε4. As various studies have suggested associations between the *APOE* ε2 allele and the occurrence of hyperlipoproteinemia and lipoprotein glomerulopathy, new research has been initiated into the relationship between this APOE variant and the risk of renal failure in diabetic patients, known as "diabetic nephropathy" (DN). One of these studies was a case-control study of 223 DN patients and 192 controls. The DNA analysis of the *APOE* alleles showed that carriers of the ε2 allele had a highly increased risk of developing DN, compared with individuals who did not have the ε2 allele (OR = 3.1, 95% CI 1.6–5.9).

7.3.2   Linkage disequilibrium

During meiosis – the cell division process in which reproductive cells are generated – the two homologous chromosomes come together and recombine because of the "crossing-over" between two chromatids (the half of a replicated chromosome). If two DNA markers are far apart there is a good chance that a crossing-over will take place between them, resulting in a recombination. If two markers are very close together on the chromosome (linked) a crossing-over between them is unlikely. DNA variants found in the current population that are located very near an unknown causal DNA variant will thus also display linkage disequilibrium (LD) with the phenotype. This Bach4aal means that the specific alleles of nearby variants, like the causal alleles themselves, will be more common among patients. The LD approach in association studies uses a high number of single nucleotide DNA variants (SNVs) spread across the genome. SNVs of which the minor alle frequency is higher than 5% are also called single nucleotide polymorphisms (SNPs, called "snips"). By looking at the size of the associations between the SNV alleles and the phenotype in a case-control setup we can track down that part of the genome where the actual causal variant is most likely to be found. This is the locus where the size of the associations peak. Case 7.5 gives an example of such an association.

7.3.3   Linkage equilibrium

In genetics, we assume that each allele of a gene developed thousands of generations ago in one of the ancestors. We can thus assume that there has been sufficient opportunity for crossing-overs to occur between a locus of interest and nearby loci, and recombination has therefore occurred. The prevalence of the combination of alleles at two random locations on a chromosome (haplotype) in a population is therefore, in principle, equal to the product of the separate allele frequencies. The population is then in equilibrium for these loci and the alleles of the two loci are not associated: this is referred to as linkage equilibrium (LE). If an allele developed more recently, however (hundreds

7

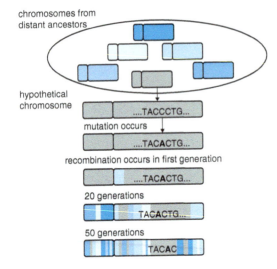

chromosomes from distant ancestors

hypothetical chromosome

....TACCCTG...

mutation occurs

....TACACTG...

recombination occurs in first generation

....TACACTG...

20 generations

TACACTG...

50 generations

TACAC

Figure 7.4 Situation where six haplotypes for a genomic region occur in a population. A new allele is introduced into the grey haplotype. After a few generations (and therefore meioses) crossing-over causes haplotypes comprising a mix of the six original haplotypes (recombinants) to develop. Because of lack of recombination between nearby variants, however, after 50 generations, the new variant allele A still occurs only on a grey haplotype background (haplotype TACAC).

rather than thousands of generations ago), or if the places on the genome are very close together (as we have seen above), it may be that little or no recombination has taken place for this marker and for nearby locations in the population (see Figure 7.4). Combinations of particular alleles of these markers and/or genes will then be more common, or less common, than we would expect based on the separate allele frequencies. This dependency between nearby alleles is referred to as allele association or correlation between alleles. The strength is often expressed as the measure r^2, which can range from 0 to 1, where 0 means complete LE and 1 complete LD (see Figure 7.5).

Case 7.5 Variants in TCF7L2 and Risk of Type 2 Diabetes

In 2003, Icelandic researchers showed in a linkage analysis that the chromosomal region 10q is linked to type 2 diabetes (DT2). This region was studied more closely in 2006 in a genetic association study among the Icelandic population (and in two other

case-control studies). Associations were found between DT2 and markers in the gene "transcription factor 7-like 2" (*TCF7L2*), which is located in the 10q region. These markers were DG10S478 and five SNVs that displayed moderate to strong LD with DG10S478. *TCF7L2* codes for a transcription factor that plays a role in the "Wnt signaling pathway," an important regulatory mechanism in cell development and growth. Other researchers subsequently carried out a replication study on *TCF7L2* in a Finnish population. Of the five SNVs that emerged from the Icelandic study, rs12255372 and rs7903146 displayed the strongest association. Twelve additional SNVs were selected in *TCF7L2*, as these were able to indirectly measure (or "tag") all of the 63 SNVs that showed LD with rs12255372 in the HapMap data, the SNV that displayed the strongest association with DT2 in the Icelandic study. However, the twelve additional SNVs displayed a weaker association with DT2 than rs12255372. The researchers therefore concluded that rs12255372 and rs7903146 in *TCF7L2* display the strongest – indirect – association with DT2. They could not rule out the possibility that other variants in *TCF7L2* influence the risk of DT2, as the twelve selected SNVs were only able to tag some of the variants located in *TCF7L2*. In a subsequent study of the association signal of SNVs in *TCF7L2* among other populations, the Icelandic researchers found the strongest signal for rs7903146. To ascertain whether this signal was actually a direct or an indirect one, Palmer et al. sequenced the gene region in DT2 patients and controls of African ethnicity in 2011. In this control population with a relatively long population genetic history, the LD between variants is relatively weak, promoting the discovery of the causal variant. The results of this study again pointed to variation in rs7903146 as the explanation for the association between gene *TCG7L2* and DT2.

7.3.4 Genome-wide association studies

Microarrays contain SNVs (often hundreds of thousands spread across the genome) that can be used for LD analyses in association studies, also called GWAS. In a GWAS, the entire genome is searched for disease

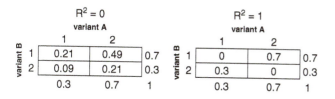

Figure 7.5 Numerical example of pairwise linkage disequilibrium (LD) where LD is expressed as r^2. This measure can range from 0 to 1, where 0 means linkage equilibrium and 1 linkage disequilibrium. Where $r^2 = 1$ there is perfect correlation: by measuring the genotype of variant A we can perfectly predict the genotype for variant B. In this example, for instance, we know that if we find genotype 11 for variant A the genotype for variant B will be 22 the numbers in the boxes are the combined alle frequencies.

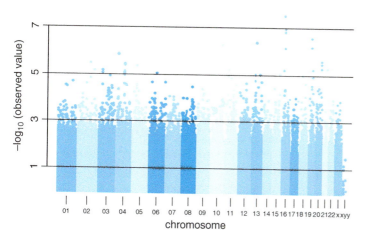

Figure 7.6 The Manhattan plot.

variants, without a prior hypothesis. It is possible, based on the measured SNVs and knowledge of patterns of correlation between variants in the human genome, to make a probabilistic estimate of the genotypes for unmeasured SNV. Case 7.6 gives an example of one of the first GWASs. The principles underlying GWASs or LD studies and linkage studies are related. Whereas in a linkage study we follow the segregation of the health outcome and the marker within a family, in an LD study we only look at the association between the marker and the health outcome in the current generation (of a virtual enormous family). For these GWASs, we therefore need far more markers, as the region over which LD extends in populations is far smaller than the region that displays linkage in families, because of the many meiosis that have taken place before the current population. Whereas a few thousand markers will suffice for a linkage study within families, GWASs require a minimum of hundreds of thousands of SNVs to map most of the existing variation in the human genome. These results are often shown in a scatter plot with the loci of the SNV on the x-axis and the negative logarithm of the p-values of the markers on the y-axis: a Manhattan plot (see Figure 7.6). The result of a GWAS is one or more candidate regions each containing a genetic variant that influences the risk of the health outcome occurring. We can zoom in on the candidate region using even more markers to track down the actual causal variant. Sequencing techniques enable genomic regions to be looked at in detail. This method can be used to track down the actual causal susceptibility variants, guided by the results of GWASs. Molecular biology and bioinformatic methods can also be used for this purpose. Past GWASs have shown, however, that it is not always easy to determine an underlying causal mechanism from an associated variant. The search for genetic factors of multifactorial disorders is gradually being supplemented with or replaced by next-generation sequencing techniques (which are still relatively expensive at present), providing researchers with a complete picture of all the variants, including very rare ones. While not substantially changing the study design, this technique has brought with it some new challenges, such as dealing with potential genotyping errors and processing the large quantities of data generated.

Case 7.6 GWAS for type 2 Diabetes

One of the first large-scale case-control GWASs was conducted by the Wellcome Trust Case Control Consortium (WTCCC), a partnership of various research groups in the UK. It looked at seven different disorders, including type 2 diabetes (DT2). The DNA of 2,000 DT2 patients and 3,000 controls was studied using an array of over 500,000 SNVs. Twelve SNVs showed an association with DT2 based on a probability threshold (p-value) of below 0.00001. Three of these association signals were SNVs in genes which had already been shown in previous linkage and association studies to be linked to the risk of DT2. The GWAS also revealed an association with TCF7L2, as the strongest association signal was found for rs4506565. This SNV displayed strong LD with rs7903146 (which had not been measured directly), the variant located in *TCF7L2* that had been detected in previous linkage and association studies. The nine additional signals were SNVs, of which, some were located in or near candidate genes for DT2. Some of these SNVs have now been confirmed in additional case-control populations.

7.3.5 Population stratification

The association between a genetic variant and a health outcome can be confounded if those affected and the controls have different genetic backgrounds of which the researcher is not aware. This phenomenon is known as population stratification. Suppose we want to investigate the causes of prostate cancer. We take a group of 100 prostate cancer patients and compare them with a group of 100 controls. As people of African ancestry have a higher risk of prostate cancer than those of European ancestry, there is a high likelihood that there are more individuals of African ancestry in the prostate cancer group. After analyzing the

DNA of all the participants, it was found that 70 of the 100 patients had specific allele 1, as against only ten of the controls. The OR of $(70/30):(10/90) = 21$ suggests that people with allele 1 are at a much higher risk than those without it. It is quite possible, however, that allele 1 does not have anything to do with the disease but is simply more common in individuals of African ancestry. Other random markers could also be associated with the disease, merely because the allele frequency differs for different ancestries. This, of course, is a classic example of confounding (see Chapter 5). While an epidemiologist will never make the mistake of not taking such an obvious factor as ancestry into account, genetic ancestry goes back many generations and is not easy for researchers to trace. It is often impossible to clearly classify the underlying genetic backgrounds of participants. If we are unsure about the presence of population stratification, we can take a group of SNVs known to be not associated with the health outcome of interest, run an association analysis, and confirm that there is indeed no association.

7.3.6 Collaboration

An untargeted search for genes associated with health outcome in the entire genome, i.e. without any specific prior hypotheses, as is the case with GWASs, entails some particular problems. For example, conducting hundreds of thousands or millions of association tests of minor genetic effects (involving low-penetrance variants, possibly measured with some errors) requires large samples of thousands of people to achieve sufficient power and not miss findings. When performing 1,000,000 standard statistical tests with an α (type 1 error) of 0.05 you would expect 50,000 false positive associations. To reduce the type 1 error, much smaller critical values are chosen. Even then, the results of the study need to be replicated in other samples to distinguish false positive from true positive associations. The need for large-scale studies and replication of results in independent samples has vastly encouraged collaboration between research groups in consortia and the creation of biobanks. An example of a consortium is the WTCCC (see Case 7.7). To date (June 2021), 50 research groups are involved. The original study population comprised 14,000 patients (2,000 each for seven different disorders) and two control samples of 1,500 controls each, but it has now grown much larger.

The term biobank refers to a collection of biological material (e.g. blood, DNA, tumor material) linked to detailed descriptions of the characteristics of a large number of people. Biobanks provide a rich source for genetic epidemiological research. The importance of integrating knowledge and data from various "omics" (genomics, transcriptomics, proteomics, metabolomics) to clarify the genetic etiology and pathophysiology of multifactorial disorders is becoming increasingly clear, and here too biobanks can play an important role. Most biobanks are based on a cohort design and include a sample of the population (e.g. of a geographical region) or a group of patients. The data collected and managed by consortia and biobanks are often made available (subject to certain conditions) to other researchers. This is also true of some important large-scale cross-sectional studies designed to describe genetic variation in human populations, for example, the 1,000 Genomes Project mentioned earlier.

7.4 Precision medicine

GWASs have rapidly increased our knowledge of genetic factors of multifactorial disorders. Some of these factors are genes whose involvement in pathophysiological mechanisms was previously unknown. This knowledge provides an important basis for the development of new preventive measures and treatments, and the detection of biomarkers for diagnosis and prognosis. Particularly important is research into effect modification between genetic factors and modifiable behavioral and environmental factors, as knowledge from these studies enables selection of people who are likely, given their genetic profile, to benefit more from preventive and treatment measures designed to influence those behavioral and environmental factors. This is referred to as personalized prevention and precision medicine. Pharmacogenetic epidemiological research, for instance, focuses specifically on identifying genetic factors of a patient's drug response. The hope is that there will ultimately be enough affordable genetic tests available to determine, before the start of treatment, which patients will benefit from a particular drug, and which will not or will need a different dosage. Today, there are only few examples of this in clinical practice. One is the use of a genetic test for the *thiopurine methyltransferase* (*TPMT*) gene in patients eligible for treatment with thiopurines. These are inactive prodrugs with an immunosuppressive effect used for various disorders (e.g. rheumatoid arthritis and Crohn's disease). Certain genetic variants in the gene that codes for thiopurine methyl – transferase (TPMT) – an enzyme important in converting thiopurines into active metabolites – are known to reduce TPMT activity. Adjusting the thiopurine dose before the start of treatment based on the results of this genetic test can avoid many of the undesirable side effects of thiopurines.

7.5 Mendelian randomization

Genetic factors contributing to an explanatory factor (e.g. vitamin D or low-density lipoprotein [LDL] cholesterol) can be used for generating evidence for or against a causal association between that explanatory factor and the occurrence of a health outcome. This principle, known as Mendelian randomization, is based on the idea that various types of bias that can occur in epidemiological research (see Chapter 5) do not occur when the association between the genotype and a health outcome is examined. Information bias is unlikely, for instance, and there will be no doubt as to what is cause and what is effect (as there will be no reverse causality as the genotype is fixed at conception and precedes the health outcome). More importantly, confounding is unlikely when examining the association between a genotype and a health outcome, because of the randomization of alleles that takes place during meiosis. This natural randomization process is also known as Mendel's law of independent assortment. It makes no sense, for instance, for a genotype studied in the context of the occurrence of cardiovascular disease as substitute for exposure to cigarette smoking to be correlated with another genotype associated with the amount of dietary cholesterol intake. Indeed, genotypes contributing to different explanatory factors are likely physically distanced from each other on the genome, which will render these genotypes uncorrelated even when the explanatory factors are correlated, as could, for instance, be the case for smoking and high dietary cholesterol intake as part of an unhealthy lifestyle. Using a genetic factor as a substitute for exposure to that explanatory factor thus produces the same effect in an observational setting as randomization does in a clinical trial (see ◻ Figure 7.7). In both settings, the groups contrasted for occurrence of the health outcome are rendered comparable on all factors other

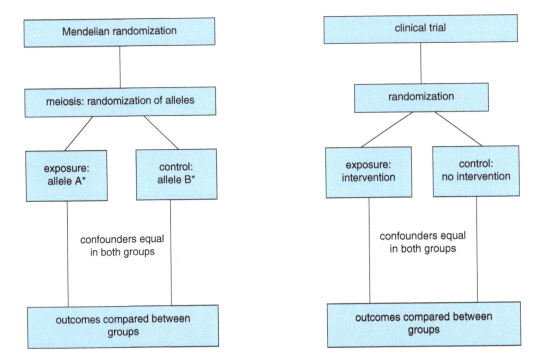

* is a proxy for exposure to an environmental factor

Figure 7.7 Simulating a randomized trial using the principle of Mendelian randomization.

than the genotype or exposure of interest because of (Mendelian) randomization. Thus, if there is a difference in occurrence of the health outcome between the groups, this difference can only be ascribed to being exposed to the explanatory factor of interest. This assertion holds in the context of Mendelian randomization provided the genotype contributing to the explanatory factor is solely associated with the health outcome through this factor (i.e. there should be no horizontal pleiotropic effect of the genotype).

Those contemplating undertaking a Mendelian randomization study should realize that selection (or collider bias) may still be possible and that this type of study typically has lower statistical power than observational or intervention studies. A single genetic factor contributing to an explanatory factor explains little of the variability in exposure to this factor. Even with strong genetic factors, it is rare that these explain more than 1% of the variability in the exposure. Therefore, most genetic factors are considered weak instruments in the context of Mendelian randomization, and it is common to rely on multiple genetic

factors contributing to an explanatory factor rather than one. An estimate of the causal effect can be arrived at by scaling the association between the genotype and the health outcome on the association between the genotype and the explanatory factor. Where the association between the genotype and the health outcome provides evidence for the presence or absence of a causal effect, the causal effect estimate gives an estimation of the strength of association between the explanatory factor and the health outcome. The causal effect estimate can be biased in the presence of weak instruments. Therefore, evidence from Mendelian randomization studies is best used in triangulation with evidence from observational and intervention studies and can be particularly useful in situations where exposure to a certain explanatory factor is difficult to measure observationally or cannot be intervened on. Genetic factors contributing to an explanatory factor also likely represent more of a lifelong predisposition to, for instance, a higher body mass index (BMI), which can be of interest depending on the research question underlying the study.

7.6   Reporting guidelines

There are reporting guidelines available on the publication of genetic epidemiological studies similar to the CONSORT (Consolidated Standards of Reporting Trials) statement for randomized controlled trials (RCTs). STREGA (STrengthening the REporting of Genetic Association studies) builds upon the STROBE (STrengthening the Reporting of Observational studies in Epidemiology) guidelines on the publication of observational studies (see Chapter 4). The STREGA guidelines provide specific advice on the elements that should be included in an article on genetic association research.

Recommended reading

Khoury, M.J., Bedrosian, S.R., Gwinn, M. et al. (2010). *Human Genome Epidemiology: Building the Evidence for Using Genetic Information to Improve Health and Prevent Disease*, 2e. Oxford: Oxford University Press.

Chan, B.K.C. (2018). *Biostatistics for Human Genetic Epidemiology.* Springer.

Source references (cases)

Claus, E.B., Risch, N.J., and Thompson, W.D. (1990). Age at onset as an indicator of familial risk in breast cancer. *Am J Epidemiol.* 131: 961–972. (Case 7.1).

Polderman, T.J.C., Benyamin, B., De Leeuw, C.A. et al. Meta-analysis of the heritability of human traits based on fifty years of twin studies. *Nature Genetics* 47: 702–709. (Case 7.2).

Hall, J.M., Lee, M.K., Newman, B. et al. (1990). Linkage of early-onset familial breast cancer to chromosome 17q21. *Science* 250: 1684–1689. (Case 7.3).

Miki, Y., Swensen, J., Shattuck-Eidens, D. et al. (1994). A strong candidate for the breast and ovarian cancer susceptibility gene BRCA1. *Science.* 266: 66–71. (Case 7.3).

Newman, B., Austin, M.A., Lee, M., and King, M.C. (1988). Inheritance of human breast cancer: evidence for autosomal transmission in high risk families. *Proc Natl Acad Sci U S A.* 85: 3044–3048. (Case 7.3).

Araki, S., Dariusz, K.M., Hanna, L. et al. (2000). APOE polymorphisms and the development of diabetic nephropathy in type 1 diabetes. *Diabetes* 49: 2190–2195. (Cases 7.4 and 7.7).

Grant, S.F.A., Thorleifsson, G., Reynisdottir, I. et al. (2006). Variant of transcription factor 7-like 2 (TCF7L2) gene confers risk of type 2 diabetes. *Nat Genet.* 38: 320–323. (Case 7.5).

Helgason, A., Pálsson, S., Thorleifsson, G. et al. (2007). Refining the impact of TCF7L2 gene variants on type 2 diabetes and adaptive evolution. *Nat Genet.* 39: 218–225. (Case 7.5).

Palmer, N.D., Hester, J.M., An, S.S. et al. (2011). Resequencing and analysis of variation in the TCF7L2 gene in African Americans suggests that SNP rs7903146 is the causal diabetes susceptibility variant. *Diabetes.* 60: 662–668. (Case 7.5).

Scott, L.J., Bonnycastle, L.L., Willer, C.J. et al. (2006). Association of transcription factor 7-like 2 (TCF7L2) variants with type 2 diabetes in a Finnish sample. *Diabetes* 55: 2649–2653. (Case 7.5).

Wellcome Trust Case Control Consortium (2007). Genome-wide association study of 14,000 cases of seven common diseases and 3,000 shared controls. *Nature.* 447: 661–678. (Case 7.6).

Knowledge assessment questions

1.   Genetic Terminology
     What is a phenotype?
     a.   the genetic make-up (code)
     b.   the physical trait
     The passing of genetic traits from parents to offspring can also be called
     a.   gene
     b.   trait
     c.   heredity
     d.   allele
     An alternative form of a gene can also be called
     a.   marker
     b.   heterozygous
     c.   DNA
     d.   allele
     The minor allele variant of a polymorphism has a frequency of
     a.   at least 1% in the population
     b.   at least 5% in the population
     c.   maximum 1% in the population
     d.   maximum 5% in the population
     If two alleles are in linkage disequilibrium. This means that
     a.   the DNA variants of two loci are equal
     b.   the DNA variants of two loci are not equal
     c.   the DNA variants of two loci are correlated
     d.   the DNA variants of two loci are not correlated

2.   Describe what a GWAS Manhattan plot looks like and what the peaks on this plot represent?

3.   Previous twin studies have estimated that the narrow-sense heritability of endometriosis is 51%, 75%, and 87%. Do you interpret these three estimates as consistent with each other? If so, explain why. If not, explain possible reasons for this inconsistency. What additional pieces of information could help you jointly interpret these results?

4.   Genomic data were used to determine genetic ancestry, and only samples of 95% or more European ancestry were included in statistical analysis. Why did the investigators do this?

Outbreak Epidemiology

This chapter has been extensively revised and partly rewritten by Gowri Gopalakrishna and Marino van Zelst

Textbook of Epidemiology, Second Edition. Lex Bouter, Maurice Zeegers and Tianjing Li.
© 2023 John Wiley & Sons Ltd. Published 2023 by John Wiley & Sons Ltd.
Companion website: www.wiley.com/go/Bouter/TextbookofEpidemiology

8.1 Introduction

An outbreak is an unexpected and rapid increase in the occurrence of a health outcome in a specific geographical region and time. The words epidemic and pandemic are often used interchangeably with the term outbreak. Any sudden increase in the incidence of a disease in a large population or area is referred to as an epidemic. A pandemic is an epidemic occurring worldwide, or over a very wide area, crossing international boundaries and usually affecting many people. To define an increased incidence as an outbreak, we need to know the usual number of cases that can be expected in a particular period, place, and population, and what incidence and variability is normal. Proper surveillance is key to recognizing and investigating outbreaks.

The aim of investigating outbreaks is to identify their characteristics and explanatory factors. Ideally, we will want to track down both the agent (the main explanatory factor) and its source as soon as possible, as both are critical for interventions and disease control, for example:

1. Detecting or treating the disease faster and better.
2. Taking steps to halt the spread of the disease, or
3. Recommending measures to prevent similar outbreaks locally or elsewhere in future.

Usually, the aim for outbreak investigation is *not* to discover new explanatory factors of the disease but to find out what has caused a particular time, person, and place-related outbreak (and what species and type of microorganism is involved in the case of an infectious disease outbreak). Based on this knowledge, it may be possible to take steps locally to halt the outbreak and prevent similar ones. If the investigation also brings novel insights, e.g. of a transmission route not previously identified, new (acquired) properties of a microorganism (e.g. resistance or escape mutants), or new risk groups, it will also produce useful knowledge that can improve public health elsewhere. Sometimes the primary aim is to gather this knowledge as epidemiological research can only be carried out during an outbreak when people are exposed, for example, a study on measles during an outbreak in a religious community with a low vaccination rate. In this case, gaining knowledge of how to fight the disease is not the primary aim of the study, as we already have a good deal of knowledge of measles transmission and prevention. An investigation into

the outbreak can contribute to new knowledge. A measles outbreak in a group of this kind, for instance, provides an opportunity to carry out behavioral studies into the effect of interventions to promote the acceptance of vaccination against, e.g. mumps, measles, and rubella (MMR) in unvaccinated children.

When we talk about the explanatory factors of outbreaks, we are usually referring to infectious disease outbreaks (e.g. foodborne infections such as Salmonella, open tuberculosis, Q fever, methicillin resistant *Staphylococcus aureus* [MRSA] on livestock farms, measles in populations with religious objections to vaccination, mumps among students, severe acute respiratory syndrome [SARS], Middle East respiratory syndrome [MERS], Ebola or influenza pandemics). An outbreak can also be caused by an environmental incident (e.g. children playing on contaminated land, unintentional emissions of toxic substances or contaminated drinking water), or errors in the treatment and care of patients, also called iatrogenic outbreaks (e.g. congenital abnormalities due to the use of thalidomide during pregnancy, or eye abnormalities due to excessive oxygen levels in premature babies' incubators). Thus, not all outbreaks are infectious, and not all infectious diseases cause outbreaks.

As these two types of epidemiology – infectious disease epidemiology and the epidemiology of outbreaks – often coincide, this chapter will focus mainly on infectious disease outbreaks. A specific feature of infectious disease epidemiology is that a microorganism (virus, bacterium, parasite, prion, fungus, etc.) is involved. Many microorganisms that are pathological in humans can only survive if they are transmitted from one host to another.

This transmission can take place directly from one human to another (e.g. in measles, COVID-19), through an "intermediate host" (e.g. an insect, as in malaria and in Lyme disease: see ▢ Figure. 8.1), or directly from animal to human (zoonosis, e.g. Q fever and psittacosis). Zoonosis can also transform later into human-to-human transmission, such as in the cases of novel corona viruses (SARS and SARS CoV-2) jumping species from bats to humans with intermediatory hosts. The term "contagious disease" is only used if there is direct human-to-human transmission. Other microorganisms infect humans through the environment, e.g. water (*Legionella*, for instance). In such cases, the human is usually a "dead-end" host; humans cannot infect other humans.

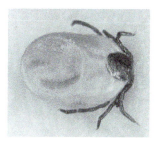

Figure 8.1 Disease transmission from animal to human (e.g. in Lyme disease). Source: Henrik Larsson / Adobe Stock.

The infectious agent's tendency to reproduce is countered by the host's tendency to defend itself. For this purpose, a host body has a general innate immune system, supplemented by acquired specific resistance (immunity) to agents. This acquired immunity can result from previous exposure to the agent (or a related microorganism in the case of cross-immunity) or vaccination. An impaired immune system or lack of resistance makes the host particularly susceptible to infections. The behavior, virulence and "dose" of the infectious agents, and the efficacy of potential hosts' immune responses are not the only explanatory factors of an epidemic, however. Unlike noninfectious diseases, the likelihood of an infection in an individual also depends on the presence of infections and immunity in other members of the population, as the following example shows. A microorganism such as the polio virus can only cause an epidemic if it is able to circulate in a community of people who are not yet immune to it. Interventions against infectious diseases (e.g. polio vaccination) therefore have effects not only on the people receiving them, but also on the other individuals in the population. Once "herd immunity" has been developed (enough people are immune or have been immunized), the spread of the disease is halted. A complicating factor in infectious disease epidemiology is that it is not always clear who is infected, as people often can spread the disease without being ill (asymptomatic).

Thus, infectious disease epidemiology differs from chronic disease epidemiology in four important ways:

- It is essential to differentiate between exposure, colonization, infection and disease due to a potentially pathogenic microorganism. The aim of infection control is to reduce the disease frequency; the actions taken can focus on reducing the number of cases, the number of infected people, or the number of exposed people.
- An infected person (with or without symptoms) is a potential risk factor as infectious disease risk depends on whether there are other people in the vicinity who have the infection. The network of contacts in the population is therefore also important when studying the transmission of infectious diseases.
- People can be immune to infection or disease to varying degrees depending on their immunological responses.
- Microorganisms can have a protective effect. In a normal situation, people live in symbiotic equilibrium with these microflorae on the skin and mucosa such as in the throat and in the intestines, and they are an important line of natural defense against external threats.

From time to time, a new disease previously unknown will emerge: HIV/AIDS was unknown before 1983, SARS before 2003, MERS before 2012, and COVID-19 before 2020 for instance. A disease may emerge due to a variety of causes:

- Changes in human behavior (e.g. intravenous drug users sharing needles, increasing international tourism, or increasing contact between humans and animal carriers of pathogens). Since 2009, for instance, a new malaria species has been found in Asia due to increasing contact between humans and monkeys.
- Wars and natural disasters (e.g. rapes and resulting HIV infections in children during the Rwandan civil war).
- Changes in the environment (e.g. pollution, climate change, urbanization where animal reservoirs are in closer contact with humans).
- Changes in the agent itself (e.g. the development of resistance, or mutations in the microorganism's genetic material, as in the case of bird flu and COVID-19).
- Changes in healthcare (e.g. interventions that severely impair immune response, or relaxing preventive measures).
- Changes in food preparation or the food chain (e.g. the variant form of Creutzfeldt-Jakob disease that emerged in 1996 due to the contamination of food with prions which cause bovine spongiform encephalopathy [BSE or mad cow disease], or the use of growth-promoting antibiotics).

In addition to carrying out surveillance and developing outbreak management plans, various preventive measures can be taken to reduce the risk of new diseases. These measures usually target the causes listed above, e.g. improving food and water hygiene, responsible use of antibiotics, developing new vaccines, reducing human exposure to animal reservoirs, protecting susceptible groups (children, the elderly, pregnant women), addressing climate change and environmental change, and combating bioterrorism.

Infectious disease epidemiology is exciting because outbreaks usually develop quickly and society is deeply involved. Infectious disease epidemiology can also be very gratifying for researchers, especially when the results can be used to prevent new cases of the disease. On the other hand, time pressure to produce useful results leaves less opportunity to design and execute studies meticulously. Investigators and policy makers must often work with data of lower quality than they otherwise demand.

8.1.1 Terms in infectious disease epidemiology

Because of the nature of infectious disease epidemiology, some additional concepts are needed to describe and explain the frequency and patterns of infectious diseases.

A person's infection often follows a pattern. When a person becomes infected, clinical symptoms may develop after a certain period (the incubation period). These symptoms usually disappear, with or without treatment, but the infected individual usually remains infectious for some time after the infection (the infectious period) and can pass the disease on to other people in the case of human-to-human transmission. The infectious period usually comes to an end too, but it is important to note that the start and end will typically not coincide with the period when the clinical symptoms are manifest (Figure 8.2).

Thus, an individual may be infectious before displaying any symptoms of the disease (as in the case of childhood chickenpox, SARS-CoV-2, and HIV), whereas contagiousness may persist for years after the symptoms have disappeared (as in the case of hepatitis B). Individuals can therefore be infectious before the symptoms develop, the asymptomatic stage following the symptoms, or during an infection that runs a completely asymptomatic course.

$$\text{Attack rate} = \frac{\text{Number of diseases or infected individuals}}{\text{Total population at risk}\,(\text{non} - \text{immune})}$$

$$\text{Secondary attack rate} = \frac{\text{Number of diseases or infected individuals}}{\text{Number of individuals exposed to an infected individual}}$$

The probability of a person becoming infected, given a particular source of infection, is referred to as the transmission rate (p). This will depend on the nature of the source (often an infected individual, animal, or other infected source), any vector providing transmission (mosquito, food, airborne particles), how the contact takes place and for how long, the virulence and number of microorganisms to which the person is exposed, and the characteristics (genetic, immunological, behavioral) of the host being infected. The simplest ways of representing the transmission rate are (i) the attack rate (the number of cases or infected persons divided by the total population at risk) and (ii) the secondary attack rate (the number of cases or infected persons divided by the total number of people who have been in contact with an infected individual). The basic reproduction number (R_0) is the average number of new infections that a contagious individual can produce in a population in which everyone can contract the infection. The dispersion parameter (K) indicates the percentage of infected people who are driving the epidemic. Both concepts are elaborated on in Section 8.6.2.

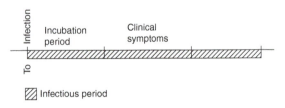

☐ **Figure 8.2** Incubation period, clinical symptoms, and infectious period.

8.2   Surveillance for early warning

Almost every outbreak begins with an unusual disease-related finding in the population. Sometimes, a single case of the disease provides sufficient warning (e.g. a case of botulism, paralysis due to shellfish poisoning or anthrax). In many cases, however, an outbreak will be suspected when observing two or more cases in close chronological and geographical proximity. This is referred to as a disease cluster (see Section 8.6). Usually astute doctors – or, in some cases, alert citizens may raise the red flag on a possible cluster of cases. Independent of vigilant individual professionals and citizens, we need systems designed to give early warning of unusual clusters of cases. Various types of surveillance have been developed to provide ongoing monitoring, analysis and reporting of disease data. Surveillance has been going on for centuries and has demonstrated its usefulness in revealing trends in health. Back in the seventeenth century, John Graunt (see ▣ Figure 1.6) published a weekly survey of causes of death in London. William Farr (see ▣ Figure 8.3) analyzed and published regular disease and mortality data

for England and Wales in the mid-nineteenth century. After World War II, designated institutions, such as the World Health Organization (WHO), the Center for Disease Control and Prevention (CDC) in the United States, the European Centre for Disease Prevention and Control (ECDC), and regional CDC in Southeast Asia and WHO regional centers in many other parts of the world were established. In 1983, the Chinese CDC was set up as an independent agency of the Chinese government's National Health Commission. In 2016, the African CDC was established to provide technical support to the African member states and to strengthen the capacity of the public health institutions of these member states.

Due in large part to active surveillance, we have succeeded in eliminating smallpox worldwide – an unparalleled achievement. During the smallpox campaign, there was active surveillance for new cases throughout the world and, after each case identification, the patient was isolated and all his/her contacts vaccinated.

The principles of surveillance do not only apply to infectious diseases; they also apply to cancer, congenital abnormalities, and traumas (▣ Figure 8.4). Surveillance is not designed primarily as a type of epidemiological research but as a tool for identifying changes in trends quickly, and to enable actions and interventions to nip an outbreak in the bud. Promptness is usually more important than validity and precision here.

Many countries have statutory surveillance notification requirements for some infectious diseases. Authorities can impose a requirement on doctors, microbiological laboratories, and heads of institutions to report on cases of infectious diseases as soon as they

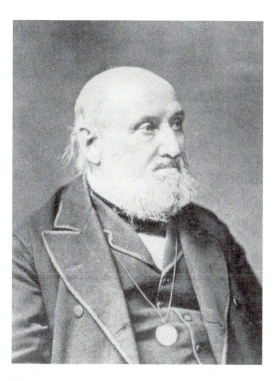

▣ **Figure 8.3** William Farr (1807–1883), British epidemiologist and one of the founding fathers of today's medical statistics. Source: Unknown / Wikimedia Commons / Public domain.

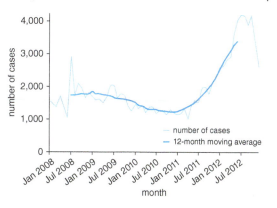

▣ **Figure 8.4** Overview of confirmed cases of reported whooping cough in Europe, 2008–2012.

are discovered. As a result of these notifications, the regional and national authorities responsible for infectious disease control can take timely action in the event of an outbreak. Up-to-date information on the notification requirements can usually be found on the national public health institutes' websites. National healthcare registries – death registers, hospital registries, and cancer registries – can be used for this purpose, but they do not usually analyze the data to identify outbreaks.

General practitioners play a very important role in surveillance. In some countries, this is done by reporting the number of new cases of certain conditions (e.g. influenza) each week by a group of general practitioners. This type of surveillance, in which data are collected from specific geographical locations, healthcare institutions, or populations during defined time periods, is referred to as a sentinel system. Sentinel surveillance systems have also been developed for the surveillance of infectious diseases in nursing homes, for instance.

Because the aim is to identify changes in disease frequency and clusters of disease in time and place as quickly as possible, a surveillance system needs to pick up most of the cases and therefore have high sensitivity, if necessary, at the expense of specificity (see Chapter 9). This can result in many false positives, which need to be followed up and verified. In some cases (e.g. polio), even a mere suspicion is sufficient to warrant notification.

To understand the course of infectious diseases, it is important to keep both cases and microorganisms under surveillance. As part of influenza surveillance, for instance, a nose or throat swab is taken from patients with flu symptoms regularly (once a week) to see which, if any, microorganisms are present. The virology laboratories document the number of positive diagnoses of selected viruses.

Computerized surveillance systems are also available for local outbreaks involving resistance to antibiotics such as The European Antimicrobial Resistance Surveillance Network (EARS-Net) and the WHO AMR Surveillance and Quality Assessment Collaborating Centres Network.

Establishment of international disease surveillance systems requires political will and cooperation, and can be sometimes tricky, especially for new and emerging diseases. Testing methods and policies can affect data comparability across surveillance systems. A recent example of such a disease is COVID-19. The ECDC outlines issues in setting up a surveillance system across EU countries and the requirements needed to allow for data comparison and monitoring.

The value of international surveillance is illustrated in detecting cases of Legionnaires' disease among tourists returning from holiday. This infection is often spread by bacteria in showers or air conditioning systems in hotels. Patients would only fall ill after returning home, making them look like isolated cases. Pooling data internationally enables outbreaks of Legionnaires' disease to be identified and possible sources tracked down and dealt with. The value of a surveillance system relies on the consistency and quality of the data. As these data are usually supplied by healthcare providers, it is important to involve them closely in the surveillance and provide them with regular feedback to optimize data quality and usage.

Surveillance systems can also be utilized to assess and monitor the efficacy of public health measures. Ongoing surveillance of infectious diseases is used to assess the impact of vaccination programs. An increase in the number of cases of childhood whooping cough, for instance, may be a reason to change the vaccination schedule, use a different vaccine, or shift focus to the underserved populations.

Case 8.1 Surveillance of and Vaccination against Whooping Cough

Whooping cough is an acute infectious lung disease usually caused by the bacterium *Bordetella pertussis*. The typical coughing fits are caused by the toxins produced by these bacteria. It is transmitted from person to person via air. Patients are most infectious during the period preceding the coughing fits, but contagiousness continues for a few weeks thereafter. Whooping cough is highly contagious. On average, 90% of susceptible members of a family with a whooping cough patient will contract the infection. In countries with high vaccination rates, adolescents and adults play a major role in spreading it. Having whooping cough does not confer lifelong immunity. Immunity declines 4–20 years after a whooping cough infection. Vaccination does not provide protection for life, only for 4–12 years.

Whooping cough occurs throughout the world, with an estimated 45 million cases and 400,000 deaths a year. Reported incidence differs widely, partly due to differences in prevention and control strategy, and partly due to different diagnosis and reporting criteria (see e.g. the Surveillance Atlas on Infectious Diseases [SAID] on the European Centre for Disease Prevention and Control).

The number of whooping cough cases rose sharply in Europe around 2012, a year when 40,000 confirmed cases were recorded, as against 20,000 cases in previous years (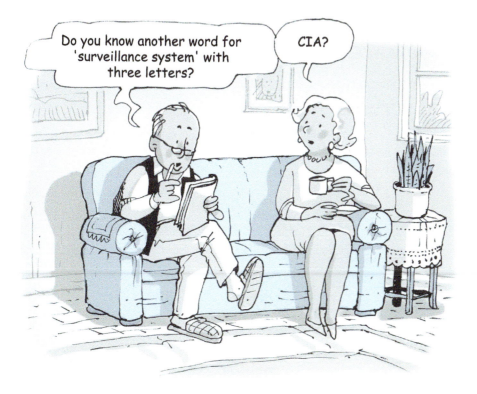 Figure 8.5). Hospitalization is needed in fewer than 10% of cases, mainly young infants. Deaths due to whooping cough are fortunately very rare, less than 0.2% of the cases.

Both cellular and non-cellular vaccines are available to prevent whooping cough. Cellular vaccines are made from dead bacteria. They contain large quantities of antigens and sometimes cause mild to severe side effects. Non-cellular vaccines contain combinations of protein components taken from the surface of the bacterium. These also, albeit to a lesser extent, can cause mild side effects, such as redness, pain and swelling at the injection site, as well as crying and listlessness.

Since 1950, infants in many European countries have been given a combined vaccine containing a cellular whooping cough vaccine and vaccines against, e.g. diphtheria, tetanus and poliomyelitis. The efficacy of whooping cough vaccination in infancy declined about a decade into the second millennium and there were repeated substantial epidemic waves of whooping cough in Europe, possibly due to a change in the *Bordetella pertussis* bacteria in circulation. In response, most European countries decided to introduce an additional whooping cough vaccination at nursery school. A non-cellular vaccine was chosen in most cases, as the cellular vaccine had too many side effects for that age group. Many countries nowadays also use a non-cellular whooping cough vaccine in the first year of life. 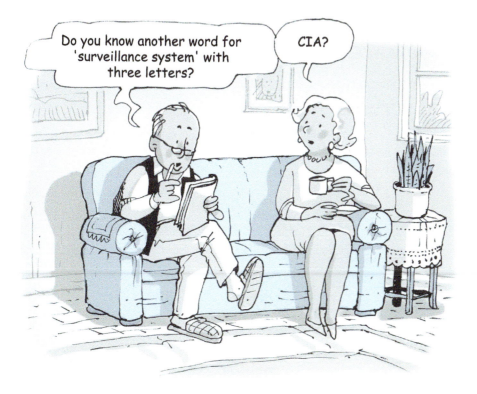 Figure 8.5 shows a clear outbreak of whooping cough in Europe around 2012, which has again brought the efficacy of vaccination using the non-cellular vaccine into question.

Figure 8.5 Surveillance systems are not only for infectious diseases.

Following the recent pandemic of COVID-19 (see Case 8.1), and epidemics of SARS, H5N1 bird flu virus, and the threat of bioterrorism, the need has grown to identify unusual rises in non-specific signs and symptoms (and combinations thereof). This syndrome surveillance involves studying the frequency of early non-specific signs or symptoms reported by General Practitioners, hospitals, pharmacists, or occupational health services (absenteeism figures). Syndrome surveillance definitions are based on combinations of symptoms without a single diagnosis. Increased incidence of a syndrome may then warrant further investigation or even actions.

An increase in the number of cases does not always mean that there is an outbreak: the size or composition of the population may have changed, or there may have been changes in healthcare, the insurance system, or the way cases are detected, diagnosed or recorded. Case definition is extremely important in outbreak investigations and also therefore in surveillance systems. The clearer the definition, the lower the likelihood of misclassification and the better the quality of the data. A case definition in outbreak investigation should always include the following four elements:

- Symptoms.
- Characteristics of the persons affected.
- Geographical factors (where the outbreak is taking place).
- Chronological factors (when did the associated cases occur).

It is often worthwhile to differentiate between confirmed, probable, and suspected cases (see Case 8.5). Europe has uniform definitions of confirmed and probable cases for most infectious diseases of public health importance, which enable international comparisons.

Once an outbreak or a developing epidemic is established, the next step is to investigate the possible causes. A whole range of information on each case is needed for this purpose, for example:

- Name, age, sex, ethnicity.
- Place of residence.
- Social network and movement pattern.
- Date and time when the disease first manifested itself.
- Symptoms and their duration, and date of death when relevant.
- Possible transmission routes, high-risk behavior.
- Microbiological data (type/serotype, sequence, load).
- Any other relevant information (vaccination status, occupation, etc.).

The more a surveillance system has recorded, the more effectively it can be used for additional investigation once an outbreak is established (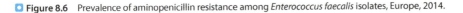 Figure 8.6).

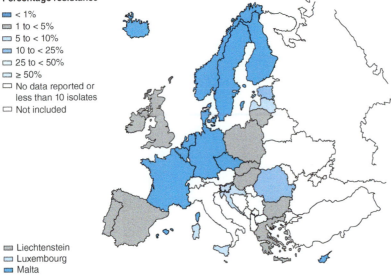

Percentage resistance
- < 1%
- 1 to < 5%
- 5 to < 10%
- 10 to < 25%
- 25 to < 50%
- ≥ 50%
- No data reported or less than 10 isolates
- Not included

- Liechtenstein
- Luxembourg
- Malta

Figure 8.6 Prevalence of aminopenicillin resistance among *Enterococcus faecalis* isolates, Europe, 2014.

8.2.1 Rapid warning without false alarms

Timely identification of an outbreak or potential outbreak involves the ongoing comparison of the number of cases observed with the number of cases that would be expected from a chronological comparison or comparison with other regions. It goes without saying that false alarms should be avoided as much as possible. Before concluding there is an outbreak, other explanations, such as chance, incorrect estimation of the baseline level, changes in demography (e.g. a baby boom), or changes in diagnostic and recording procedures, should be ruled out. Although we cannot rule out false alarms completely, statistical techniques can reduce the number of warnings due solely to random variation to an acceptable level. The principle underlying these methods is that random variation over time and place is a less likely explanation if cases occur in successive periods or neighboring areas.

Before using various statistical techniques, we can graphically display the disease frequencies, for example, a graph of the cumulative numbers of cases observed and the numbers that would be expected (assuming that the incidence of the disease remains stable) plotted against time. The time axis should ideally be based not on the date of notification or diagnosis but on the first day of the illness. Local variations can be studied by making a map of the disease frequencies (incidence densities: see Section 2.6.2; ☐ Figure 8.6).

Autocorrelation coefficients are correlations between disease frequencies in neighboring areas, which can be used to show patterns in the area. The problem is that an outbreak may not be the only possible explanation for such a correlation. Densely populated areas, for instance, will have more stable incidence densities (IDs) and therefore stronger correlations. Recording methods will be more similar between neighboring areas compared with areas further apart. Lastly, neighboring areas will also display greater similarities in other explanatory factors of the disease. To avoid being misled by random variation between areas, we can "smooth" the disease frequencies, that is to calculate adjusted frequencies based on the information in the neighboring areas. This technique is referred to as "empirical Bayes estimation." These methods enable us to detect underlying patterns in disease frequencies better than when using unsmoothed figures. An example of how (spatial) autocorrelation can be used to analyze epidemiological characteristics of Hand Foot and Mouth Disease, an infectious disease with the highest incidence in China can be found in the further reading section (Zhang et al. 2019).

Geographical information systems (GIS) can be used to plot cases on a map and facilitate the analysis. Geographical methods often rely on information from surveillance systems, which only record the locations where the cases were diagnosed. Because of high mobility of the population, these locations often differ substantially from the locations where the infections were contracted. The first international map of the distribution of AIDS cases, for instance, coincided with the main airline routes rather than any epidemiological pattern. These geographical methods, however, are highly suitable for, for example, a local outbreak caused by a shared water supply.

Special software (e.g. SaTScan™), which provides combined analysis of time and place data, enables time and place-related outbreaks to be detected simultaneously, making it a very powerful tool in surveillance. The software records the time and place of each case and calculates the numbers of observed and expected cases for each location at each time. Statistical procedures considering multiple testing enable the detection of clusters not due to random fluctuation.

8.3 Study designs for research into outbreaks

An outbreak is an unexpected event and can only be studied once it has begun or sometimes after it has stopped, making an adequate study design challenging. Usually there is substantial time pressure, as outbreaks can be of limited scope and duration, making it difficult to differentiate between the effects of suspected risk factors and random variation in the incidence of the disease. To learn as much as possible from an outbreak, including identification of the most effective preventive measures as well as effective interventions during and after an outbreak, we need to be properly prepared for outbreak investigations before they may occur. Obtain, for example, ethical approval for generic study protocols, establish partnerships (e.g. between national health authorities, hospitals, laboratories, and General Practitioners, and between regional and international public health authorities).

Legislations and policies may also need revision, for instance, to enable the identification of new and emerging infectious disease during an outbreak and to promote adequate surveillance and clinical vigilance. These coordinated steps are important for rapid identification and confirmation of possible outbreaks locally, regionally, and/or internationally and for effective prevention of further spread. Historical cohort studies and case-control studies are typically used for outbreak investigations.

8.3.1 The epidemic curve: learning from the time dimension

The epidemic curve plots the number of cases detected against the time when the symptoms of the disease emerge. The scale used for the x-axis (the time when the symptoms began) depends on the nature of the disease, in particular, the incubation period (see 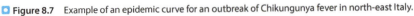 Figure 8.2). The x-axis may also include a period preceding the outbreak showing the normal incidence of the disease. As a rule of thumb, one quarter of the incubation period is often used as the unit of measurement for the x-axis. Occasionally, you may need to draw an epidemic curve of an unknown disease with an unknown incubation period. In such cases, it is useful to draw several curves with variations in the units of the x-axis. ◻ Figure 8.7 gives an example of an epidemic curve for an outbreak of fever caused by the Chikungunya virus (CHIKV) in a few villages in north-east Italy in summer 2007.

For each day, the figure shows all the reported new cases of CHIKV fever in Castiglione di Cervia, Castiglione di Ravenna, and in other or unknown locations in the Cervia during the July–September 2007 period (205 cases).

If the average incubation period of the disease is known and all the cases were exposed at about the same time (as may be the case in an outbreak of food poisoning, for instance), the most likely time of exposure can be deduced from the figure. Note, however,

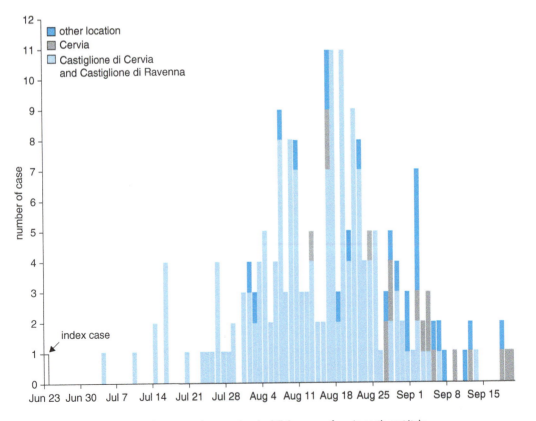

◻ **Figure 8.7**　Example of an epidemic curve for an outbreak of Chikungunya fever in north-east Italy.

that the shape of the epidemic curve can be influenced not only by case number, but also by delays in reporting, reporting fatigue, changes in process for the notification of new cases, case definition, and changes in care-seeking behavior.

The epidemic curves drawn at an early stage of the outbreak are particularly useful. They usually form the first analyses once the case definition has been decided upon and the cases have been identified.

The shape of the epidemic curve often provides information on the most likely mode of transmission. A point source outbreak in which all cases were infected at a single time point by the same source usually produces a sharply rising curve with an early peak followed by a gradual decrease in the number of new cases. If the population has been exposed to the same source of infection over a lengthy period (e.g. where a food product contaminated with Salmonella has stayed on the supermarket shelf or has been traded for a long time, or where people have been exposed to an air conditioning system containing *Legionella*), the curve will have a longer tail. An outbreak caused by person-to-person transmission (e.g. in the case of influenza or measles) produces an epidemic curve with several smaller peaks, the distance between two adjacent peaks is the average incubation period. In practice, however, a pattern of this kind is often difficult to visualize because of variation in the latent period following infection, which blurs the pattern of peaks.

An epidemic curve provides information on the course of the outbreak. If it remains in the rising part of the curve, transmission is likely to be continuing, whereas a falling curve indicates that the outbreak may have already been halted. The epidemic curve informs whether actions need to be taken, and if so, what measures.

8.3.2 Cohort studies

Cohort studies are best for outbreaks confined to a group that is well-defined and, within which, both cases and non-cases may be identified. Cohort studies are therefore, most useful for the investigation of outbreaks of common events such as outbreaks at a school, or among attendees at a social event. Table 8.1 shows the suitability of using cohort studies for investigating certain types of outbreaks. Such a cohort design compares disease risks in two groups defined according to exposure (i.e. the exposed group compared with the non-exposed group). Outbreak investigation using the cohort design allows the calculation of attack rates.

In general, cohort studies can be more straightforward than case–control studies as all cohort members are eligible based on exposure status regardless of outcome. There is no need to identify and recruit controls, which may introduce selection bias.

Table 8.1 Suitability of cohort design in different outbreak situations.

Outbreak type	Study suitability
Common event (an outbreak where cases are grouped by place and time and exposure is brief)	Cohort studies are well-suited to the epidemiological investigation of common event outbreaks, because the "at risk" population can be easily defined, e.g. outbreak at a dinner party
Common site or source (an outbreak where cases have exposure at the same site or source but not necessarily at the same time)	cohort studies are generally not applied to common site outbreaks, unless full lists of those exposed (e.g. complete lists of diners at a restaurant, hotel guests) are available
Dispersed (an outbreak in the community due to a common exposure which may not be grouped in place or time)	Cohort studies are not well suited to the investigation of dispersed outbreaks as such outbreaks have wide exposures (e.g. environmental source contamination) and may or may not be grouped in time and place making it difficult to enumerate the exposed group
Community-wide (an outbreak where transmission occurs through direct exposure of susceptible persons to infectious persons in the community)	Cohort studies are not well suited to the investigation of community-wide outbreaks due to wide exposures making enumeration of the exposed group challenging
Institutional (an outbreak confined to an institutional setting)	Cohort studies are well-suited to the investigation of institutional outbreaks. These are similar to common event outbreaks in that the site of transmission is known at the outset. Investigation should involve hazard identification and collection of environmental specimens

8

8.3.3 Attack rates

As outbreaks typically span a short period of time, the changes in the composition of the population at risk are negligible. Disease frequencies are therefore generally expressed in the form of attack rates. An attack rate is a cumulative incidence, i.e. a proportion, and consequently strictly speaking is not a rate (see Section 2.6.2). The difference in attack rates between people exposed and people not exposed to an explanatory factor is therefore the attributable risk (Section 3.2.1). Similarly, the ratio between attack rates is the relative risk (see Section 3.2.2). By comparing attack rates in cohorts of exposed and non-exposed persons, we can test hypotheses concerning potential causes of the outbreak. ❑ Table 8.2 gives an example of a salmonellosis outbreak among 226 people who attended a large buffet.

From ❑ Table 8.2, we can conclude that the Russian salad was the most likely source of the outbreak. Although in this example, eating kiwi fruit also entailed an increased relative risk of 1.8, only 9% of the patients had eaten it, as against 90% who had eaten the Russian salad. The relative contribution of an exposure to the epidemic is expressed as the population attributable risk (see Section 3.2.6). We find that eating kiwi fruit was responsible for only $0.09 \times (1.8 – 1)/(0.09 \times (1.8 – 1) + 1) = 0.07$, i.e. 7% of the cases, compared with 60% for the Russian salad. Once we have tracked down the most likely source, for further investigation, we need to know what microorganism caused the cases. Identifying the source is not always easy, even in the case of a point source outbreak, as there can be interaction between factors (human, environmental, microbiological).

8.3.4 Case–control studies

In the example shown in ❑ Table 8.3, it was possible to obtain the guest list of the attendees at a large buffet.

❑ **Table 8.3** Suitability of case–control design for different types of outbreaks.

Outbreak type (see ❑ Table 8.1 for definitions)	Case–control study suitability
Common event	Case–control studies may be applied to the investigation of common event outbreaks if the size of the cohort is unfeasibly large
Common site	Case–control studies are well suited to the investigation of common site outbreaks when cases can be clearly identified but the potentially exposed group cannot be completely listed, e.g. outbreak at a supermarket or geographical area
Dispersed	Case–control studies are well suited to the investigation of dispersed outbreaks as the exposed group cannot be completely listed
Community-wide	A case–control design would be appropriate for the same reasons as a common site outbreak
Institutional	Case–control studies are generally not applied to institutional outbreaks but may be necessary if the potentially exposed group cannot be easily enumerated. Why?

Source: https://surv.esr.cri.nz/episurv/Manuals/GuidelinesForInvestigatingCommDiseaseOBs.pdf

Based on this information, a cohort of potentially exposed individuals and cases could be defined, but that was an exception. Usually, it is not possible to assemble a cohort of potentially exposed individuals. If an outbreak of Q fever is confirmed in a rural area, for instance, it will not be possible to identify everyone who has been exposed, so a case–control study will be needed. Another situation is when the incidence of the

❑ **Table 8.2** Numbers of cases and attack rates for foods eaten by 226 attendees at a cold buffet.

	Eaten (attack rate)	Not eaten (attack rate)	Difference in attack rate	Relative risk
Russian salad	116 (73%)	18 (27%)	+46%	2.7
kiwi fruit	12 (100%)	123 (57%)	+43%	1.8
prawn cocktail	34 (74%)	101 (56%)	+18%	1.3
French cheese	46 (53%)	89 (64%)	−11%	0.8
stuffed tomatoes	49 (82%)	86 (52%)	+30%	1.6

isease in an outbreak is low and cases are spread throughout the population. In these situations, case–control design is the most efficient design to study the causes of an outbreak. ◻ Table 8.3 summarizes the suitability of a case–control study design.

As an investigation into an outbreak will usually include only cases occurring over a particular period and in a particular area (in other words, the case definition will be restricted in terms of time and place), the same restriction will need to be applied to the control group. Controls should ideally be selected from the population who would have been included in the case group if they had developed the disease (see Section 4.3.2). So, in the case of an outbreak among visitors to a music festival, the controls should also be sought among those festival attendees. However, their selection should be independent of exposure to the suspected explanatory factor(s) of the disease. For example, if we want to find out whether playing on contaminated land could be the cause of an outbreak of poisoning among children, playing or not playing on contaminated land must

not influence the likelihood of being included in the control group.

The longer we wait before investigating possible exposures, the more difficult it becomes to obtain accurate data. If we are interviewing patients and controls, for instance, and controls remember less about possible exposures than patients, there is a risk of information bias. Unlike in epidemiological research into chronic diseases, in a case–control study of an outbreak, we are rushed to collect the data, and that poses a threat to the quality of the study. It is important, therefore, to plan properly and use standard instruments and trained personnel for data collection, analysis, and interpretation, to achieve adequate quality in studies of this kind. Standard study materials include study protocol, consent information, study leaflet or brochure, data collection forms, data management and analysis plans, and outbreak investigation toolkits such as Epidata and Epi Info™. Many examples of such standard documents can be found on government websites for re-purposing such as at the US CDC website on surveillance and reporting.

Case 8.2 Example of a Case–Control Study Design: Toxic Shock Syndrome

The first cases of toxic shock syndrome (TSS) were identified in seven adolescents by Todd et al. in 1978. Symptoms of TSS are sudden high fever, low blood pressure or shock, and a bright red skin rash that persists for one or two weeks. TSS patients also feel miserable and often have gastrointestinal and muscular problems. The kidney and liver may also be affected. TSS can be caused by *Staphylococcal* and *Streptococcal* bacteria.

In 1980, various young otherwise healthy women were brought into Emergency Departments of hospitals in Wisconsin and Minnesota with the signs and symptoms described above. Remarkably, the disease had begun in these women at the start of an otherwise normal menstrual period. As the number of cases among menstruating women did not go down, it was decided to report women with these menstruation-linked symptoms to the Center for Disease Control (CDC) to enable an investigation. The first case–control study was carried out in Wisconsin on 35 patients with TSS during menstruation and 105 controls. For each patient, three controls from the same area, of the same age, and with a normal menstrual pattern were selected

through GPs. Data on marital status, sexual health, sexual practices, history of sexually transmitted diseases, length and intensity of menstrual periods, contraceptive use and use of tampons were collected through telephone interviews. It was found that patients were more likely to use tampons (97%) than controls (76%). There was also a difference in contraceptive use. No difference was found in the type or brand of tampons used. Both cases and controls often reported using "highly absorbent" Rely® tampons. A subsequent case–control study by the CDC in Atlanta confirmed the association with tampons (100% use among patients, as against 80% among controls) but not with contraception. The CDC carried out a further study in summer 1980 among 50 patients with recent TSS patients and 150 controls recruited by the patients. In this study, all the women were asked to find the box containing the tampons that they had recently used and report the brand and serial number. As 100% of the patients used tampons (83% of them Rely brand), as against 75% of the controls (26% Rely brand), the study concluded that the cause of the TSS in these young women probably lay in the use of this brand of tampons. Rely tampons had been introduced in 1975 as "super tampons" with high absorption and ease of use, as they only needed to be changed after a few days. Although they did indeed absorb more blood, they were also found to cause more mucosal irritation and higher growth of microorganisms when used for a longer period. Women with *Staphylococcus aureus* were indeed found to be at greater risk of TSS if they used these Rely tampons. The

manufacturer took these tampons off the market on September 22, 1980, and the absorption capacity of tampons was reduced across the board. As ◻ Figure. 8.8 shows, TSS disappeared almost entirely. Subsequent cases of TSS were usually due to wound contamination with *S. aureus*. As this case shows, three relatively small case–control studies can provide enough information to halt an epidemic.

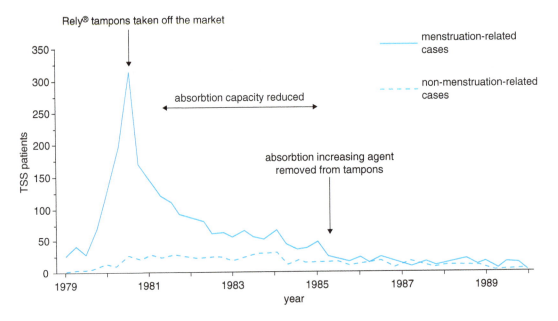

◻ **Figure 8.8**   Numbers of TSS cases in the United States between 1979 and 1990.

8.3.5   Risks to individuals and populations

Infectious diseases are caused by microorganisms transmitted to a host where they can multiply. An individual can be infected by a source in the vicinity or by another infected person. Many microorganisms can be transmitted from person to person, thus creating transmission chains in the population – a typical characteristic of infectious diseases.

Over time, this person-to-person transmission of pathogens leads to dynamic changes in transmission rates. Because of these time-dependent events, which are unique to infectious diseases, we need to distinguish between different levels of disease risk.

An individual encountering a source has a certain likelihood of exposure to the infectious agent. Once

this exposure has taken place, the person has a certain likelihood of infection by the agent. The infected individual then has a certain likelihood of getting the disease, and finally a certain likelihood of dying from the disease. Identifying and reducing these risks is in the interest of the individual and his or her contacts, and this is what the prevention and treatment of cases focuses upon in an outbreak investigation. Minimizing an individual's risk to being exposed, ensuring that if exposed, the risk of becoming infected is minimized, preventing the disease from developing if infected by prompt treatment with post-exposure prophylaxis and preventing further transmission of the infection to others ("treatment as prevention"), and lastly ensuring that cases are cured as quickly as possible.

From a population perspective, the likelihood of infected persons in the population being infectious and the likelihood of them transmitting the pathogen to other people during the infectious period is more important. These factors determine the likelihood of an outbreak in the population, as well as the likelihood of the epidemic increasing, decreasing, or disappearing completely.

Epidemiologists study the epidemiological function at each of these levels: the likelihood of infection at various levels of exposure, the likelihood of disease given an infection, the likelihood of contagiousness, the actual transmission at various levels of infection, and so on. Knowledge of these factors enables targeted interventions. Data might be used and interpreted for different purposes, depending on whether one is concerned with preventing the likelihood of disease in an individual with a particular risk profile or with the prevention of the likelihood of an outbreak in the population from a public health context.

Transmission by infectious persons, for instance, depends on how long cases are contagious, the degree of contagiousness, and the number of susceptible persons they have been in contact with. So, given a particular degree of contagiousness, transmission depends on patients' and their contacts' behavior. In the COVID-19 pandemic of 2020–2022, social distancing, use of face masks, hand hygiene, and ventilation of indoor spaces were key National Provider Identifiers (NPIs) in limiting and preventing spread of the SARS-CoV2 virus. Individual patients who have been treated for bacillary dysentery (shigellosis) will sometimes excrete Shigella bacteria in their feces for several months, even after their symptoms have cleared up. An outbreak can therefore easily develop, for instance, among children at a nursery school where hygiene rules are not implemented sufficiently.

8.4 Stepwise approach to outbreak investigation

Although no two outbreaks are the same, the response to an outbreak or potential outbreak will nevertheless usually involve the same steps. Various international organizations such as the CDC, ECDC, and WHO have developed roadmaps to guide outbreak investigations and responses.

A formal outbreak investigation may not always be needed: if it is immediately clear what is going on, what the source or cause is, and which control measure is suitable, the standard approach based on existing plans and protocols will suffice. If not, a systematic, structured outbreak investigation is needed to prevent unnecessary mistakes (e.g. time wasting, wrong measures, missed opportunities to gather unique information, loss of support among administrators, policymakers and healthcare providers, and panic in the population). The roadmaps or stepwise approach can be very useful in these situations.

The persons investigating the outbreak should have relevant knowledge and expertise to recognize the diseases in an outbreak and the possible explanatory factors that could be involved. Bring in experts who have this knowledge at their fingertips if necessary. Proper administrative and logistics procedures must be in place in advance, including the names and contact information of relevant authorities and people. It must be clear from the outset who is responsible for what, including who is in charge of the outbreak investigation and in developing the control measures. In practice, this will often be a physician expert in infectious diseases from the regional public health authority. If an outbreak covers more than one region, the national center for prevention and control of infectious disease will usually be in charge.

The various steps in an outbreak investigation are as follows:

■ Step 1: Establish that there is an outbreak

Determining the existence of an outbreak involves comparing the observed number of cases with the expected number, the latter being based on the number of cases reported during other periods or at other sites. Even if the observed number of cases is higher than the expected number, this does not necessarily mean that there actually is an outbreak. First, we need to verify, for example, that the disease diagnosis and recording system remained unchanged, that the definition of a case is the same, or that the population size was stable. Random fluctuation also needs to be ruled out as much as possible. Whether an apparent cluster of cases should be investigated further not only depends on verifying the existence of an outbreak (more cases than expected) but also on other factors. Severity of the illness, the potential for spread, availability of control measures, political considerations, public relations, and available resources can all influence the decision on whether or not to launch a field investigation.

Case 8.3 Example on Establishing an Outbreak

For the month of August, 12 new cases of tuberculosis and 12 new cases of West Nile virus infection were reported to a local US health county department. You are not sure if either group of cases is a cluster or an outbreak. What additional information might be helpful in making this determination?

First, you should check the dates of onset rather than dates of report. The 12 reports could represent 12 recent cases but could represent 12 cases scattered in time that were sent in as a batch. Assuming that all 12 reports of tuberculosis and the 12 of West Nile virus infection represent recent cases in a single county, both situations could be called clusters (several new cases seen in an area during a relatively brief period of time). Classifying the cases as an outbreak depends on whether the 12 cases exceed the usual number of cases reported in August in that county.

Tuberculosis does not have a striking seasonal distribution. The number of cases during August could be compared with: (i) the numbers reported during the preceding several months; and (ii) the numbers reported during August of the preceding few years.

West Nile virus infection is a highly seasonal disease that peaks during August to October months. As a result, the number of cases in August is expected to be higher than the numbers reported during the preceding several months. To determine whether the number of cases reported in August is greater than expected, the number must be compared with the numbers reported during August of the preceding few years.

■ Step 2: Verify the diagnosis

This step ensures that there is no misdiagnosis or laboratory error, which can be an explanation for the increase in the number of cases. This step is often closely linked to Step 1. Specifically, this step involves studying the medical records and lab results for the reported cases. In order to control the outbreak, the pathogenic microorganisms need to be ascertained quickly. Regional (or other) laboratories can provide fast diagnosis of many but not all infectious diseases using the polymerase chain reaction (PCR). The sooner the outbreak is detected and confirmed by microbiological diagnosis, the sooner steps can be taken to control it. It may also be wise at this stage to interview patients with the disease to form hypotheses of the nature of the outbreak. Tabulating the frequencies of the clinical signs and symptoms is also recommended. Are the clinical features consistent with the diagnosis? Frequency distributions of the signs and symptoms are useful in characterizing the spectrum of illness, verifying the diagnosis, and developing case definitions (see Step 3). They are frequently presented in an investigation's report or manuscript.

■ Step 3: Construct the case definition

A case definition is a standard set of criteria for deciding whether an individual should be classified as having the health condition of interest. The aim of a good case definition is to include as many true cases of the outbreak as possible and as few unrelated cases as possible, as the latter group causes misclassification, thus reducing the likelihood of tracking down the cause of the outbreak. Beginning with a broad definition so as not to miss any cases, and collecting as much information as possible on patients, will be helpful in making sense of what may be at play. Soon afterwards, we may apply a more restricted case definition including symptoms, signs, lab results, specific personal characteristics, places and times. National (or international) agreed case definitions strengthen comparability and facilitate interpretation.

If necessary, cases can be divided into "probable" cases, "possible" cases, and cases "confirmed" by laboratory results. Classifications such as confirmed-probable-possible are helpful because they provide flexibility to the investigators. A case might be temporarily classified as probable or possible while laboratory results are pending. Alternatively, a case may be permanently classified as probable or possible if the physician decided not to order the confirmatory laboratory test because the test is expensive, difficult to obtain, or unnecessary. Epidemiologists strive to ensure that a case definition includes most, if not all, of the actual cases, and very few or no false-positive cases; this may not be possible since mild or those with no symptoms may not get tested.

In essence, four aspects should be covered in a good case definition: clinical criteria and restrictions by time, place, and person. The clinical criteria should be based on simple and objective measures such as "fever ≥ 40°C," "three or more loose bowel movements per day," or "myalgias (muscle pain) severe enough to limit the patient's usual activities." The case definition should be restricted by time (for example, to persons with onset of illness within the past two months), by place (for example, to residents of a certain province or area or to employees of a particular plant), and by person (for example, to persons with no previous history of a positive tuberculin skin test, or to premenopausal women). Whatever the criteria, they must be applied consistently to all persons under investigation. The case definition must not include the exposure or risk factor you are interested in evaluating, which is a common mistake. For example, if one of the hypotheses under consideration is that persons who worked in an office in wing B were at greater risk of disease, do not define a case as "illness among persons who worked in wing B with onset between. . ." Instead, define a case as "illness among persons who worked in the office building with onset between. . ." Then, conduct the appropriate analysis to determine whether those who worked in wing B were at greater risk than those who worked elsewhere in the office.

■ Step 4: Identify the "right" cases

Find the "right" cases that meet the definition decided upon in Step 3 and list them in a table. This should include at least data on the date of the first symptoms, the date of diagnosis, age, gender, geographical location, specific symptoms, and proof of infection (from laboratory results). Active detection of all cases forms the basis for determining the extent of the outbreak. One way of achieving this is to actively request local GPs, specialists, and clinical laboratories to notify cases known to them and watch out for new cases. The public can also be asked to report new cases (without creating panic).

■ Step 5: Describe the incidence of the cases in terms of time, place, and personal characteristics

Initial descriptive analysis can be carried out using the table from Step 4. First draw and interpret the epidemic curve: this may provide indications of the nature of the outbreak when exposure took place and about the course of the outbreak (see Section 8.3.1). If all cases are plotted on a map, this will show at a glance whether there are any geographical similarities that suggest a possible source of infection or transmission. Case 8.2 shows how this can be used to develop hypotheses about the possible cause. It was in this way that John Snow discovered the source of contamination in the

London cholera epidemic (see Case 1.3). In some outbreaks, this descriptive step will lead to hypotheses about factors that could explain the outbreak.

■ Step 6: Formulate hypotheses

Interviews with the patients may produce further ideas about the possible nature and source of the infection. If it is a "standard" outbreak, where the pathogen is known but not the source, a standard questionnaire should be used for the interviews. If the pathogen is unknown, the interviews will need to be more exploratory. Experts and the medical literature may provide insights about the possible cause of the outbreak. Cases that do not fit in with the characteristic pattern of the epidemic curve can be a valuable source of information. An isolated case where the incubation period occurred earlier than in the other cases could, for instance, identify the cook who unwittingly contaminated a food product. Many countries' national centers for prevention and control of infectious diseases carry out recurrent questionnaire surveys of a sample of the general population about possible risk factors. This sample can serve as "controls" for patients possibly having been exposed to sources. Hypotheses should ideally include the source, the mode of transmission, and the explanatory factor that is causing the disease. This step will often be the last one in a small-scale outbreak investigation (with a known microorganism and source). In other words, not all the steps will be required for every outbreak. It is also worth mentioning that while this step may be a "last" one theoretically, practically, an investigator may have already started formulating a working hypothesis from Step 2. The epidemic curve in Step 5 can offer useful clues.

■ Step 7: Conduct an initial analytical study

The hypotheses on possible causes of the outbreak can be further tested in analytical studies. The initial study will often utilize a case–control design (see Section 8.3.3). The initial studies will elucidate the likelihood of the possible explanations and enable the planning of next steps.

■ Step 8: Adjust the hypotheses and carry out additional research

The hypotheses that remain intact or were modified during the previous step provide the basis for further research. This could take the form of epidemiological studies or visits to sites where outbreaks occur. A visit to the location of the presumed pathogen (inspection of the kitchen, or a visit to the company, or neighborhood from which the patients come) can provide rich information and secure relevant "evidence." It is critical to take samples from patients, food, animals, and the environment as soon as possible, as otherwise the causative agent may have disappeared. In addition, people are more likely to cooperate while the outbreak is still going on. Incoming data should be checked for completeness and consistency and entered in a database. As outbreaks are usually short-lasting and the changes in the population at risk is negligible, the disease frequency is generally expressed in the form of attack rates (see Section 8.3.3).

■ Step 9: Implement control and prevention measures

In most outbreak investigations, the primary goal is to control outbreak and prevent additional cases. In practice, these activities should be implemented as early as possible. The health department's first responsibility is to protect the health of the public, so if appropriate control measures are known and available, they should be initiated even before an epidemiologic investigation is launched. For example, a child with measles in a community with other susceptible children may prompt a vaccination campaign before an investigation on how that child became infected is launched.

Confidentiality and privacy are important issues in implementing control measures. Healthcare workers need to be aware of the confidentiality and privacy issues relevant to the collection, management, and sharing of data. For example, in managing stigmatized diseases like STIs or tuberculosis, the relationship between the patient and the healthcare worker has to be trustworthy. If sensitive information is disclosed to unauthorized persons without the patient's permission, the patient may be stigmatized or experience rejection from family and friends, lose a job, or be evicted from housing. The healthcare worker may lose the trust of the patient, which can affect adherence to intervention.

In general, control measures are usually directed against one or more segments in the chain of transmission (agent, source, mode of transmission, portal of entry, or host). For some diseases, the most appropriate intervention may be directed at controlling or eliminating the agent at its source such as food poisoning outbreaks, vector-borne diseases like dengue or malaria. Some interventions are aimed at blocking the mode of transmission. Interruption of direct transmission may be accomplished through quarantine of primary cases and contacts of primary cases. Similarly, to control an outbreak of an influenza-like illness in a nursing home, affected residents could be put together in a separate area to prevent transmission to others. Efforts may also be focused on changing behaviors, such as promoting hygiene through hand washing or use of face masks (COVID-19). For air-borne diseases, strategies may be directed at modifying ventilation or air pressure, and filtering or treating the air. To interrupt vector-borne transmission, measures may be directed toward controlling the vector population, such as spraying insecticides to reduce the mosquito population that carries West Nile virus. Some interventions aim to increase a host's defenses. Vaccinations promote development of specific antibodies that protect against infection. Similarly, prophylactic use of antimalarial drugs, recommended for visitors to malaria-endemic areas, does not prevent exposure through mosquito bites but prevents infection from taking root.

■ Step 10: Initiate or maintain surveillance

Once control and prevention measures have been implemented, they must continue to be monitored. If surveillance has not been ongoing, now is the time to initiate active surveillance. If active surveillance was initiated as part of case-finding efforts, it should be continued. The reasons for conducting active surveillance at this time are twofold.

First, one must continue to monitor the situation and determine whether the prevention and control measures are working. Are the number of new cases slowing down or, better yet, have they gone down to zero? Or, are new cases continuing to occur? If so, where are the new cases? Are they occurring throughout the area, indicating that the interventions are generally ineffective, or are they occurring only in pockets, indicating that the interventions may be effective but that some areas were missed?

Second, it is important to know whether the outbreak has spread outside its original area or the area where the interventions were targeted. If so, effective disease control and prevention measures must be implemented in these new areas, or control measures should be revised. For example, in the case of COVID-19 control and prevention, in March 2020, many countries in Europe focused on contact tracing with the aim of halting the spread, later measures involved massive public health education campaigns around hand hygiene, social distancing, and limiting indoor gatherings as spread of the virus increased. Eventually, nationwide lockdowns were necessary when community widespread in many parts of a country was detected.

■ **Step 11: Make the findings known to the public**

Effective, clear, and timely information is vital in any investigation of an outbreak, for example:

- Informing the public of the nature of the disease and how it can be identified, treated, and prevented. Press releases and social and other media can be used to disseminate this information. It goes without saying that the information should be phrased in language that is clear and easy to understand. It may be necessary to adapt it for subgroups or to convene public information campaigns to target particular groups.
- Informing the investigation team. All staff involved should be briefed regularly with up-to-date information on the course of the outbreak and the investigation into the causes.
- Informing the administrators. To enable them to fulfill their responsibilities, the public health officials should be given information on the progress of the investigation regularly.
- Informing local GPs, specialists (insofar as relevant to the particular disease) and other healthcare workers who could come into contact with patients or people suspected of having the disease.
- Informing other authorities who could become involved with the outbreak: institutions or areas elsewhere with similar exposures, and also authorities indirectly involved, e.g. authorities in environmental health, transportation, consumer products, and others.
- Informing fellow researchers. National infectious disease control centers will often have an electronic messaging network in place for this purpose.

8.5 Interpreting data on supposed outbreaks remains difficult

In practice, there may be disagreement as to whether there is an outbreak and whether the correct source has been identified, as many forms of bias can creep in, hindering the interpretation:

- How is the affected population and/or outbreak area defined? False alarms may occur if definitions are based on unverifiable or inaccurate observations. Narrowing down the boundaries of the area or population will reduce the number of expected cases. Consequently, excess cases will become more apparent and might even produce significant results, even in situations of normal variation in disease incidence.
- How is the outbreak period defined? There may be seasonal variation, and this too can vary from one year to another, which makes it difficult to interpret a temporary increase in disease frequency. If the outbreak is observed over a longer period, random variation will be less concerning, but important signals may be missed. Consider, for instance, the situation where an outbreak leads to earlier deaths among individuals who are at increased risk of death. Mortality rates covering a longer period might miss this phenomenon ("early harvest") because a temporary mortality peak is counter-balanced by a period of lower mortality.
- What led to the hypotheses about possible causes? A poorly formulated hypothesis is likely to result in false alarms or missing the actual risk factors.
- How good are the data? Inaccurate data on cases and missed cases make it difficult to identify the causes of outbreaks. Cases that emerge once a suspected cause of the outbreak has been identified can also cause bias. Lastly, the absence of high-quality data on the nature and duration of exposure to risk factors will limit this kind of investigation. The exposure data will be impossible to obtain once the source of the exposure disappears.
- Have all the confounders been taken into account? Confounding can cause serious bias, just as in other types of epidemiological research.
- Are the researchers being given enough time and opportunity to carry out the outbreak investigation?

8

There is almost always public pressure to take actions quickly, leaving fewer resources and attention for systematic assessment of the problem and the impact of the measures taken.

Case Study 8.4 A more Transmissible Variant of COVID-19 in the United Kingdom

SARS-CoV-2 (Severe Acute Respiratory Syndrome – CoronaVirus-2) is a coronavirus that was first detected in Wuhan, China and is associated with severe outcomes such as pneumonia, multi-organ failure, and death. The initial outbreak in Wuhan spread globally in 2020 and caused the largest pandemic in a century. In the fall of 2020, concerns about a more transmissible variant (mutation of the original strain) arose in the United Kingdom (UK), as the number of cases started rising rapidly in certain areas. While public health measures such as stay-at-home orders and intensive "test and isolate" policies were in place, the number of cases still rose daily in certain regions.

Researchers in the UK used genetic sequencing to track mutations. They realized in late 2020 that the PCR tests used for the detection of RNA viral particles in test individuals were not responding the same as earlier. As viruses mutate, their genetic structure changes over time. In this case, a specific gene target ("S-gene") did not test positive for viral RNA, when the N-gene target would still be positive. Soon, scientists started to hypothesize that the variant with this mutation might be more transmissible.

The hypothesis arose from mathematical modeling studies (using hospital admissions/occupancy, deaths, and prevalence), which led to discussions on whether the variant was more transmissible or whether confounding factors could explain the increased growth in cases. For example, people's behavior could have changed or the virus was hitting more susceptible populations by chance.

Researchers used data from the Office of National Statistics (ONS), which regularly conducted seroprevalence studies of random samples. The survey randomly selects households from address lists to generate a representative sample of the UK population on a continuous basis. They

used features of PCR tests to conclude whether people were infected with the new variant or not, and subsequently estimated relative growth rates (between the old and new variants) using iterative sequential Poisson regression. Growth rates are expressed in rate ratios per day. On average, they found that the new variant had a relative growth rate of 1.06 (CI: 1.04–1.09) compared to the old variant, implying that the new variant was more transmissible.

The main study strength is its design, being a large-scale community survey with a robust sampling frame across all ages. The survey also included asymptomatic infections, providing direct population-level estimates of positivity. These findings allowed the researchers to draw definitive conclusions about the transmissibility of the new variant.

8.6 Other approaches to studying outbreaks and clusters

While the foregoing has been specifically concerned with outbreaks, infections can have major effects on public health. Outbreaks can develop insidiously, not only due to human-to-human transmission but also to contamination of food or the environment or to the use of unsafe material in the health service. Outbreaks of this kind can go unnoticed, as the time dimension is different (i.e. the outbreak will cease to exist once the source is removed), and the effects are less pronounced. Carefully designed epidemiological research should ensure that these signals are discovered.

When analyzing data from outbreak investigations, classic statistical methods can be used. We translate the epidemiological problem into a regression model and estimate the regression coefficients as a measure of the association of the explanatory factor on the occurrence of the disease, adjusting for confounders. As the classic epidemiological methods are not always adequate when studying infectious diseases, researchers sometimes have to apply special methods and techniques, the most common of which are briefly discussed below.

8.6.1 Surveillance using non-medical data

Epidemiological studies have relied on medical data for a long time. However, for many infectious diseases, the outbreak takes time to develop. Surveillance through medical data, such as infections or hospitalizations, is time consuming. Researchers can utilize non-medical data, such as mobility data to study whether people have visited high-risk places and whether interventions have limited such behavior. Behavioral researchers can track the mobility of populations by using mobile devices. The integration of behavioral research, mobility data, and medical data also leads to improved insights for epidemiological modeling, which is often used to study outbreaks.

8.6.2 Simulation models if reality is too complex

Models can be very useful in both outbreaks and situations of equilibrium. The advantage of modeling is that problems due to random variability can be manipulated through simplifying assumptions. This can also be a disadvantage if the model becomes too simple and ignores relevant variations.

Infectious diseases behave dynamically in the population, and while these processes follow certain principles, they sometimes cannot be captured in a simple model. Section 8.6.3, for instance, examines the basic reproduction number, a vital concept in explaining the rise and fall of outbreaks and infectious disease epidemics over long periods. This process is influenced by so many factors that complex infectious disease models are needed to describe it fully. The models can be deterministic (the chance of occurrence of the variable involved is ignored), but more often dynamic transmission models (with random elements) provide more realistic estimates of the effects of interventions and people's behavior. Take the average age at which an infection is contracted, for example. If many people are immunized against an infectious agent, the incidence of the disease will drop, thus increasing the average age at which infections occur among people who are susceptible. Some diseases (e.g. mumps, measles and rubella), however, are relatively serious when they occur in later life. A vaccination campaign can therefore reduce the total number of cases while increasing the number of severe cases. Complex processes of this kind are studied using dynamic transmission models, which can subsequently be used to evaluate various intervention scenarios. Additional models can then be used to estimate the cost-effectiveness of various interventions before taking decisions on the matter.

Models also need to account for contact patterns in a population. Simple models are based on the assumption that the distribution of susceptible individuals in a population are random. The risk of anyone coming into contact with an infectious individual and becoming infected is the same. This assumption is usually wrong, of course, so that more complex contact patterns in a population need to be described. For nearly all infectious diseases, there is considerable heterogeneity in the disease transmission rate in a population. As population subgroups come into close contact with one another to a greater or lesser extent, the mathematical models for the spread of a disease need to take different contact and transmission rates into account for different groups. Sexually active homosexual men played a major role in the initial spread of HIV/AIDS in Western countries, for instance. In the case of influenza outbreaks, on the other hand, nursery schools play a major role in spreading the disease, as they bring children from different neighborhoods into close contact with one another. This heterogeneity in disease transmission can be accounted for by using different transmission rates in the models for the different subgroups.

A model that is often used to study the course of a directly transmissible infectious disease (e.g. polio, mumps, measles, rubella, whooping cough) is the SEIR model. This is based on dividing the population into four compartments, which represent the four possible stages that a person can occupy: susceptible (S), exposed (E: infected but not yet infectious), infectious (I), and resistant (R: recovered and sometimes immune). The SEIR model is a dynamic model for studying the likelihood of transitioning from one stage to the next. The model is described by a system of differential equations based on the characteristics of the infectious disease, the demographic characteristics of the population, the likelihood of contact between infectious and susceptible individuals, and the microorganism's transmission rate when contact takes place. The likelihood of transitioning from one stage to the next is modeled and estimated using empirical data from the literature or the researchers' own work. Various subgroups can be included in the models separately so as to reflect the heterogeneity in disease transmission. For example, people could be placed in quarantine during parts of the infectious period. An additional compartment quarantine (Q) can be included in the model to represent people who are not yet recovered but do not contribute to the ongoing outbreak.

In addition to the classic SEIR model, which is based strongly on population averages and various assumptions, there are other types of approach, such as microsimulation. This simulates an epidemic in a hypothetical population, with realistic parameters entered for the behavior of microorganisms, people and so on. Given these assumptions, infectious disease risks can be estimated with great precision.

Case 8.5 A Meningitis Outbreak in Sudan

An epidemic of meningitis emerged in north-west Sudan in January 1999. The first case was diagnosed in mid-January, and in the ensuing weeks the disease spread rapidly throughout the country and neighboring areas. The climatic conditions in Sudan are ideal for the spread of meningococcal meningitis for a large part of the year. Given the rapid spread and the country's experience of previous epidemics, Médecins sans Frontières (MSF) was soon called in to provide assistance. One of the MSF teams was sent to West Darfur, an area with a population of around 550,000 that had been hit badly by civil wars and was cut off from the rest of the country during a few months of the year because of poor infrastructure. The first cases were seen in this area at the beginning of February. By Week 8, the number of cases had risen to 15 per 10,000 per week. This area was therefore regarded as suffering an epidemic, in line with the WHO threshold of 15 per 100,000 per week. The MSF team arrived to carry out an exploratory mission that week, including taking lumbar punctures. *Neisseria meningitidis* group A was isolated from the samples, and preparations for a vaccination campaign began in Week 10.

Within a few days, eight vaccination teams had been trained and fully equipped with vaccination supplies. The public were informed via the radio, newspapers, mosques, and public address systems. Meningitis patients were treated effectively with chloramphenicol

in oil, administered intramuscularly. Vaccination started in Week 11, with up to 12,000 people a day being vaccinated in the urban areas. Health workers in rural areas were trained in using the case definition and the medication, and in providing information to the public. They also completed surveillance forms, which were sent to the coordination center once a week. This enabled the epidemic to be mapped out and further vaccination activities to be organized effectively.

The case definition was as follows:

- Suspected in the event of rapid-onset fever, stiff neck, or rash of small red patches since February 1999 in the province of West Darfur (symptom in infants: bulging fontanelle)
- Probable if a suspected case has a cloudy lumbar puncture
- Confirmed if a suspected case has a positive culture or antigen detected in the lumbar puncture.

Despite the poor infrastructure, this effort suppressed the epidemic in the province. The epidemic was brought under control within eight weeks of the start of the campaign, by which time 200,000 people had already been vaccinated. Of the 755 cases diagnosed, 106 died, representing an attack rate of 0.02% and a case fatality rate of 14%. Without vaccination, the attack rate could have risen to 1 or 2%.

8.6.3 The basic reproduction number

The basic reproduction number (R_0) is the average number of newly infected individuals that one contagious individual can produce in a population in which everyone is susceptible to the infection. Measles is an example of a highly contagious disease, with an R_0 of approximately 16 (see ▢ Table 8.4).

This means that during the period of contagiousness a child who has measles can, on average, infect 16 new individuals in a population who are all still susceptible to the disease. Ebola, on the other hand, is a far less contagious disease, with an R_0 of 2. To be able to cause an outbreak, R_0 must be greater than 1. R_0 is the product of the transmission rate (p), the number of contacts between infected and uninfected people

Table 8.4 The basic reproduction number for some familiar infectious diseases.

Disease	R_0
Measles	12–18
Whooping cough	12–17
Diphtheria	6–7
Smallpox	5–7
Polio	5–7
Rubella	5–7
Mumps	4–7
HIV/AIDS	2–5
SARS	2–5
Influenza	2–3
Ebola	1–4

per unit of time (c), and the duration of the infectiousness (D).

$$R_0 = p \times c \times D$$

The basic reproduction number is difficult to interpret because R_0 is based on the assumption that all contacts will produce potential patients whereas, in reality, some contacts will be with people who are immune, or partially immune, to the pathogen. This leads us to the effective reproduction number (R):

$$R = R_0 \times x$$

where x is the proportion of people susceptible to the disease in a well-mixed population. If the basic reproduction number for measles is 16 and half of the children in the population are immune, a child who has measles will only be able to infect eight new (contagious) cases of the disease.

It is important to note that R describes the average number of infections that an infected person produces. In reality, there is a lot of heterogeneity where R might be higher for younger age groups (due to contact patterns) while lower for older age groups. Further, heterogeneity may exist due to the nature of the pathogen. For example, air-borne diseases such as measles are known to follow the general "20/80" rule, where 20% of cases cause 80% of transmission. Dispersion parameter K, which describes how variable

the infection can be, quantifies the heterogeneity. A low value of K implies that a small number of cases is responsible for a large amount of subsequent transmission. When R is high and K is low, we tend to observe superspreading events which can drive a new outbreak of a pathogen.

It is not easy to estimate the basic reproduction number directly, so R_0 is usually estimated indirectly. In a stable situation, where the incidence and prevalence of the infectious disease do not change, each case will produce one new case on average. In this case, the basic reproduction number is the reciprocal of the proportion of people susceptible to the disease times the effective reproduction number. We can also take advantage of the fact that, in a stable situation, the average age at which the infection occurs depends on the basic reproduction number: the lower R_0, the higher the average age. The reverse is true of life expectancy: the higher the average life expectancy, the higher R_0. A rough indication of R_0 can be gained by these indirect methods.

The basic reproduction number is a complex concept that includes various important characteristics of the behavior of an infectious agent in a population. It helps to understand many important features of the prevention and control of epidemics. To halt an outbreak of an infectious disease, the reproduction number needs to be brought below 1. Suppose $R_0 = 5$ for HIV infection in a population and use of condoms reduces the transmission rate (p) by 90%, the basic reproduction number could be reduced to 0.5 if condom use was frequent. Without public health interventions, an outbreak will also halt if the proportion of people who have become immune is large enough. The size of the immunized fraction (f) needed to prevent an epidemic can be calculated in this way: $f = 1 - x$:

$$R = R_0 x (1-f)$$

To prevent an outbreak R must be less than 1. This means that:

$$R_0 x (1-f) < 1$$

In the measles example with $R_0 \approx 16$. $16*(1-f) < 1$ yields $f > 0.94$. In other words, 94% of the children at risk of initial infection must have been immunized (naturally or by vaccination) to prevent a measles outbreak. This is only true if the immunized children are evenly distributed in the population. The foregoing leads us to an important concept in infectious disease control, namely group protection ("herd immunity"). This describes the protection status of the population (as opposed to that of an individual) with regard to a particular infectious agent. A population is "immune" if the reproduction number R is less than 1. This does not necessary require all the individuals in the population to be immune: the more people have been vaccinated against the agent in question or have been become immune as a result of infection, the higher the population protection.

Source references

European Centre for Disease Prevention and Control. (2014). Annual epidemiological report 2014 – vaccine-preventable diseases (Case 8.1).

Holland, W.W., Olsen, J., and du Florey, V.C. (2007). *The Development of Modern Epidemiology: Personal Reports from those Who were there*. Oxford: Oxford University Press (Case 8.2).

Press, D.J., McKinley, M., Deapen, D. et al. (2016). Residential cancer cluster investigation nearby a superfund study area with trichloroethylene contamination. *Cancer Causes Control* 27: 607–613. (Case 8.4).

Personal communication from R. Appels, University Medical Center Groningen (Case 8.5).

Sarah, W.A., Pritchard, E., House, T. et al. (2021). Ct threshold values, a proxy for viral load in community SARS-CoV-2 cases, demonstrate wide variation across populations and over time. *eLife* 10: https://www.cdc.gov/csels/dsepd/ss1978/Lesson6/Section2.html#step2.

References

Zhang, H., Yang, L., Li, L. et al. (2019). The epidemic characteristics and spatial autocorrelation analysis of hand, foot and mouth disease from 2010 to 2015 in Shantou, Guangdong, China. *BMC Public Health* 19: 998. https://doi.org/10.1186/s12889-019-7329-5.

Recommended reading

Bonita, R., Beaglehole, R., Kjellström, T., and World Health Organization (2006). *Basic Epidemiology*, 2e. World Health Organization https://apps.who.int/iris/handle/10665/43541.

Elliott, P., Wakefield, J.C., Best, N.G., and Briggs, D.J. (2001). *Spatial Epidemiology: Methods and Applications*. Oxford: Oxford University Press.

Giesecke, J. (2002). *Modern Infectious Disease Epidemiology*, 2e. London: Arnold Publishers.

Gregg, M.B. (2008). *Field Epidemiology*, 3e. New York: Oxford University Press.

European Centre for Disease (2021). COVID-19 surveillance guidance. https://www.ecdc.europa.eu/sites/default/files/documents/COVID-19-surveillance-guidance.pdf (accessed 11 May 2022).

Institute of Environmental Science & Research Limited (2012). Guidelines for the. Investigation and Control of Disease Outbreaks. https://surv.esr.cri.nz/episurv/Manuals/GuidelinesForInvestigatingCommDiseaseOBs.pdf (accessed 11 May 2022).

Koepsell, T.D. and Weiss, N.S. (2003). *Epidemiologic Methods: Studying the Occurrence of Illness*. New York: Oxford University Press.

Lauffer, S. and Walter, J. (2020). *Control. A Practical Handbook for Professionals Working in Health Emergencies Internationally*. Berlin: Robert Koch Institute ISBN: 978-3-89606-307-6 https://doi.org/10.25646/7125.

Morabia, A. (2004). *A History of Epidemiologic Methods and Concepts*. Basel: Birkhäuser Verlag.

Nelson, K.E. and Masters, W.C. (2013). *Infectious Disease Epidemiology: Theory and Practice*, 3e. Boston: Jones and Bar-tlett Learning.

Rezza, G., Nicoletti, L., Angelini, R. et al. (2007). For the CHIKV study group. Infection with chikungunya virus in Italy: an outbreak in a temperate region. *Lancet* 370: 1840–1846.

Rothman, K.J., Greenland, S., and Lash, T.L. (2008). *Modern Epidemiology*, 3e. Philadelphia: Lippincott, Williams & Wilkins.

Thomas, J.C. and Weber, D.J. (ed.) (2001). *Epidemiologic Methods for the Study of Infectious Diseases*. New York: Oxford University Press.

Webb, P. and Bain, C. (2011). *Essential Epidemiology: An Introduction for Students and Health Professionals*, 2e. Cambridge: Cambridge University Press.

World Health Organization (2004). The global epidemiology of infectious diseases. In: (ed. C.J.L. Murray, A.D. Lopez and C.D. Mathers). World Health Organization https://apps.who.int/iris/handle/10665/43048 (accessed 12 June 2022).

Knowledge assessment questions

1. An outbreak of diarrheal illness occurred following a birthday party held at a petting zoo in Aurora, Colorado on June 10. One person has tested positive for Salmonella indicating that this outbreak was likely caused by *Salmonella*. There were cows, goats, sheep, and llamas present at the petting zoo. Most ill people reported petting the llamas.
   a. Construct a case definition for the outbreak. Assume you are constructing an outbreak case definition early in the outbreak investigation.
   b. How might your outbreak case definition change later in the outbreak? Give 1–2 examples of how the case definition might change.
2. Health workers reported an increased number of diarrhea cases at Hapsvil village beginning on June 17. They notified the local Ministry of Health (MOH) Office on June 19. Hapsvil is a remote village in rural southern India. Many villagers lack access to electricity, toilets, and potable water.

a. Do you think this could be an outbreak? Why or why not?
b. What additional information would help you in making this determination?
c. What other explanations might explain the increase in cases (other than an outbreak)?

3. *Let's continue with the same case from question 2, now...* MOH staff visited the local clinic and reviewed health clinic records for diarrhea cases over the previous three years. The number of cases reported on June 17–19 was three-times that reported during the same week in the previous two years. There were no reported changes in the composition of the village population, healthcare seeking behaviors, or the case definition used; therefore, you consider this to be a real outbreak.
a. How would you define a case? Provide a case definition.
b. How would you find additional cases? Describe two ways in which you would do this.
c. Name one other thing you would do at this early stage in the outbreak investigation.

4. *Let us continue with the same case from question 3, now...* Laboratory tests confirmed cholera in three villagers. Cholera is an acute, diarrheal illness caused by infection of the intestine with the bacterium *Vibrio cholerae*. Symptoms can include profuse watery diarrhea, vomiting, and leg cramps. It can take anywhere from a few hours to five days for symptoms to appear after infection. Symptoms typically appear in two to three days. It is typically spread by water or food that has been contaminated with human feces containing the bacteria.

After interviewing some villagers, you hypothesize that contaminated surface water from the local pond was the source of the outbreak. Villagers use pond water for washing utensil and garments, bathing, and preparation of foods.
a. What type of epidemiological study would you conduct to test the hypothesis that contaminated pond water was the cause of the outbreak? Why?
b. Explain how you would go about identifying people for your epidemiological study?
c. What exposure period would you ask about?

5. *Let's continue with the same case from question 4, now...* The investigators decided to undertake a case–control study. In the case–control study, 30 of 41 cases reported the pond water used for fermented rice preparation, compared with 15 of 41 controls.
a. Based on the data provided above, calculate the appropriate measure of association for using the pond water for fermented rice preparation.
b. Interpret what the measure of association means.
c. Is this finding statistically significant?

Diagnostic and Prognostic Research

Textbook of Epidemiology, Second Edition. Lex Bouter, Maurice Zeegers and Tianjing Li.
© 2023 John Wiley & Sons Ltd. Published 2023 by John Wiley & Sons Ltd.
Companion website: www.wiley.com/go/Bouter/TextbookofEpidemiology

9.1 Introduction

This chapter describes epidemiological research for diagnostic and prognostic purposes. Diagnosis and prognosis are two central concepts in medicine. The Greek word "diagnosis" means "distinction," and the aim of the diagnostic process is indeed to distinguish, or discriminate, between the absence or presence of a specific health outcome in individuals, between different health outcomes that appear similar in signs and symptoms, or between different stages of a particular condition in patients. The aim of prognosis is to predict the course or outcome of a disease process after a patient has been diagnosed. In many cases of prognostic research, outcomes are dichotomous as we are interested in predicting the probability of a future event, such as the occurrence of a pregnancy complication, or the 30-day mortality after surgery. Other frequent outcomes are time-to-event outcomes, such as time-to-recurrence after treatment (censored at 5 years), or time-to-death (censored at 10 years). Outcomes measured on interval or ratio measure (i.e. continuous outcomes) can also be predicted, but fall beyond the scope of this chapter. An example of a continuous outcome in prognostic research is predicting the number of days until discharge from the hospital after surgery, or blood pressure in millimeter mercury after taking antihypertensives.

The main difference between this chapter and the other chapters is that, in diagnostic and prognostic research, we are not particularly interested in investigating causal relationships. Instead, we are interested in identifying a test or a set of predictors that are strongly associated with the presence (diagnosis) or future occurrence (prognosis) of an outcome. Taking it to extremes, if we were to find that the length of the big toe shows whether a person will recover completely from a cerebral infarction, the length of the big toe would have major prognostic value. Whether the length of the big toe is also a causal factor is irrelevant. This chapter is about predicting whether a particular health outcome is present at this moment (diagnosis) or will occur in the future (prognosis) in an individual given their diagnostic or prognostic factors.

9.1.1 Diagnostic and prognostic information

Epidemiological research in this field usually concerns the performance of a diagnostic or prognostic test or model (i.e. a combination of tests and/or characteristics associated with the outcome). However, diagnosis and prognosis are not an end in themselves; they provide information for patients and health professionals to take actions and decisions. Diagnostic and prognostic information is vital when deciding whether to initiate treatment or preventive strategies, and if so, what kind. Even if there is no suitable or acceptable treatment, diagnostic and prognostic information may be useful to patients, for example, to assist with coping processes or behavior modifications. Diagnostic or prognostic information can also be useful when deciding whether the patient should undergo further diagnostic testing. For instance, based on the outcome of a diagnostic test to identify symptomatic sarcoidosis patients, a physician may decide whether the patient should undergo a subsequent positron emission tomography (PET) scan. The outcome of diagnostic tests and prognostic models can be categorical (e.g. positive/negative, or low-/intermediate-/high-risk), or continuous (e.g. the probability that a health outcome is present or will occur in the future). A high likelihood of a certain health outcome may lead to treatment, for example, or treatment can be withheld from someone with a low likelihood of that health outcome. Therefore, it is essential that the findings of diagnostic tests and prognostic models are accurate. We do not want to miss serious diseases or undesirable outcomes (i.e. have a false-negative result), but nor do we want diagnostic tests and prognostic models to give rise to incorrect suspicions that the patient has a condition or will have an undesirable outcome (i.e. have a false-positive test result) (◘ Figure 9.1).

When used in healthcare, diagnostic and prognostic tests or models must not only be of good quality, meaning that they are accurate and distinguish well between different health outcomes, they must also be efficient and convenient: the use of invasive tests must be minimized, results must be produced quickly, and the cost to the individual and the community must be kept low. The requirement of good quality and the desire to reduce burden and cost are often incompatible, as improving quality in many instances means increasing patient burden or costs.

In order to develop a diagnostic or prognostic model, researchers aim to find the minimum set of diagnostic (or prognostic) factors by which to distinguish individuals who have or will develop (or are likely to have or develop) a particular health outcome from individuals who do not have or will not develop

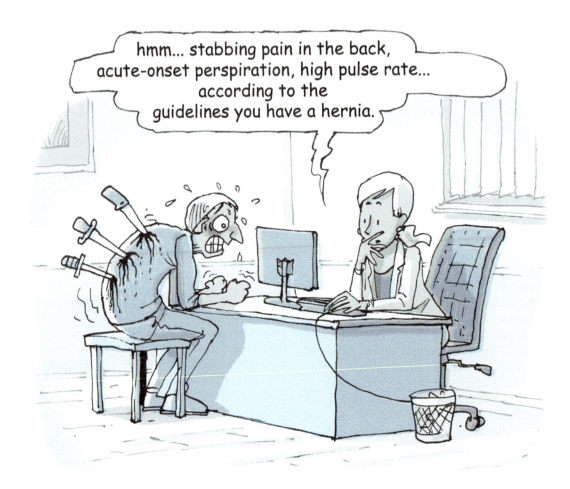

Figure 9.1 The practice of diagnosis.

(or are not likely to have or develop) that outcome. Variables can be selected based on their contribution to the model's accuracy, but others may be omitted if found too burdensome or invasive, costly, or otherwise impractical to use in the intended setting. In other words, diagnostic and prognostic research is research into (i) the probability of a health outcome and (ii) the minimum set of factors needed to calculate that probability with sufficient accuracy.

Diagnostic and prognostic factors generally fall into three categories:

1. Symptoms and signs.
2. Results of laboratory and other tests.
3. Patient characteristics (e.g. age and sex).

The purpose of medical history-taking is to identify and record symptoms experienced by the patient. Often, the practitioner also carries out a physical examination to look for signs. This clinical investigation – history-taking and physical examination – can be supplemented with observations using imaging techniques such as X-rays, computed tomography (CT), magnetic resonance imaging (MRI) or ultrasound, and lab tests such as hematological tests of blood parameters (e.g. hemoglobin), biochemical tests of the molecular composition of body fluids, tissues, and excreta (e.g. serum, urine, feces, fatty tissue, liver tissue, nails, hair, saliva, and cerebrospinal fluid).

Diagnostic research has traditionally been confined to the performance of a single test or a single measurement, instead of a diagnostic model containing multiple variables of which the combined performance is measured. The methodology for diagnostic research has been developed and expanded extensively in recent years. Prognostic research has gained a lot of popularity in public health and medicine in the first decade of this millennium. We will discuss diagnostic and prognostic research separately in the following sections. Note, however, the epidemiological techniques of both types of research have considerable overlap; the most profound difference between them is the timing of the health outcome: concurrently in time as the test or predictive factors (diagnostic research) or at some time later during follow-up (prognostic research).

9.1.2 Diagnostic research phases

Just as research into the efficacy of pharmaceutical products is not a single-step process, careful assessment of the quality and clinical utility of a diagnostic test may require a series of studies. The research required when developing a diagnostic test may include four phases:

- Phase I: comparing the test results of patients with the health outcome of interest with healthy controls without the health outcome of interest (a case–control study with diseased and healthy participants).
- Phase II: comparing the test results of patients with the health outcome of interest and controls with a variety of other health outcomes (a case–control study with related conditions).
- Phase III: comparing test results over the entire spectrum of the health outcome being diagnosed, i.e. those with or without symptoms, mild and severe, with and without comorbidity, with different anatomical, microscopic, and etiological characteristics.
- Phase IV: carrying out the diagnostic test on a large series of consecutive patients whose clinical presentation warrants it (a prospective cohort study of patients representative of the target group).

This classification shows how important it is to select the study population for diagnostic research carefully.

9.1.3 Predicting Prevalence

Research questions for diagnostic studies relate to the likelihood of a health outcome or a particular stage of a disease being present. As a result, diagnostic research always describes the prevalence of a health outcome as a function of one or more factors. Diagnostic research is always cross-sectional in nature as it aims to quantify the likelihood of an outcome at the exact time the relevant factors are taken (see Chapter 4). This feature also distinguishes diagnostic research from prognostic research as, by definition, outcomes in prognostic research have yet to occur. Diagnostic research also differs substantially from etiological research, where the aim is to find causal explanatory factors of the development of a disease. Etiological research focuses on incidences and therefore a longitudinal design is more suitable. Prognostic research, as described above, is not interested in causal associations but predictive factors. In this regard, prognostic research also differs substantially from etiological research.

9.2 Validity and reproducibility of diagnostic tests

9.2.1 Sources of diagnostic variability

Many diagnostic tests are based on measurements of continuous variables. Examples include using temperature to diagnose the presence of an infection or measuring fasting blood glucose to diagnose diabetes mellitus. The variability observed in the results of such a test can be due to several sources (see ☐ Table 9.1). Variability of a parameter being measured can be due to several measurement conditions: the number of different observers taking measurements, whether

☐ **Table 9.1**   Sources of variability in a measured diagnostic parameter.

Source		Notes
Actual (biological) variability	Within individuals	Changes in individuals in relation to time and measurement condition
	Between individuals	Biological differences between individuals
Apparent variability (measurement errors)	Measuring device	Measuring device lacks precision
	Observer	Random errors on the part of the person using the measuring device or interpreting the test results

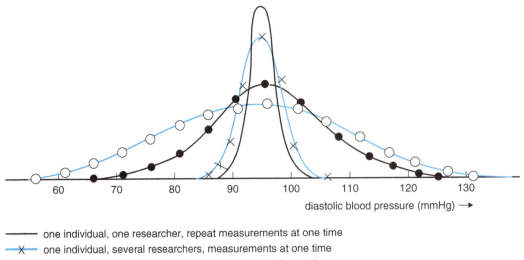

one individual, one researcher, repeat measurements at one time
one individual, several researchers, measurements at one time
one individual. one researcher, measurements at different times
several individuals (population)

Figure 9.2 The cumulative effect of various sources of variability on the observed distribution of test results for a biological parameter (diastolic blood pressure).

measurements are taken at a single point in time or over a period of time, and whether measurements are taken from an individual or from a sample of persons from the source population (see **Figure 9.2**).

Test results thus reflect actual (biological) variability in the parameter being measured in the population as well as random or systematic errors (see Chapter 5). As the aim of a diagnostic test is to distinguish individuals with abnormal values from those with normal values of a parameter, taking into account both within-person and between-person variability, measurement errors need to be eliminated as much as possible. Even within the same individual, parameters can take on different values over time and are dependent on the measuring condition. Most biological parameters have a normal distribution, with most values around the middle and relatively few extreme values.

The next question is which values of a diagnostic parameter should be regarded as normal and which as abnormal. When, for example, should creatine phosphokinase – the blood level of which is an indicator of myocardial infarction – be considered too high or too low? This question implies that there is a cut-off point in the distribution of the diagnostic parameter that marks the transition from normal to abnormal. Ideally, the distribution of a diagnostic parameter would be bimodal and non-overlapping (i.e. there would be two

clearly distinguishable distributions of values without overlap, one for those with the health outcome of interest, one for those without), but this is rarely the case. The distribution of the parameter for persons with the outcome usually substantially overlaps the distribution for those without it. This makes selecting a suitable cut-off point far from simple, especially since the distribution of a biological parameter often depends on other characteristics, e.g. age, sex, and diet, making it ever more difficult to decide on a single value as cut-off.

To enable us to interpret the result of a diagnostic test, we need to investigate properly how the biological parameter of interest relates to the presence of the health outcome. Abnormal values on the test are those associated with the presence of the health outcome; normal values are those where the health outcome is absent. Some biological parameters, however – e.g. serum cholesterol – display a continuous rise in morbidity and mortality risk over the entire range of possible test results, with each increase in the measured value being associated with additional risk. In such cases, there are no normal values, strictly speaking. In practice, we will often nevertheless select a cut-off point for action (e.g. initiating a treatment to manage high serum cholesterol). The cut-off point chosen should exert more benefits than harms to patients. We should also realize that these cut-off points may need

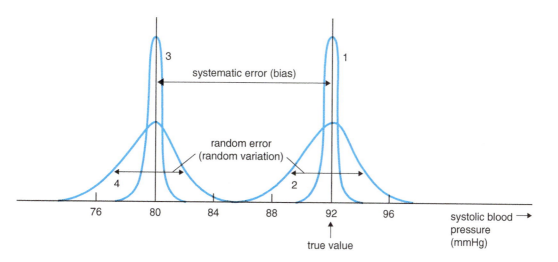

◻ **Figure 9.3** Systematic and random error when measuring a diagnostic parameter (blood pressure), 1: Measurement is valid and reproducible. 2: Measurement has poor reproducibility, but sufficient repeat measurements average out the random errors, giving a valid estimate of the actual blood pressure. 3: Measurement is reproducible but not valid. 4: Measurement is neither valid nor reproducible.

to be adjusted later in the light of discoveries and innovations in medicine, or that different cut-off points need to be selected for different populations (e.g. different cut-off points of hemoglobin values for men and women when testing for anemia).

Measuring errors cloud our view of the true value of a diagnostic parameter and of biological variability in that parameter. Systematic measurement errors – due for example to incorrect calibration of the device – cause bias: values are systematically under- or overestimated. When there are no systematic errors in the diagnostic measurement, the measurement is valid. The validity of a measuring procedure thus refers to the extent to which a test result corresponds to the true value of the measured parameter. We can correct for systematic errors if we know the magnitude and direction of the errors. If, for instance, we know our sphygmomanometer on average overestimates blood pressure by 10 mm Hg, we only need to subtract the systematic error from the observed findings to get to the "truth."

Random measurement errors that produce a random distribution of the test results around the true value of a diagnostic parameter are unavoidable and may pose a bigger problem. They affect reproducibility of the test, i.e. the extent to which two measurements on the same individual produce the same result. Those two measurements may be performed by a single person, or by multiple persons (e.g. when two radiologists separately judge the same CT scan).

Repeating the measuring procedure and taking the average of the test results reduces random measurement errors and improves reproducibility. That is why a patient's blood pressure is usually measured more than once and an average is calculated. ◻ Figure 9.3 illustrates the measurement of diastolic blood pressure in an individual with low pressure (measured intra-arterially) of 92 mmHg.

9.2.2 Reproducibility of diagnostic tests

One measure of the quality of a diagnostic test is the consistency of the results obtained through repeated tests of the same individual. If the measuring conditions remain constant, and the parameter being measured does not change, a repeat test should give an identical result. Many different terms are being used to describe the amount of agreement between repeated measurements and the absence of random errors in measurements. In Chapter 5, we introduced the term "precision" to refer to the amount of agreement between the results of repeated cause-and-effect research based on samples of limited size. In the case of diagnostic tests, the standard term is reproducibility, i.e. the extent to which consistent results are obtained when the test is repeated by the same or different observers. The term "accuracy" is not recommended, as there is no unequivocal definition of this concept, and it is moreover also associated with validity.

◘ Table 9.2   Examples of conditions along with diagnostic tests that can be used to detect them and the respective external criteria (gold standards).

Condition	Diagnostic parameters or test	Gold standard
Gallstones	Dyspepsia, pain	Ultrasound
Appendicitis	specific pain in the abdominal region	Histological test after appendectomy
High blood pressure	External blood pressure measurement (sphygmomanometer)	Intra-arterial blood pressure measurement
Breast cancer	Palpation (breast lump), mammogram, thermogram	Histological test after biopsy
Cervical cancer	Contact bleeding, pain, cytological test after smear	Histological test after biopsy
Coronary heart disease	Specific symptoms, exercise electro-cardiogram, serum enzymes	Coronary angiogram
Fever	Taking temperature using hand on forehead	Taking temperature using a clinical thermometer

Reproducibility of a diagnostic test can relate to a situation where a single observer repeats the test on the same participants (intra-observer variability, stability, test–retest reliability). If the time interval between them is too short, the precision of the diagnostic test could be overestimated because the observer remembers the previous result which may influence subjective observation. If the interval is too long, on the other hand, the measurements could be affected by actual changes in the biological parameter and reproducibility could be underestimated. As mentioned above, reproducibility of a diagnostic test can also relate to a situation where two or more observers carry out the test on the same participants around the same time (interobserver variability, interobserver agreement, inter-rater reliability).

9.2.3   Validity of diagnostic tests

Reproducible test results are a necessary but insufficient precondition for the quality of a diagnostic test. The results should also give a valid representation of the health outcome by correctly classifying participants into categories of severity or stage of a condition. The closer a diagnostic test reflects the underlying clinical condition, the greater the validity of the test. Systematic differences (bias) between the test result and the clinical condition result in the diagnostic test having imperfect validity. In healthcare, valid and reproducible diagnostic tests that are also quick, simple, inexpensive, and non-invasive are preferred.

To assess the validity of a diagnostic test, we need to compare the results of the test with the results from a different measuring tool (the external criterion). This is referred to as criterion validity. Ideally, there will be a gold standard that can serve as the external criterion; the gold standard measures the outcome objectively and that is certain (or almost certain) to give a correct picture of reality.

As the gold standard is usually expensive, labor-intensive, or invasive, and not suitable for routine diagnostic testing, a good deal of diagnostic research focuses on comparing the results of a simpler, quicker, less expensive, or less invasive test with the gold standard. The results of this comparison can then be used to justify using the simple test in the future. ◘ Table 9.2 shows examples of conditions, along with commonly used diagnostic tools, and their respective gold standards.

For many conditions, there is no suitable gold standard, e.g. complaints such as angina pectoris (chest pain), low back pain, migraine, and most psychiatric conditions. Sometimes, it is possible to draw a conclusion as to the validity of the test by waiting to see how the symptoms progress (without intervention). This is predictive validity, a special type of criterion validity.

In other cases, the only way of gaining an idea of validity is to assess whether the measurement tool is likely to measure what it is supposed to measure through subjective assessment (face validity), to check whether it takes account of all relevant aspects based on theoretical considerations (content validity), or to submit it to the scrutiny of one or more outside experts (expert validity).

9.3 Measures of validity of diagnostic tests

9.3.1 Sensitivity and specificity

Two common parameters for quantifying the validity of a diagnostic test are sensitivity and specificity. The sensitivity of a test indicates what percentage of the participants with a particular health outcome are correctly classified as positive by the test (see ◻ Figure 9.4). Sensitivity therefore gives some indication of how "sensitive" the test is in recognizing cases of the health outcome of interest. If the test detects all the participants who have the health outcome – i.e. all of them test positive – it has maximum sensitivity, 100%, and we can say that the percentage of true positive test results is 100%. Note that this does not mean that all patients who received a positive test result have the health outcome! The probability of a positive test result, given the presence of the heath outcome of interest, is generally not equal to the probability of the presence of the health outcome given the positive test result. The latter can be computed as a positive predictive value (or a posterior probability, which takes into account the prior probability, i.e. the prevalence of the health outcome in the population as well as a positive test result). The term "positive" can be confusing to patients: patients often get mixed up and think that it is a favorable result, and incorrectly conclude that they do not have the health outcome according to the test.

The specificity of a test indicates what percentage of the participants without the health outcome are correctly classified as negative by the test (see Figure 9.4). Specificity, then, gives some indication of the test's ability to correctly identify people with that health outcome, and correctly classifies those with similar health outcomes to differentiate from those who are negative. If all individuals without the health outcome are tested negative, the specificity will be 100%.

Using a diagnostic test with two possible results – positive (health outcome is present) and negative (health outcome is not present) – in a population containing both people with and without the health outcome produces a total of four categories:

- True positives (TP).
- False positives (FP).
- True negatives (TN).
- False negatives (FN).

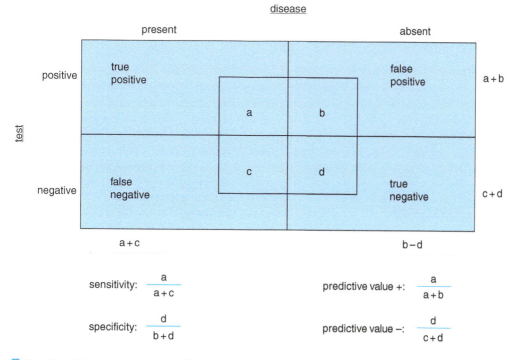

The two-by-two table in ◘ Figure 9.4 can only be filled in if we know with certainty which of the participants have the health outcome. This means that there must be a gold standard (see Section 9.2.3) and that the outcome status of each person has been assessed using both the diagnostic test and the gold standard. Case 9.1 illustrates the calculation of sensitivity and specificity based on hypothetical data from diabetes diagnostics.

Case 9.1 Diagnosing Diabetes – a Hypothetical Example

Diabetes can be detected using the oral glucose tolerance test (OGTT). This involves orally administering a standard quantity of glucose in solution (50 g of glucose in 200 ml water) and then taking blood samples every half hour for a few hours to measure the blood sugar level. The levels measured can be plotted on a graph. If the blood sugar curve does not fall sufficiently during the observation period, the patient is diagnosed with diabetes. Diabetic patients have a hormone dysfunction (insulin deficiency) which makes it difficult for cells to absorb glucose from the blood. The question is whether diabetes could be diagnosed more simply, for example, by looking at the blood glucose level two hours after eating a meal, i.e. a glucose test (GT).

To assess the quality of the GT method, the results of the GT and OGTT methods for 1,000 successive patients suspected of having diabetes are compared in a diagnostic study. The OGTT is treated as the gold standard, although there is some doubt as to whether the OGTT measures the presence of diabetes correctly in every case. For the GT method, a blood glucose level of $\geq$100 mg/ml two hours after a meal is regarded as indicative of diabetes. Based on the OGTT results, 250 persons are classified as diabetic and 750 as non-diabetic. The distribution of the results of the quick test among them is shown in ◘ Table 9.3.

The comparison between the two methods shows that the GT correctly detects 90% of the diabetics. Its sensitivity is therefore:

$$\frac{a}{a+c} = \frac{225}{250} \times 100\% = 90\%$$

The GT correctly classifies 70% of the non-diabetics (specificity):

$$\frac{d}{b+d} = \frac{525}{750} \times 100\% = 70\%$$

In total, 75% (([225 + 525]/1,000) × 100%) of the participants are classified correctly. The GT produces a "false negative" (FN) diagnosis in 25 cases and a "false positive" (FP) diagnosis in 225 cases.

So, what does this say about the value of the GT as a diagnostic tool in day-to-day practice? For this, we need to look at the predictive value (PV). Prior to the diagnostic study, 25% of the people in the population were thought to be diabetic (P(O)) and 75% non-diabetic (P(O)). After the diagnostic test, we know that 50% of the people who test positive are indeed diabetic (positive predictive value, PV+) and moreover that 95% of those who test negative are indeed non-diabetic (negative predictive value, PV−). In the case of people who test positive, then, the probability of having the disease has gone up from 25% to 50%, whereas that probability has gone down from 25% to 5% in the case of people who test negative, as shown in ◘ Figure 9.5. Thus, the test has provided more information on the likely presence of diabetes, but it has not been found capable of distinguishing diabetics from non-diabetics completely. The question is whether this increased knowledge is sufficient to base treatment decisions or other follow-up activities on.

◘ Figure 9.5 shows that the positive and negative predictive values of a test result depend on the sensitivity (a/[a + c]) and specificity (d/[b + d]) of the test. Higher sensitivity (a goes up and c goes down) is associated with a lower positive predictive value and a higher negative predictive value of the test. This may seem counterintuitive, but if we select a low cut-off point for which sensitivity is 100%, many without the health outcome will also receive a positive test result, thereby decreasing the positive predictive value. Conversely, as no patients with the health outcome are missed by the test, the negative predictive value is 100% as none of those with a negative test result actually have the health outcome. The prevalence (P(O)), or prior probability of the health outcome in the underlying population also affects the positive and negative predictive values of a diagnostic test, which can be considered the posterior probabilities given the test result.

◘ Figure 9.6 shows differences in predictive values when the same blood glucose test (with 90% sensitivity and 70% specificity) is used as a screening test on a predominantly healthy population of 100,000 in which the prevalence of diabetes is estimated to be 0.25%. The increase in the negative predictive value (PV⁻) due to the screening test is minimal, but the positive predictive value (PV⁺) decreased considerably. The number of people with a false positive result is far higher than the number of diabetics detected. In a predominantly healthy population, the test turns out to be worthless in detecting diabetes, in spite of the fact that the test conditions remain the same: hardly any of the people who test positive have diabetes. A negative test result is almost certainly indicative of the absence of diabetes, but that was already highly likely anyway.

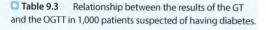

Table 9.3 Relationship between the results of the GT and the OGTT in 1,000 patients suspected of having diabetes.

Test	Diabetes	No diabetes	
≥100 mg/ml	225	225	450
<100 mg/ml	25	525	550
	250	750	1,000

9.3.2 Receiver operating characteristic (ROC) curve

It is not difficult to develop a test that is 100% sensitive. If we blindly label everyone as having the health outcome, i.e. select a very low cut-off point for a diagnostic test, everyone with the outcome will be correctly classified as diseased. The price we pay for this is

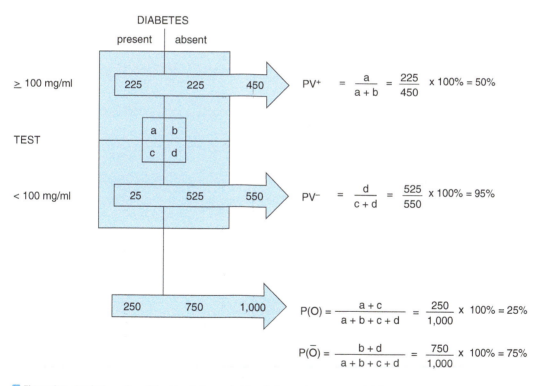

Figure 9.5 Predictive value of the blood glucose test in relation to the presence of diabetes in 1,000 patients suspected of having diabetes in a general practice situation. *P(O):* Prior probability of diabetes = prevalence of diabetes in the population being tested for the presence of the disease outcome. P(Ō):Prior probability of the absence of diabetes = prevalence of non-diabetes in the population being tested for the presence of the disease. *PV⁺:* Posterior probability of diabetes in persons who test positive = predictive value of a positive test result. *PV⁻:* Posterior probability of the absence of diabetes in persons who test negative = predictive value of a negative test result.

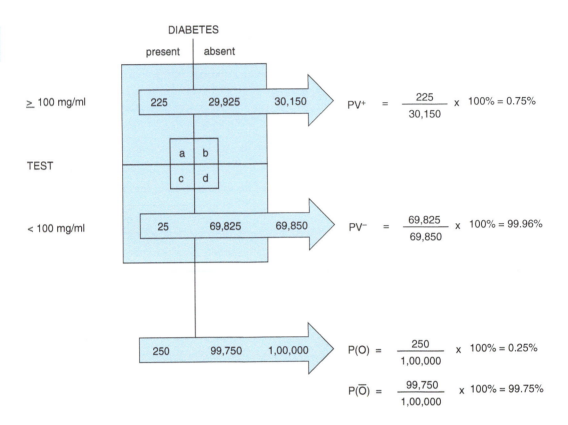

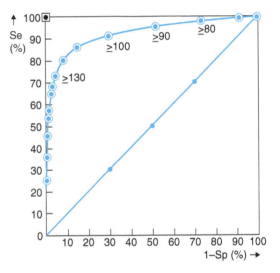

Figure 9.6 Predictive value of the GT for the presence of diabetes in 100,000 people in a predominantly healthy population.

that everyone who does not have the health outcome will also be classified as having it, i.e. specificity is 0%. Conversely, we could develop a test that is 100% specific but does not detect a single person with the outcome. It is always important, therefore, to look at the test's sensitivity and specificity in combination, as the higher one is, the lower the other.

All combinations of sensitivity and specificity for different cut-off points in a diagnostic test can be represented by an ROC (Receiver Operating Characteristic) curve, as exemplified by ▣ Figure 9.7.

Each dot in the graph represents a pair of sensitivity and specificity for a different cut-off point on the test. The closer the curve approaches the top left corner of the graph (where both sensitivity and specificity approach 100%), the discriminative ability of a test increases. The discriminative ability is expressed by calculating the area under the ROC curve and dividing it by the maximum area (the entire rectangle). The result – the proportion of the area under the ROC curve – is referred to as the area under the curve (AUC), the value of which lies between 0.5 and 1. Note that an AUC of 0.5 means that the ROC coincides with

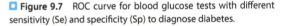

Figure 9.7 ROC curve for blood glucose tests with different sensitivity (Se) and specificity (Sp) to diagnose diabetes.

the diagonal line in ▣ Figure 9.7. This is the 50/50 chance line, where the number of true positives is the same as that of false positives and the number of true negatives the same as that of false negatives. In other words, a test with an AUC of 0.5 has no discriminatory power; only at AUC values substantially higher than 0.5 does the test begin to have diagnostic value. The AUC – a measure of the discriminative ability of the diagnostic procedure independent of the cut-off point chosen – can only be improved by improving the current test, using a different test, or by using a combination of tests in series or in parallel.

Many diagnostic factors (e.g. blood pressure, lab results and function tests) are not dichotomous (positive/negative, abnormal/normal, unhealthy/healthy) but on a scale (ordinal, interval, or continuous). From the range of possible values on that scale, a cut-off value can be selected to dichotomize the diagnostic factor into abnormal/normal orssssss any other dichotomization. But what are the rationales for selecting a cut-off point? In the blood glucose test described in Case 9.1, the cut-off point was set at 100 mg/100 ml. Based on that cut-off, 225 of the 250 diabetic patients were recognized as such (true positives, sensitivity = 90%) and 25 were missed (false negatives). Of the 750 patients without diabetes, 525 were classified correctly (true negatives, specificity = 70%) and 225 incorrectly (false positives). Was the correct cut-off selected?

Figure 9.8 shows the full range of the glucose test in the diabetics and non-diabetics. Each time the cut-off point between positive and negative test results is moved, the number of diabetics and non-diabetics detected change, illustrating the phenomenon mentioned earlier that the sensitivity and specificity of the test should be considered jointly.

This distribution of blood glucose values among diabetics and non-diabetics can also be shown graphically in a histogram (see Figure 9.9) or frequency polygon (see Figure 9.10).

In Figure 9.9, the distributions for diabetics and non-diabetics are projected "back-to-back" here, showing that they overlap. Hence, no cut-off point exists with which we can separate those with diabetes from those without. If we want to use the diagnostic test only to detect cases of diabetes, the cut-off point should be set at a very high blood sugar level of 180 mg/100 ml, and if the test is positive, we will know for sure that the patient is diabetic. We will miss most diabetes cases, however. If we want to use the test only to exclude people without diabetes, we should set a cut-off point of 70 mg/100 ml, and only people who are not diabetic will test negative. A lot of non-diabetics will be identified as having diabetes,

however. The optimum cut-off point lies somewhere between these two values.

Figure 9.10 shows that a cut-off point of 100 mg/100 ml yields approximately equal numbers of people with a true positive and a false positive test result. By increasing the cut-off point to 120 mg/100 ml we can reduce the number of false positives substantially, while the number of false negatives increases relatively little. At first sight, this cut-off would therefore seem to be a better option.

As in this example, it is not possible to find a cut-off point that discriminates completely between diabetics and non-diabetics (no false positives and no false negatives), it is impossible to reach 100% sensitivity and 100% specificity at the same cut-off point). The perfect test situation is shown in Figure 9.11, where a cut-off point can be found that distinguishes perfectly between people who have and do not have the health outcome.

Given a particular type of test, we can never increase sensitivity and specificity at the same time by moving the cut-off point. As we saw when introducing the ROC curve, we increase sensitivity at the expense of specificity and, conversely, increasing specificity means sacrificing sensitivity (see Figure 9.12).

There is no generic answer to the question of whether more weight should be attached to high sensitivity or to high specificity when selecting a cut-off point. Two considerations are important when weighing this up:

- The consequences of incorrect diagnosis (false positive and false negative).
- The prevalence of the health outcome in the population where the test will be used, as this is a factor in the numbers of false positive and false negative diagnoses, and greatly affects positive and negative predictive values.

A sensitive test is called for particularly if we do not want to miss a single case of the health outcome (and thus has a high negative predictive value): for example, a health outcome that has a poor prognosis if left untreated but that is treatable if discovered early (e.g. Hodgkin's disease or phenylketonuria). A sensitive test can also be useful at the start of the diagnostic process to eliminate people who almost certainly do not have the health outcome in question (those who test negative), as it provides the greatest certainty if the result is negative. A sensitive test has the effect, how-

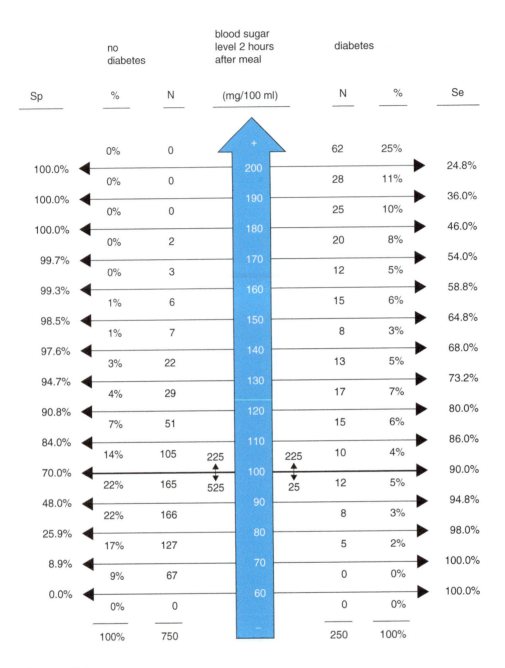

Sp	%	N	blood sugar level 2 hours after meal (mg/100 ml)	N	%	Se
	0%	0	+	62	25%	
100.0%			200			24.8%
	0%	0		28	11%	
100.0%			190			36.0%
	0%	0		25	10%	
100.0%			180			46.0%
	0%	2		20	8%	
99.7%			170			54.0%
	0%	3		12	5%	
99.3%			160			58.8%
	1%	6		15	6%	
98.5%			150			64.8%
	1%	7		8	3%	
97.6%			140			68.0%
	3%	22		13	5%	
94.7%			130			73.2%
	4%	29		17	7%	
90.8%			120			80.0%
	7%	51		15	6%	
84.0%			110			86.0%
	14%	105	225	225	10	4%
70.0%			100			90.0%
	22%	165	525	25	12	5%
48.0%			90			94.8%
	22%	166		8	3%	
25.9%			80			98.0%
	17%	127		5	2%	
8.9%			70			100.0%
	9%	67		0	0%	
0.0%			60			100.0%
	0%	0	−	0	0%	
	100%	750		250	100%	

Se = sensitivity
Sp = specificity

Figure 9.8 Distribution of the results of the glucose test in 250 diabetics and 750 non-diabetics. Sensitivity and specificity for various cut-off points for a positive/negative test result.

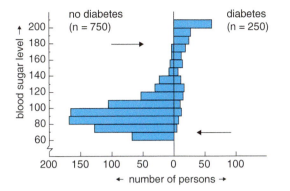

Figure 9.9 Frequency distribution of people with different results in the blood glucose test among diabetics and non-diabetics respectively.

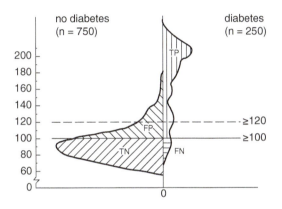

Figure 9.10 Distribution curves of the results of the blood glucose test in diabetics and non-diabetics (P(O) = 25%).

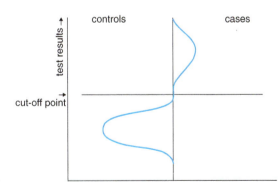

Figure 9.11 Example of a perfect diagnostic test.

ever, of incorrectly labeling healthy people as "unhealthy" (stigmatization). This is a problem particularly if further investigation or treatment is stressful and risky and could result in physical, emotional, or financial burden to the patients. An oversensitive test overconsumes healthcare resources.

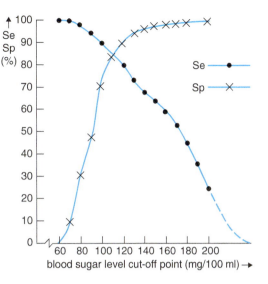

Figure 9.12 Relationship between sensitivity (Se) and specificity (Sp) for various cut-off points for a positive/negative result of the blood glucose test.

9.3.3 Likelihood ratio

The ROC curve (see Section 9.3.2) nicely illustrates how the sensitivity and sensitivity of a test depend on each other and on the cut-off point selected. The likelihood ratio is another way of combining information on persons with and without the health outcome and can be used to compare various cut-off points.

The likelihood ratio of a positive test result (LR$^+$) is the ratio between the probability of a positive test result in people with the health outcome and the probability of a positive test result in people without the health outcome:

$$LR^+ = \frac{P(T^+|O)}{P(T^+|\bar{O})} = \frac{a/(a+c)}{b/(b+d)}$$
$$= \text{sensitivity} / (1-\text{specificity})$$

The likelihood ratio of a negative test result (LR$^-$) is the ratio between the probability of a negative test result in people with the health outcome and the probability of a negative test result in people without the health outcome:

$$LR^- = \frac{P(T^-|O)}{P(T^-|\bar{O})} = \frac{c/(a+c)}{d/(b+d)}$$
$$= (1-\text{sensitiviy}) / \text{specificity}$$

A likelihood ratio can be regarded as a yardstick of how much weight can be attached to a particular

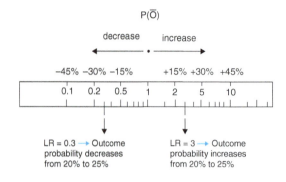

Figure 9.13 The likelihood ratio as a diagnostic yardstick.

test result in the diagnostic process (see Figure 9.13). A likelihood ratio of around 1 means that the test result does not add anything when gauging whether the health outcome is present or absent. The higher LR$^+$ is and the closer LR$^-$ approximates zero, the more information the diagnostic test provides. An LR$^-$ below 0.3 means a reduction of at least 20%–25% in the probability of the health outcome compared with the prior probability (prevalence), whereas an LR$^+$ higher than 3 means an increase of at least 20%–25% in that probability. For example, if the prevalence of a health outcome in the general population is 4%, the estimated probability of the health outcome is 5% if the LR+ of the test result is approximately 3. Diagnostic tests with LRs higher than 10 or below 0.1 are generally rated as "good."

In addition to being a yardstick – i.e. how much a test adds in the diagnostic process - another benefit of the likelihood ratio is that it can also be used for tests that have more than two outcome categories. An example of this can be seen in Table 9.4.

Table 9.4 Likelihood ratios for different categories of blood glucose for the diagnosis of diabetes.

mmol/l	Absent N	Absent %	Present N	Present %	LR
≥150	11	1.5	162	64.8	44.2
120–150	58	7.7	38	15.2	2.0
100–120	156	20.8	25	10.0	0.48
80–100	331	44.1	20	8.0	0.18
<80	194	25.9	5	2.0	0.08
Total	750	100	250	100	

9.3.4 Predictive value

The predictive value of an abnormal or positive test result (PV$^+$) indicates the probability that a person with this test result has the health outcome. The predictive value of a normal, or negative, test result (PV$^-$) indicates the probability that a person with this test result does not have the health outcome (see Figure 9.4). This is also referred to as the posterior probability of the presence or absence of the health outcome, i.e. the likelihood once the test result is known. We can then compare this posterior probability with the prior probability of the health outcome, which is the same as the prevalence of the health outcome in the population (see Section 9.3.6). Case 9.1 illustrates this based on hypothetical data on how useful blood sugar levels are when diagnosing diabetes.

A higher prevalence of the health outcome in the population studied results in a higher positive predictive value and a lower negative predictive value. A lower prevalence results in a lower positive predictive value and a higher negative predictive value. This point has important consequences for the interpretation of diagnostic tests as it depends on the population the test is applied to (see Section 9.3.6).

The predictive value of a test is thus highly dependent on prevalence. Let's quantify this relationship: Table 9.5 shows the predictive values (PV$^+$ and PV$^-$) calculated for three different diagnostic tests (1: sensitivity = 0.90, specificity = 0.70; 2: sensitivity = 0.80, specificity = 0.90; 3: sensitivity = 0.70, specificity = 0.60) used in populations with different prevalence of the health outcome (P(O)). You can also calculate these values for yourself by using a hypothetical sample of, for example, 10,000 patients. The prevalence then determines the number of those with and without the health outcome, sensitivity and specificity, which are not dependent on prevalence, and can be used to complement all cells of a two-by-two table.

Figure 9.14 shows the relationship between the prevalence of the health outcome, the sensitivity and specificity of the test, and the predictive values of a positive or negative test result in graph form. The diagonal in the graph shows the situation for a test with both a sensitivity and a specificity of 50%. A test of this kind does not produce any information: we

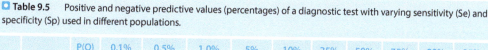

Table 9.5 Positive and negative predictive values (percentages) of a diagnostic test with varying sensitivity (Se) and specificity (Sp) used in different populations.

		P(O)	0.1%	0.5%	1.0%	5%	10%	25%	50%	75%	90%	95%	99%
Test 1	Se 90%	PV⁺	0.30	1.49	2.9	13.6	25.0	50.0	75.0	90.0	96.4	98.3	99.7
	Sp 70%	PV⁻	99.99	99.93	99.86	99.25	98.4	95.0	87.5	70.0	43.8	26.9	6.6
Test 2	Se 80%	PV⁺	0.79	0.79	7.5	29.3	47.1	72.7	88.9	96.0	98.6	99.4	99.9
	Sp 90%	PV⁻	99.98	99.98	99.78	98.84	97.6	93.1	81.8	60.0	33.3	19.2	4.4
Test 3	Se 70%	PV⁺	0.17	0.87	1.7	8.4	16.3	36.8	63.7	84.0	94.0	97.1	99.4
	Sp 60%	PV⁻	99.95	99.75	99.50	97.44	94.7	85.7	66.7	40.0	18.2	9.5	2.0

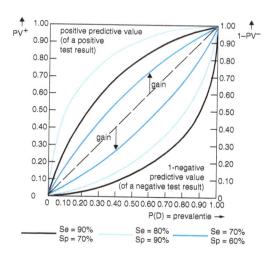

Figure 9.14 The effect of the prevalence of the disease and the sensitivity (Se) and specificity (Sp) of a test on the positive and negative predictive values of the test result.

know just as much after it as we did before it. Clearly, the predictive value of a positive test result increases the more common the health outcome is (i.e. increasing prevalence).

Another interesting point is that the test provides the most additional information in situations where the health outcome is common (prevalence = 20–80%). A test that performs moderately is generally less suited to detecting a condition in populations where that condition is rare. Nor is there much point in using a test of that kind on a population where virtually everyone has the condition. Most diagnostic tests produce the most information when used if there are indications that the health outcome is present, but they are not particularly strong. The degree of certainty needed regarding the presence of a health outcome to justify a treatment intervention based on the test result (the posterior probability) in fact differs from one health outcome to another, depending on the severity of the condition and the risks associated with the treatment.

One problem is that the information on the prevalence of the health outcome in the group to which a person belongs is often inadequate, in which case, a sensitivity analysis is called for. Broadly speaking, this involves calculating the PV⁺ and PV⁻ for various prevalence (prior probabilities) within the range in which the actual prevalence is likely to be found. We then examine whether the results obtained lead to different diagnostic or treatment decisions. In this case, then, sensitivity analysis is used to find out how sensitive a diagnostic or treatment strategy is to changes in the assumptions regarding the occurrence of the health outcome in the study population. Sensitivity analysis can also be used to examine the consequences of different assumptions regarding the sensitivity and specificity of a diagnostic test.

9.3.5 Bayes' theorem

Bayes' theorem can be very helpful to understand the relation between prevalence of an outcome, or prior probability, and predictive values, or posterior probabilities.

In effect, diagnosis is nothing more nor less than the estimation of likelihoods (the prior and posterior probability of the presence or absence of the health outcome). The aim of diagnostic tests is to reduce uncertainty in these estimates. ☐ Figure 9.15 shows the spectrum of diagnostic uncertainty.

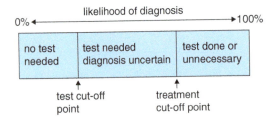

Figure 9.15 When is a diagnostic test required?

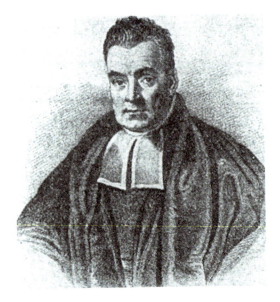

Figure 9.16 Thomas Bayes (1702–1761). Source: Unknown author / Wikimedia Commons / Public domain.

If there is no suspicion of the health outcome (low prior probability) or it is patently obvious that the health outcome is present (high prior probability) there is no point in carrying out further investigation. In the gray area of diagnostic uncertainty, a test can have added value: this is the range of indications for the test. The result of this test can be used to calculate the posterior probability, enabling health outcome probabilities to be better estimated and with less uncertainty. This is Bayes' theorem (see ◻ Figure 9.16).

Bayes' theorem states that the posterior probability of health outcome given a particular test result $P(O|T^x)$ can be calculated by multiplying the prior probability $P(O)$ by the additional evidence from the diagnostic test $P(T^x|O)/P(T^x)$.

As a formula:

$$P\left(O \,|\, T^x\right) = P\left(T^x \,|\, O \frac{P(O)}{P\left(T^x\right)}\right)$$

As we have already seen, the posterior probability is synonymous with the predictive value of a test (PV^x). If we replace the general test result T^x in the formula with a positive or negative test result, this brings us back to our classic measures of validity (sensitivity = Se and specificity = Sp):

$$P\left(O^+ \,|\, T^+\right) = P\left(T^+ \,|\, O^+\right) \times \frac{P\left(O^+\right)}{P\left(T^+\right)}$$

$$PV^+ = \frac{Se \times prev.}{\left(Se \times prev\right) + \left[\left(1 - Sp\right) \times \left(1 - prev\right)\right]}$$

$$P\left(O^- \,|\, T^-\right) = P\left(T^- \,|\, O^-\right) \times \frac{P\left(O^-\right)}{P\left(T^-\right)}$$

$$PV^- = \frac{Sp \times \left(1 - prev\right)}{\left[Sp \times \left(1 - prev\right)\right] + \left[\left(1 - Se\right) \times prev\right]}$$

In these formulas, we also notice that the PV of a test depends on the prevalence of the health outcome.

Further application of Bayes' theorem shows the relationship between the prevalence of the health outcome (the prior probability $P(O)$), the likelihood ratio (LR) and the predictive values of a test result (the posterior probability PV):

$$\frac{P(O)}{1 - P(O)} \times LR^+ = \frac{PV^+}{1 - PV^+}$$

And

$$\frac{P(O)}{1 - P(O)} \times LR^- = \frac{1 - PV^-}{PV^-}$$

Since (note that a similar derivation can be made for LR^-):

$$LR^+ = \frac{a / \left(a + c\right)}{b / \left(b + d\right)} = \frac{a \times \left(b + d\right)}{b \times \left(a + c\right)}$$

$$= \frac{a / \left(a + b\right)}{b / \left(a + b\right)} \times \frac{\left(b + d\right) / \left(a + b + c + d\right)}{\left(a + c\right) / \left(a + b + c + d\right)}$$

$$= \frac{PV^+}{1 - PV^+} \times \frac{1 - P(O)}{P(O)}$$

Generally speaking, the following is true of test result x (which is + or −):

$$\frac{P(O)}{1 - P(O)} \times LR^x = \frac{PV^x}{1 - PV^x}$$

9.3.6 Diagnostic odds ratio

Another way of examining diagnostic questions is to start from our familiar epidemiological function. The aim of epidemiological research into diagnostic questions is to estimate a function that describes, as accurately as possible, what diagnostic factors are related to the likelihood of the presence of a particular health outcome. For practical purposes, it is important to restrict the set of factors to a minimum to predict the probability of the outcome.

The diagnostic function indicates the likelihood of the presence of health outcome O (prevalence P(O)) in relation to the set of diagnostic factors D_i (symptoms, signs, tests, personal characteristics). Note that there are no confounders or effect modifiers in the diagnostic function, as it is a descriptive function, not an explanatory one.

Logistic functions are used mainly to describe the likelihood of the health outcome dependent on the diagnostic parameters.

$$P(O) = \frac{1}{1 + e^{-(b_0 + b_1 D_1 + b_2 D_2 + \cdots + b_k D_k)}}$$

This function covers a range from 0 to 1 and produces an S-shaped curve, with a sharp increase in probability in the middle.

In the model, P(O) represents the probability of the health outcome being present given a combination of diagnostic factors. b_0, b_1, b_2 etc. are weights that can be estimated based on the data, and D_1, D_2 etc. are the values for a set of diagnostic factors for a participant. From the function above, we can derive the following:

$$\ln\left[\frac{P(O)}{1 - P(O)}\right] = \ln \text{odds}(O)$$

From this, we can infer the following: for people who test positive for factor D_1 (value = 1) compared with people who test negative for factor D_1 (value = 0), with the values of all the other factors remaining the same, their relative increase in odds, expressed as odds ratio (OR), can be calculated as:

$$\frac{\text{odds}(O)}{\text{odds}(O)} = OR_1 = e^{b_i}$$

The contribution made by each relevant diagnostic factor can thus be estimated based on the logistic regression model. When diagnosing diabetes (Case 9.1), for example, we can use this approach to

◻ **Table 9.6**   Distribution of test scores (positive/negative) among persons with and without the health outcome.

	Health outcome +	Health outcome −
Test +	a	b
Test −	c	d
Total	a+c	b+d

examine the unique contribution of fasting blood sugar level, having considered factors such as age, the pattern of symptoms and waist-hip ratio.

Another measure of the validity of a test can easily be derived from the above, namely the diagnostic odds ratio (DOR). Just like the likelihood ratio, the DOR can also be used for tests with more than two outcome categories. The DOR reflects the added value of a diagnostic factor in a diagnostic function. It is, in fact, the diagnostic counterpart of the odds ratio that can be calculated in etiological research (see Section 3.2.4). There is a difference, however, in that the OR values regarded as relevant to a diagnostic factor are higher than for an etiological factor and the DOR does not permit interpretation in terms of causality. ◻ Table 9.6 shows the distribution of the test scores for a diagnostic test with regard to a hypothetical health outcome as a contingency table.

Here, the DOR is defined as the ratio between the odds of the health outcome for a positive test result (a/b) and the odds (c/d) of the health outcome for a negative test result.

$$DOR = \frac{\dfrac{a/(a+b)}{b/(a+b)}}{\dfrac{c/(c+d)}{d/(a+d)}} = \frac{\dfrac{a}{b}}{\dfrac{c}{d}} = \frac{ad}{bc}$$

Thus, the DOR combines the information contained in both the abnormal (positive) and normal (negative) test result. In Bayesian terminology, the odds of the health outcome are also referred to as the "posterior odds" since they are the odds once the result (positive/negative) is known.

$$DOR = \frac{\text{posterior odds}^+}{\text{posterior odds}^-}$$

The DOR also indicates the relationship between LR$^+$ and LR$^-$:

$$DOR = \frac{TP/FP}{FN/TN} = \frac{Se}{1-Se} \bigg/ \frac{1-Sp}{Sp}$$

$$= \frac{a/(a+c)}{c(a+c)} \Big/ \frac{b/(b+d)}{d(b+d)}$$

$$= \frac{(a/a+c)/(b/b+d)}{(c/a+c)/(d/b+d)} = \frac{LR^+}{LR^-}$$

A DOR of 1 indicates that the test does not discriminate between persons with and without the health outcome; a DOR of less than 1 means that the test is useless (a negative test result is more likely among people with the health outcome); a DOR of more than 1 means that the test is usable (a positive test result is more likely among people with the health outcome). A useful test has a high DOR but, unfortunately, it is not possible to indicate limits for this.

9.3.7 Multiple tests

The above discussion enables us to say what strategies can be used to improve the efficiency of the diagnostic process. There are two options: ensuring that the prevalence is high in the study population or using a combination of tests to detect the condition.

The prevalence of the health outcome in the study population (and hence the prior probability of the health outcome in the individual) can be influenced in various ways:

- Through referral: this increases cases in the segment of the healthcare system to which the referral takes place.
- By carrying out the diagnostic test selectively on people with certain demographic characteristics

such as age, sex, comorbidity, etc. (the likelihood of breast cancer is higher in older women than young women, for example).

- By targeting the diagnostic test on people with certain clinical characteristics (symptoms, signs, exposure to known risk factors); these are referred to as "indications" for carrying out a diagnostic test.

Combining two or more diagnostic tests is common in practice. The tests can be carried out in two ways, either in series or in parallel.

9.3.8.1 Serial Testing

Serial testing involves carrying out independent tests successively. The second test is only carried out on people who score positive for the first test. The following decision rules are usually used: the overall result is positive if both tests are positive; in all other cases, the result is negative. The net effect is a decrease in sensitivity and an increase in specificity of the combined tests compared with separate tests. The predictive value of a positive test result goes up, whereas that of a negative test result goes down (see ○ Figure 9.17).

Serial testing is indicated where:

- A test with high specificity is needed.
- Two or more alternative tests are available, each of which is insufficiently specific on its own.
- The wait time for the final test result is acceptable.

The procedure is most efficient if the test with the highest specificity is carried out first. On the other hand, it may be decided to give priority to the least

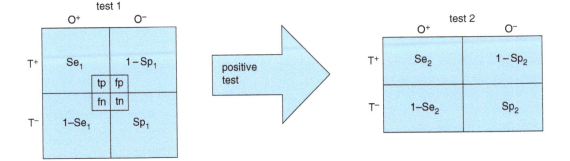

net specificity = $Se_1 \times Se_2$

net sensitivity = $Sp_1 + (1 - Sp_1) \times Sp_2$

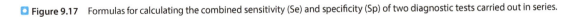

○ Figure 9.17 Formulas for calculating the combined sensitivity (Se) and specificity (Sp) of two diagnostic tests carried out in series.

Table 9.7 Using two diagnostic tests in series to detect diabetes.

A	First test 1, then test 2			B	First test 2, then test 1		
Test 1	Diabetes	No diabetes	Total	Test 2	Diabetes	No diabetes	Total
+	225	225	450	+	200	75	275
–	25	525	550	–	50	675	725
	250	750	1,000		250	750	1,000
Test 2	Diabetes	No diabetes	Total	Test 1	Diabetes	No diabetes	Total
+	180	22.5	202.5	+	180	22.5	202.5
–	45	202.5	247.5	–	20	52.5	72.5
	225	225	450		200	75	275
Test 1 + test 2	Diabetes	No diabetes	Total	Test 2 + test 1	Diabetes	No diabetes	Total
+	180	22.5	202.5	+	180	22.5	202.5
–	70	727.5	797.5	–	70	727.5	797.5
	250	750	1,000		250	750	1,000

Sensitivity = 72%	Sensitivity = 72%
Specificity = 97%	Specificity = 97%
PV⁻ = 91.22%	PV⁻ = 91.22%
Number of tests:	Number of tests:
1,000 (test 1) + 450 (test 2) = 1,450	1,000 (test 2) + 275 (test 1) = 1,275

invasive or least expensive procedure. ▫ Table 9.7 shows the hypothetical results of using two types of tests that independently measure the presence of diabetes in sequence (Test 1: sensitivity = 90%, specificity = 70%; Test 2: sensitivity = 80%, specificity = 90%).

9.3.8.2 Parallel testing

Parallel tests are independent tests carried out simultaneously on everyone in the study population. The following decision rules are often used: the overall result is positive if there is a positive result for at least one of the tests; the overall result is negative if the result of both tests is negative. If these rules are applied, the net effect is an increase in sensitivity and a decrease in specificity compared with those of each of the two separate tests. See ▫ Figure 9.18. The predictive value of a negative test result goes up, whereas that of a positive test result goes down.

Parallel testing is indicated where:

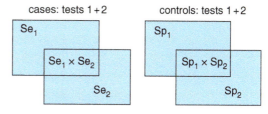

$$\text{net sensitivity} = Se_1 + Se_2 - (Se_1 \times Se_2)$$
$$\text{net specificity} = Sp_1 \times Sp_2$$

▫ **Figure 9.18** Formulas for calculating the sensitivity (Se) and specificity (Sp) of two diagnostic tests carried out in parallel.

- A sensitive test is required (i.e. where missing cases of the health outcome would have serious consequences).
- Two or more alternative tests are available, each of which is insufficiently sensitive on its own.
- The result of the test needs to be known quickly.

◻ **Table 9.8** Using two diagnostic tests in parallel to detect diabetes.

Test 1	Diabetes	No diabetes	Total	Test 2	Diabetes	No diabetes	Total
+	225	225	450	+	200	75	275
–	25	525	550	–	50	675	725
	250	750	1,000		250	750	1,000

Sensitivity = 90%   Sensitivity = 30%

Specificity = 70%   Specificity = 90%

PV^+ = 50% PV^+ = 72.73%

PV^- = 95.45% PV^- = 93.10%

P(O) = 25%   P(O) = 25%

Diabetics

Probability of positive result for both test 1 and test 2:	$0.9 \times 0.3 = 0.72$
Probability of positive result for test 1 and negative result for test 2:	$0.9 \times 0.2 = 0.13$
Probability of negative result for test 1 and positive result for test 2:	$0.1 \times 0.8 = 0.08$
Probability of negative result for both test 1 and test 2:	$0.1 \times 0.2 = 0.02$
Sensitivity of combined test	$(0.72 + 0.18 + 0.08)/1.00 = 0.98$

Non-diabetics

Probability of positive result for both test 1 and test 2:	$0.3 \times 0.1 = 0.03$
Probability of positive result for test 1 and negative result for test 2:	$0.3 \times 0.9 = 0.27$
Probability of negative result for test 1 and positive result for test 2:	$0.7 \times 0.1 = 0.07$
Probability of negative result for both test 1 and test 2:	$0.7 \times 0.9 = 0.63$
Specificity of combined test	$0.63/1.0 = 0.63$

Test 1 and test 2	Diabetes	No diabetes	Total	
+	245	277.5	5,225	sensitivity = 98%
–	5	472.5	477.5	specificity = 63%
	250	750	1,000	PV^+ = 46.89%
				PV^- = 98.95%

Parallel testing has the following disadvantages:
▪ Overdiagnosis (a larger number of false positives).
▪ Higher cost (everyone is subjected to two or more tests, whereas in serial testing only part of the study population need to take a second test).

◻ Table 9.8 illustrates the results of using two types of tests in parallel to independently measure the presence of diabetes (Test 1: sensitivity = 90%, specificity = 70%; Test 2: sensitivity = 80%, specificity = 90%).

9.4 Measures of reproducibility of diagnostic tests

Research into the reproducibility of diagnostic tests has shown that professionals' opinions of test results often differ. These differences manifest themselves not only during medical history-taking and physical examination but also, contrary to expectation, in examining and interpreting lab tests, which are often

		rater 2			
		normal test result	abnormal test result		
rater 1	normal test result	42	12		54
	abnormal test result	6	40		46
		48	52		1,000

a b
c d

$$\text{observed agreement} = \frac{\text{number of consistent observations}}{\text{total number of observations}} \times 100\%$$

$$= \frac{a + d}{a + b + c + d} \times 100\%$$

$$= \frac{42 + 40}{100} \times 100\% = 82\%$$

Figure 9.19 Calculating the observed inter-rater agreement on diagnostic tests (contingency table).

assumed to provide objective data. There are various measures to quantify the degree of consistency of a single rater (i.e. over repeated ratings) or multiple raters. The choice of which procedures and measures of association to use depends on the scale on which the diagnostic factor was measured.

9.4.1 Agreement rate

A commonly used measure is the agreement rate (between the first and second rating or the first and second rater). This is calculated mainly where there are two (or more) different test results possible (e.g. gallstones/no gallstones, no/mild/moderate/severe fatigue). Figure 9.19 illustrates the calculation of the agreement rate for a dichotomous test result, for example, a situation where two radiologists independently assess (as positive or negative) the mammograms of 100 women referred by their GP with suspected breast cancer.

The calculated agreement rate (82% in this case) is highly dependent on the prevalence of abnormal test results. In Figure 9.20, for example, the same two radiologists independently assess the mammograms of 1,000 women taking part in a breast cancer

screening program. The agreement rate is higher in this situation, even although the raters' opinions differ more often in absolute terms. The difference in agreement rate between this situation and the one in Figure 9.19 is due to the prevalence of abnormal test results in the study population, which was approximately 50% in the example depicted in Figure 9.19 and approximately 5% in the example shown in Figure 9.20.

9.4.2 Cohen's kappa

The agreement between the two ratings can be due partly to chance. Using the above examples (see Figures. 9.19 and 9.20), if rater 1 concludes that there is an abnormal test result in 46 of the 100 cases and rater 2 finds that 52 of the 100 mammograms are abnormal, hypothetically, chance alone could cause rater 2 to classify as abnormal 52% of the 46 mammograms regarded as abnormal by rater 1. The remaining 48% will be diagnosed as normal. Likewise, rater 2 will record 52% of the 54 mammograms rated as normal by rater 1 as abnormal and 48% as normal (see Figure 9.21). In other words, both raters could agree in half of the cases purely based on chance alone.

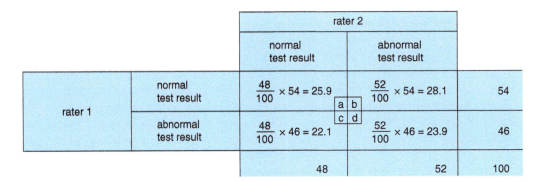

	rater 2		
	normal test result	abnormal test result	
rater 1 — normal test result	932	22	954
rater 1 — abnormal test result	16	30	46
	948	52	1,000

$$\text{observed agreement} = \frac{a+d}{a+b+c+d} \times 100\%$$

$$= \frac{932+30}{1{,}000} \times 100\% = 96.2\%$$

Figure 9.20 Calculating the observed inter-rater agreement on diagnostic tests (contingency table).

	rater 2		
	normal test result	abnormal test result	
rater 1 — normal test result	$\frac{48}{100} \times 54 = 25.9$	$\frac{52}{100} \times 54 = 28.1$	54
rater 1 — abnormal test result	$\frac{48}{100} \times 46 = 22.1$	$\frac{52}{100} \times 46 = 23.9$	46
	48	52	100

$$\text{expected agreement} = \frac{a+d}{a+b+c+d} \times 100\%$$

$$= \frac{25.9+23.9}{100} \times 100\% = 49.8\%$$

Figure 9.21 Calculating the expected agreement rate based solely on chance between two ratings or raters on a diagnostic test (contingency table).

Cohen's kappa is a measure of inter-rater and intra-rater agreement that indicates actual agreement as a proportion of potential agreement after correcting for chance agreement (see Figure 9.22).

In the example, therefore, the kappa is:

$$\frac{82\% - 49.8\%}{100\% - 49.8\%} = 0.64$$

Cohen's kappa normally has values between 0 (solely chance agreement) and 1 (perfect agreement). Agreement of 0.80 or more is regarded as strong inter-rater or intra-rater agreement, whereas agreement of 0.40 or less is regarded as low (see Table 9.9).

In clinical practice, however, diagnostic tests with a kappa of the order of 0.40–0.70 are common. It is theoretically possible that two raters agree less often

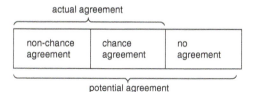

$$kappa = \frac{\% \text{ actual (observed) agreement} - \% \text{ chance agreement}}{\% \text{ potential (full) agreement} - \% \text{ chance agreement}}$$

Figure 9.22 Kappa.

Table 9.9 Interpreting Cohen's kappa.

Value of Cohen's kappa	Agreement interpretation
<0.20	None
0.21–0.39	Minimal
0.40–0.59	Poor
0.60–0.79	Moderate
0.80–0.90	Strong
>0.90	Almost perfect

than expected based on chance, in which case, the kappa is negative. Although kappa, as a relative measure of agreement between two raters or two ratings, considers the fact that the absolute agreement is due partly to chance, there are still some difficulties when interpreting it. Kappa depends on the number of rating categories (strata): the more strata, the smaller the kappa (this is also true for the agreement rate) and also depends on the prevalence of the outcome. For these reasons, and the difficulty of interpreting kappa, it has been suggested to report specific agreement, which is the agreement rate for positive and the negative test results separately. Specific agreement for a positive test result can be computed for the example as:

$$specific\ agreement^{+} = \frac{2d}{2d+b+c} * 100\%$$

$$= \frac{2*40}{2*40+12+6} * 100\% = 81.6\%$$

Conversely, specific agreement for a negative test result can be computed as:

$$specific\ agreement^{-} = \frac{2a}{2a+b+c} * 100\%$$

$$= \frac{2*42}{2*42+12+6} * 100\% = 82.4\%$$

9.4.3 Correlation coefficient

To determine the reproducibility of a diagnostic test with a continuous result, the first step is to make a scatter plot of the results of the two measurements against each other. If the measurement is reproducible, virtually all the points will be on a straight line passing through the origin (the place where both the x-axis and y-axis are zero) at an angle of 45°. The further the cloud is from that line, the less reproducible the measurement is. From this, we can derive the following agreement rates for continuous variables:

- Pearson's correlation coefficient (r) is a measure of the density of the cloud (see also Section 3.3.2). A correlation coefficient of 1 is obtained if all points would fall on a line, with no "cloud" to be seen. Note that the line does not need to go through the origin or need to have a slope of one. The lower the correlation coefficient, the poorer the reproducibility, with a value of zero indicating complete lack of correlation. The correlation coefficient does not take systematic differences between raters into account, however. If, for example, one rater systematically measures values exactly twice as high as the other observer, the correlation coefficient is still 1, but the two observers are not in agreement. Values from one rater can be perfectly calculated by knowing the value from the other rater. Also, Pearson's correlation coefficient is sensitive to the distribution of the values on the x and y-axes: an extreme value for both measurements increases the correlation coefficient dramatically. A scatter plot should therefore always be made to look at the underlying distribution. A version of the correlation coefficient that is not sensitive to extreme values (Spearman's) can be used if necessary.
- A Bland–Altman plot (see Figure 9.23) visualizes the agreement between two series of observations of a parameter measured on a continuous scale. A Bland–Altman plot can be used for a comparison of two different measuring instruments (A and B), or a comparison of the results from repeat use of the same measuring instrument (A1, A2) on a number of participants. The Bland–Altman plot plots the difference between the two measurements (e.g. A–B) against the mean value of the two measurements ([A+B]/2) for every participant. The individual difference scores are expressed in the same

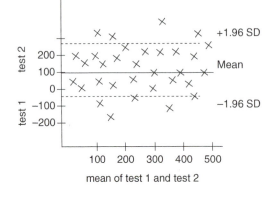

Figure 9.23 Bland–Altman plot.

dimension as the measurements. The mean difference is the estimated bias, and the standard deviation of the differences measures the random fluctuations around this mean. Assuming a normal distribution, approximately 95% of the differences found will be between the mean difference score ± approximately 2× the standard deviation of the individual difference scores. If the differences within mean ± approximately 2× the standard deviation are not clinically important, the two methods or two measures may be used interchangeably. As a way of determining the reproducibility and agreement of measurements of a continuous parameter, the Bland–Altman plot does away with some of the limitations of Pearson's correlation coefficient (r), as it shows any systematic measuring errors (the mean difference score) and provides a better picture of the size of intra-individual differences in results.

The intra-class correlation coefficient (ICC) of agreement also overcomes the problem with Pearson's correlation coefficient (r) that it does not take systematic measuring differences into account: the ICC agreement only takes on the maximum value (i.e. 1) if the test results correspond precisely at the individual level. The other problems with Pearson's r – dependency on the spread of the test results and high sensitivity to outliers – also apply to the ICC agreement, however.

9.5   Guidelines for diagnostic research

Various checklists have been developed for assessing the methodological rigor of diagnostic research. They are used in systematic reviews of diagnostic studies

and also serve as references when designing new diagnostic studies. The QUADAS-2 tool is an example of a checklist of this kind in common use. STARD guidelines (the latest version dated 2015) should be followed when reporting diagnostic research. Over 200 scientific journals require diagnostic studies to be reported in line with STARD guidelines. The STARD guidelines require a flow diagram showing the study design and the flow of participants. They also include a checklist of items with which a scientific article on diagnostic research should comply.

9.6   Prognostic research

Questions concerning the expected course of a disease differ from diagnostic questions, but the aim is the same: to produce information for healthcare providers and patients to take actions. Prognosis has a lot in common with diagnosis as described earlier in this chapter. The main difference is the dimension of time. Prognosis is about changes over time, whereas diagnosis is about what is going on right now. As it is often much more difficult to say something about a patient's prognosis compared to the presence or absence of a health outcome at that time, prognostic research generally involves not one single test but a set of prognostic factors (e.g. test outcomes, patient characteristics, disease characteristics, etc.) combined into a model. As stated in the introduction, we only discuss prognostic prediction models in this chapter, where causality or the effects of interventions are not considered.

9.6.1   Prognostic research phases

In prognostic research, the first step is to single out a set of potential prognostic factors to be studied. This may be achieved by summarizing previous literature on prognostic factors or earlier attempts to develop a prediction model. A more evidence-based approach is to perform a systematic review on previous studies (see Chapter 11). Next, the model is developed using regression models (usually logistic regression for binary outcomes or Cox proportional hazards regression for time-to-event outcomes), but other models, such as machine learning algorithms are also used. Often, the performance of a model in future patients is then tested internally using the same data as the model was developed on, such as cross-validation or bootstrapping. This is called internal validation. An important phase before adoption of the model, regardless of whether an internal validation has been performed, is external validation. In this crucial phase, the model is applied to data of participants that were not used for model development to assess how the model would perform in future patients. The last phase, which is unfortunately still relatively rare in prognostic research, is an impact study to assess whether the use of the model has the intended effect (e.g. whether patients benefit from implementation of the model).

9.6.2 Prognostic research design

To predict the prognosis of a condition or state of health for an individual, in terms of the probability of developing the health outcome of interest (e.g. death, complications, cure), similar patients from a similar setting who are at risk of developing that outcome will need to be followed over time. The cohort of participants will provide data to estimate the incidence of that outcome, and to assess what characteristics are associated with the occurrence and can be used as prognostic factors in the model. We can deduct from this that prognostic research generally takes the form of a cohort study, with the cohort consisting of people with the condition or state of health for which we want to learn the prognosis, but who are still at risk of developing the outcome. Such research only yields useful information if all prognostic factors of the members of the cohort are collected at the start of the follow-up. The use of an inception cohort (i.e. a cohort of participants that are followed from a similar point in time, e.g. diagnosis of a condition) is preferred, and all prognostic factors are measured at the time of inclusion into the cohort (e.g. the time of diagnosis). This brings us back to our familiar epidemiological function which, in this case, describes the incidence of future outcome as a function of prognostic factors. If the outcome variable (O) is a stage of disease and we wish to know the incidence of developing this outcome for an individual, the function will take the form of a logistic function with a linear set of predictors D_i:

$$P(O) = \frac{1}{1 + e^{-(b_0 + b_1 D_1 + b_2 D_2 + \cdots + b_k D_k)}}$$

Suitably modified models can be used for other types of outcomes (continuous health parameters or length of survival).

Case 9.2 provides an example of a prediction model developed to predict successful vaginal delivery after previous Cesarean section. Like diagnostic functions, a prognostic model can include prognostic factors of various domains: symptoms and signs, results of lab and other tests, and characteristics of the people. These factors must be available to be measured at the start of the follow-up, i.e. when the question of the prognosis arises, as that would be the intended setting of the prediction model.

A historical cohort can also be used for prognostic research, but this presupposes that all sorts of factors that we want to include in the function have already been measured and recorded or can still be ascertained. This is not usually possible in the case of many prognostic factors, in which case, we shall have to fall back on a prospective cohort study. If all prognostic factors have been measured, but not for all participants of the cohort, data imputation techniques may be helpful to complete the data.

The prognostic factors and the outcome must be measured accurately (validly and precisely) and independently of one another. In other words, we must not be influenced consciously or unconsciously by knowledge of the prognostic factors when determining the outcome. The converse also applies when using historical data, i.e. we must not be guided by knowledge of the outcome when assessing the prognostic factors.

Case 9.2 Prediction of Successful Vaginal Delivery after Previous Cesarean Section

To help counsel pregnant women who had a previous Cesarean section (CS) to choose between an intended vaginal birth (i.e. a trial of labor, or TOL) and an elective repeat CS, a prediction model was developed to predict the probability of a successful vaginal delivery. Compared with a vaginal delivery, elective CS is associated with more complications and longer recovery. However, an unsuccessful TOL would result in an emergency CS, which is associated with even higher risks of major complications, such as hysterectomy and operative injury.

The initial model was developed using logistic regression on a cohort of women recruited through

US academic medical centers. The prognostic factors contained in the model are shown in ☐ Table 9.10. The area under the receiver operating characteristic curve (AUC) of the model was 75.4%. The model was subsequently externally validated for usage in the US. It was unclear how this model would translate to Western European women because of significant differences in CS rates between the two regions and the lack of relevance of predictors related to ethnicity (being African-American or Hispanic). The model was also therefore externally validated in a Western European cohort. After external validation, the AUC was reduced to 68%. This could be due to the aforementioned differences between regions, but also to overfitting of the initial model that may have resulted in optimistic measures of performance (see Section 9.6.3).

To overcome this problem, a new prediction model was developed on a Western European cohort. To reduce overfitting, predictors were selected based on previously published evidence and expert opinion instead of statistical significance. ☐ Table 9.10 shows the predictors selected for the model and their regression coefficients. The AUC of the model was 70.8%, which was considerably lower than in the US model in the derivation cohort. This could be due to large differences in patient management between regions which could have resulted in different selection mechanisms for each cohort.

☐ **Table 9.10** Regression coefficients[a] for predictor variables in two prediction models for successful vaginal delivery in women with a previous Cesarean section (CS).

Predictor variable	United States model (intercept: 3766)	Western European model (intercept: 1876)
Age (years)	−0.039	
Prepregnancy body mass index (kg/m^2)	−0.060	−0.041
African-American (yes)	−0.671	
Hispanic (yes)	−0.680	
Any prior vaginal delivery (yes)	0.888	1.339
Vaginal delivery after prior (yes)	1.003	
Recurrent indication for cs (yes)	0.632	
White ethnicity (yes)		0.476
Previous CS for non-progressive labor (yes)		−0.688
Induction of labor (yes)		−0.660
Expected fetal weight ≥ 90th percentile (yes)		−0.624

[a] Positive coefficients correspond to a higher probability of a successful vaginal delivery after a previous Cesarean section. The coefficients combined with the model intercept could be used to compute a woman's individual probability of successful vaginal delivery using the logistic function.

9.6.3 The prognostic model

Practical problems arise when collecting data for a prognostic study. For example, a complete follow-up cannot be obtained for all the members of the study population (censoring), or useful information has not been obtained on all the potential prognostic factors for all the members of the cohort (missing values). Assuming that this hurdle has been overcome (e.g. the correct model has been chosen to allow for censoring, or missing data have been imputed), and all the data required to estimate the epidemiological function are available, creating the prognostic model is the next step. We create a multivariable model containing all the promising prognostic factors. The final stage is to reduce the model to obtain one that is as parsimonious as possible but can still predict the probability of the outcome accurately. The criterion applied here is that a prognostic factor can be omitted from the model if the prognostic value of the model as a whole is not reduced to any noticeable extent by the omission. The prognostic value of the model as a whole can be assessed – like that of a diagnostic study – from the AUC of the ROC curve (see Section 9.3.2).

As with diagnostic tests, the prognostic value of a parameter or test can be determined separately. Just as with the DOR (Section 9.3.7) we can calculate a prognostic odds ratio (POR) and a likelihood ratio (see Section 9.3.3). Given the nature of the question, we are particularly interested in the prognostic value (PV) of a particular result (see Section 9.6.3). The calculations are similar, as are the problems that arise when interpreting these parameters.

9.6.4 Overfitting

When interpreting the performance of a prediction model, as with PVs, we shall remember that model performance is highly dependent on the composition of the population on which the prognostic model is used. If, as recommended in this chapter, we opt for an approach in which all the relevant prognostic information is assembled in a multivariable model, we need to remember that this model is mainly suited for the population for which it was developed. The performance of the model will usually be less if we apply the same model to a different, but comparable population. Moreover, the performance of a model is generally less when it is applied in practice compared to the performance in the development cohort (and hence, why external validation is so important). This overestimation of the performance is due to chance variability in the distribution of parameters in the development cohort, and their association with the outcome, which may influence both predictor selection as well as the value of the regression coefficients that are used to compute an individual patient's probability of the health outcome. The regression coefficients in a different cohort from the same underlying population will therefore generally be slightly different, and a model will perform worse if we apply the model to new patients. This problem of optimism in model performance is worse in situations in which the model has been overfitted. Overfitting occurs when too many prognostic factors are used in the development phase, or too few participants are at our disposal. It can be solved by externally validating the model. In an external validation, the model is applied to a cohort of new patients not included in the development cohort. Subsequently, performance of the prediction model,

such as the AUC, is computed. If this corresponds closely to the performance on the development cohort, the model has demonstrated external validity and can be used with confidence on patients whose prognosis is not yet known. If the prognostic value of the model as a whole differs substantially from the original model, we can use the data about the validation cohort to see whether the model can be improved. The new model will then need to be validated again on new cohorts (see also Case 9.2).

9.7 Guidelines for prognostic research

The Prediction model Risk Of Bias ASsessment Tool, or PROBAST, can be used to assess the risk of bias and applicability of prediction models. This tool can be particularly helpful in deciding whether a published model is of sufficient quality and can be applied to the target population of interest. Just as the QUADAS-2 risk of bias tool is used for diagnostic research, PROBAST is often used in systematic reviews of prediction models.

Guidelines for reporting the development or validation of a prediction model can be found in the Transparent Reporting of a multivariable prediction model for Individual Prognosis Or Diagnosis (TRIPOD) statement. TRIPOD offers different checklists for model development, model validation, as well as combined development and validation.

9.8 An example

To conclude this chapter and illustrate the theory discussed herein, we present an example of diagnostic research. Case 9.3 shows how a well-designed study can demonstrate the limited value of a diagnostic test with the aid of an uncontroversial gold standard.

Case 9.3 Diagnostic Competence of the Alvarado Score for the Diagnosis of Appendicitis in Children

The Alvarado score is a diagnostic tool that combines signs, symptoms, and laboratory results for the diagnosis of appendicitis (see ◻ Table 9.11). In children, appendicitis is the major cause of abdominal pain and the most common indication for emergency abdominal surgery. In cases of suspected appendicitis, imaging techniques such as ultrasound and CT scanning can be used in addition to physical examination and laboratory testing. However, these imaging techniques are costly and may increase the time to final diagnosis due to variable availability, especially in low-resource countries. If accurate enough, the Alvarado score could guide patient management by helping physicians to decide which patients need surgery without the need for imaging.

A prospective observational study was performed among 588 children between 3 and 21 years of age (with a median age of 11.9 years) with abdominal pain suggestive of appendicitis. The final diagnosis was established either by the pathological report in case of surgery or by clinical review after two weeks of follow-up. This combination is regarded as the gold standard for both ruling in and ruling out appendicitis. The Alvarado scores of the participating children were not provided to the participating physicians, rendering them blind to the score's result. Of all the children suspected of appendicitis, 197 (33.5%) were ultimately diagnosed with this disease. An Alvarado score of 7 or higher has been published as the cut-off value to diagnose appendicitis and recommend surgery. Using this cut-off value yielded a sensitivity of 72.1% and a specificity of 80.8% (◻ Table 9.11). Considering the treatment is invasive surgery, the number of false-positive test results (75 out of 217 test-positives) is high, resulting in a relatively low positive predictive value. Of all the test-positive children, only about 65.4% actually had appendicitis. If the Alvarado score alone were to be used for decision-making, 34.6% of test-positives would be overtreated and would undergo unnecessary surgery. The score performs better at ruling out appendicitis, as indicated by the higher negative predictive value. However, 55 out of 371 children that scored below 7 on the Alvarado score were still falsely classified as test negative. When using the score to determine who is in need of surgical removal of the appendix, 15% of all test-negatives would not receive the necessary treatment in time. Therefore, the Alvarado score alone cannot be used to decide the need for surgery, emphasizing the importance of imaging techniques in diagnosing children with suspected appendicitis.

◻ **Table 9.11** The Alvarado score is calculated as the sum of the scores of the features that occur in a patient.

Feature	Score
Abdominal pain that migrates to the right iliac fossa	1
Anorexia (loss of appetite) or ketones in the urine	1
Nausea or vomiting	1
Tenderness in the right iliac fossa	2
Rebound tenderness	1
Fever of 37.3 °C or more	1
Leukocytosis or >10,000 white blood cells per ml	2
Neutrophilia >75%	1

◻ **Table 9.12** Distribution of Alvarado scores (test positive/test negative) among children with abdominal pain, prospectively reviewed for appendicitis.

Alvarado score	Appendicitis Yes	No	Total
≥7	142	75	217
<7	55	316	371
Total	197	391	588

Prevalence = 197/588 = 33.5%

Percentage with correct diagnosis = (142 + 316) / 588 = 77.9%

Sensitivity = 142/197 = 72.1%

Specificity = 316/391 = 80.8%

Positive predictive value = 142/217 = 65.4%

Negative predictive value = 316/371 = 85.2%

Positive likelihood ratio = (142/197)/(75/391) = 3.76

Negative likelihood ratio = (55/197)/(316/391) = 0.35

Recommended reading

Bland, M. (2015). *An Introduction to Medical Statistics*, 4e. New York: Oxford University Press.

Fletcher, R.H., Fletcher, S.W., and Fletcher, G.S. (2012). *Clinical Epidemiology: The Essentials*, 5e. Baltimore: Lippincott, Williams & Wilkins.

Grobbee, D.E. and Hoes, A.W. (2015). *Clinical Epidemiology: Principles, Methods, and Applications for Clinical Research*, 2e. Burlington: Jones and Bartlett Learning.

Harrell, F.E. Jr. (2015). *Regression Modeling Strategies. With Applications to Linear Models, Logistic and Ordinal Regression, and Survival Analysis*, 2e. New York: Springer.

Haynes, R.B., Sackett, D.L., Guyatt, G.H., and Tugwell, P. (2005). *Clinical Epidemiology: How to Do Clinical Practice Research*, 3e. Philadelphia: Lippincott, Williams & Wilkins.

McDowell, I. (2006). *Measuring Health: A Guide to Rating Scales and Questionnaires*. New York: Oxford University Press.

Newman, T.B. and Kohn, M.A. (2020). *Evidence-Based Diagnosis*, 2e. New York: Cambridge University Press.

Steyerberg, E.W. (2019). *Clinical Prediction Models: A Practical Approach to Development, Validation, and Updating*, 2e. New York: Springer.

Streiner, D.L. and Norman, G.R. (2014). *Health Measurement Scales: A Practical Guide to their Development and Use*, 5e. New York: Oxford University Press.

de Vet, H.C.W., Terwee, C.B., Mokkink, L.B., and Knol, D.L. (2011). *Measurement in Medicine: a Practical Guide*. Cambridge: Cambridge University Press.

Zhou, X.-H., Obuchowski, N.A., and McClish, D.K. (2011). *Statistical Methods in Diagnostic Medicine*, 2e. Hoboken: Wiley.

Source reference (cases)

Schoorel, E.N.C., Melman, S., van Kuijk, S.M.J. et al. (2014). Predicting successful intended vaginal delivery after previous caesarean section: external validation of two predictive models in a Dutch nationwide registration-based cohort with a high intended vaginal delivery rate. *BJOG* (Case 9.2).

Schneider, C., Kharbanda, A., and Bachur, R. (2007). Evaluating appendicitis scoring systems using a prospective pediatric cohort. *Annals of Emergency Medicine* (Case 9.3).

Knowledge assessment questions

1. From the local health authorities, you have received data of 800 participants of a study on the validity of an at-home rapid COVID-19 test kit. Participants with complaints of COVID-19 presenting at a drive-through testing site were asked to read the test kit manual and perform the at-home test in addition to the standard polymerase chain reaction (PCR) test performed by a healthcare professional. Of all participants, 187 had a positive PCR test, 128 had a positive at-home test. Only four participants had a positive at-home test, but a negative PCR test.

   a. Construct a 2×2 table and compute sensitivity and specificity of the at-home test using the PCR test as reference test. Interpret sensitivity and specificity in your own words.

   b. Compute PV^+ and PV^-. How much do the posterior probabilities (i.e. PV^+ and PV^-) differ from the prior probability (prevalence)?

   c. Given the sensitivity and specificity computed for 1a, how would PV^+ and PV^- change if the at-home test were applied in a population with a prior probability (prevalence) of COVID-19 of 1%? Verify your answer by calculating PV^+ and PV^- for a hypothetical sample of, e.g. 10,000 participants by constructing another 2×2 table given a prevalence of 1%.

   d. Compute the likelihood ratio of a positive and a negative test result using the 2×2 table of 1a. How would these change if the at-home test were applied in a population with a prior probability of COVID-19 of 1%?

2. To test reproducibility of axillary ultrasound to detect advanced axillary nodal disease in breast cancer patients, two observers rated 100 ultrasound images independent from each other. The following 2×2 table resulted from the study:

		Observer 1	
		positive	Negative
Observer 2	positive	40	10
	negative	17	33
			100

   a. Compute the agreement rate for the two observers and interpret it in your own words.

   b. Compute Cohen's kappa. What was the expected agreement based on chance alone?

   c. Compute the specific agreement for both positive and negative test results. Why are some cells counted twice in the computation?

3. As an obstetrician, you are interested in applying the prediction model for successful vaginal delivery in women with a previous cesarian section (see ◨ Table 9.10).

   a. Compute the probability of a successful vaginal delivery for a 28-year-old Hispanic woman with a body mass index of 21, who has never had a previous vaginal delivery, with no recurrent indication for a cesarian section.

   b. Would her probability of a successful vaginal delivery be lower or higher if she had a body mass index of 32 instead of 21? How can you know this using the information from ◨ Table 9.12?

   c. Using the regression coefficient for body mass index from ◨ Table 9.12, what is the odds ratio for each increase of 1 BMI-point? Interpret the odds ratio in your own words.

Intervention

Textbook of Epidemiology, Second Edition. Lex Bouter, Maurice Zeegers and Tianjing Li.
© 2023 John Wiley & Sons Ltd. Published 2023 by John Wiley & Sons Ltd.
Companion website: www.wiley.com/go/Bouter/TextbookofEpidemiology

10.1 Introduction

Has a preventive or therapeutic intervention actually achieved its intended effect? And if it has, was that because of the intervention? These are questions of cause and effect (see Chapter 6). This chapter discusses research into the outcomes of interventions that aim to have a beneficial effect on the occurrence or course of a disease, for example, vaccinations, drugs, surgical interventions, dietary changes, lifestyle and behavioral interventions, and environmental measures such as reducing air pollution or occupational risks. Note that interventions can also be associated with undesirable effects such as complications and adverse events.

Intervention studies focus primarily on the effect of interventions. As we want to establish a causal relationship between the change in health outcome and the intervention itself, we will need to take into account all the other factors that affect the health outcome in the study, and therefore in the epidemiological function:

$$P(O) = f(F_i)$$

where F_1 is the intervention and F_2, F_3, ... F_k represents the other explanatory factors of the outcome (confounders). Research into the effects of interventions is usually experimental and randomized: participants – generally patients – undergo an intervention with the aim of answering the scientific question about the benefits and harms of the intervention.

10.2 The research question

Randomized controlled trials (RCTs) can be used to answer whether an intervention is more effective than no treatment, a placebo, or another intervention (that is the comparative effectiveness of two active interventions). It is not just a question of whether the new intervention works better than the reference intervention in real life, but also whether the amount of improvement is worth the costs (cost-effectiveness). This leads us to three considerations:

1. What interventions will be compared? A new intervention will often be compared with the current standard intervention. It goes without saying that it is important to describe precisely in the trial protocol and the final report of the trial what the intervention entails (dosage/intensity, mode of delivery, personnel who deliver it, frequency, duration or timing of delivery, etc.), so that it can be replicated in future research and used in practice, if so desired. Some complex interventions, in rehabilitation or mental health care, for instance, are difficult to standardize, but have to be tailored to patients. A treatment protocol describing these adaptations will be critical to ensure the interventions are delivered as intended.

2. To which patients or populations are the interventions being given? Predefined, unambiguous eligibility criteria are a fundamental prerequisite of an RCT. Eligibility criteria, comprised of both inclusion and exclusion criteria, will determine the composition of the source population. In Case 10.1, for instance, the source population was restricted to hospitalized patients with clinically suspected or laboratory-confirmed SARS-CoV-2 infection, including pregnant or breast-feeding women.

3. Although decreasing generalizability, restricting the source population by age, gender or other prognostic factors improves homogeneity in the study sample, which, in return, will reduce the variability in the estimated effects of the interventions. If the effects are likely to be substantially different in subgroups of patients (effect modification), they will need to be studied and reported separately for each subgroup. Understanding the subgroup effects may be highly desirable by patients and providers, but it requires a much bigger sample size and therefore it is not often done in practice. Most intervention studies aim to estimate "average" effects in "standard" patients.

4. What are the relevant outcomes? The primary outcome follows the main claim for the intervention under investigation and is used for determining the sample size for a trial. A completely specified outcome (regardless of whether it's a primary or a secondary outcome) includes the: (i) domain (e.g. depression); (ii) specific measurement used to assess the outcome (e.g. Beck Depression Inventory); (iii) specific metric used to characterize each participant's results (e.g. change from baseline); (iv) method of aggregation of data within each trial arm (e.g. mean); and (v) time-points of assessment (e.g. 3 months after randomization). The choice of outcomes should be meaningful to all stakeholders: patients, clinicians, policymakers, payers, and others. Unfortunately, due to practical reasons, the outcomes chosen in trials are not

necessarily the most objective or most patient-centered outcomes. For example, quality of life, one type of patient-reported outcomes, may be a more important measure of the effect of a vascular procedure than the extent to which the arteries are actually widened. In Case 10.1, 28-day mortality was the primary outcome measure. Secondary outcomes included time until discharge from the hospital, subsequent receipt of invasive mechanical ventilation or death (among those who did not receive invasive mechanical ventilation at the time of randomization).

Case 10.1 The Effect of Dexamethasone in Hospitalized Patients with COVID-19 (Excerpt from the Abstract)

Coronavirus disease 2019 (COVID-19) is associated with diffuse lung damage. Glucocorticoids may modulate inflammation-mediated lung injury and thereby reduce progression to respiratory failure and death. In an RCT, the investigators randomly assigned patients (i) to receive usual care plus oral or intravenous dexamethasone (at a dose of 6 mg once daily) for up to 10 days, or (ii) to receive usual care alone. Hospitalized patients were eligible for the trial if they had clinically suspected or laboratory-confirmed COVID-19 infection and no medical history that might, in the opinion of the attending clinician, put patients at substantial risk if they were to participate in the trial.

The primary outcome was all-cause mortality within 28 days after randomization. Secondary outcomes were the time until discharge from the hospital and, among patients not receiving invasive mechanical ventilation at the time of randomization, subsequent receipt of invasive mechanical ventilation (including extracorporeal membrane oxygenation) or death.

A total of 2,104 patients were assigned to receive usual care plus dexamethasone and 4,321 to receive usual care only. Overall, 482 patients (22.9%) in the dexamethasone group and 1110 patients (25.7%) in the usual care group died within 28 days after randomization (age-adjusted hazard ratio [HR], 0.83; 95% confidence interval [CI], 0.75–0.93. The proportional and absolute between-group differences in mortality varied considerably according to the level of respiratory support that the patients were receiving at the time of randomization. In the dexamethasone group, the incidence of death was lower than that in the usual care group among patients receiving invasive mechanical ventilation (29.3% vs. 41.4%; HR, 0.64; 95% CI, 0.51–0.81) and among those receiving oxygen without invasive mechanical ventilation (23.3% vs. 26.2%; HR, 0.82; 95% CI, 0.72–0.94) but not among those who were receiving no respiratory support at randomization (17.8% vs. 14.0%; HR, 1.19; 95% CI, 0.91–1.55). In conclusion, in patients hospitalized with COVID-19, the use of dexamethasone resulted in lower 28-day mortality among those who were receiving either invasive mechanical ventilation or oxygen alone at randomization but not among those receiving no respiratory support.

The trial was funded by the Medical Research Council and National Institute for Health Research and others. The trial was registered with ClinicalTrials.gov (registration number: NCT04381936); the trial protocol and statistical analysis plan were published alongside the manuscript reporting the preliminary results.

Careful preparation and coordination are required to carry out an RCT. Special attention should be paid to the following points:

- A detailed trial protocol setting out the entire plan of the study. Key steps to minimize the risk of bias should be carefully considered and articulated in the protocol. Important elements in the procedures need to be tested beforehand. The minimal items that should be included in a trial protocol are described in the SPIRIT guideline and checklist, available from the EQUATOR network's website.
- A carefully planned strategy for recruiting participants, which includes a realistic recruitment plan and goal. Researchers often tend to overestimate their ability to recruit participants.
- The study personnel who will be recruiting participants and carrying out the interventions should be involved at an early stage. The trial will only be successful if they make efforts to recruit eligible

participants and provide them the intervention in line with the protocol.

- An ethics committee should assess the ethical and methodological aspects of the research proposal. The principle underlying the consent procedure is that people can decide to participate after being informed adequately about the trial.
- The proposed trial should be registered before the start of data collection. The major clinical journals require trials submitted for publication to be registered in an international trial register (e.g. clinicaltrials.gov) before they commence. The purpose of publishing the trial protocol in the register in advance is to prevent selective reporting and to assure replicability of the study.
- When the trial ends, guidelines for reporting trial results, e.g. the CONSORT guidelines, should be followed (see Section 4.2.1).

The decision to approve a pharmaceutical product is almost always based on data from RCTs. Drug development, the process of bringing a new pharmaceutical product to the market, is strictly regulated, for example, by the Food and Drug Administration in the United States and the European Medicines Agency in Europe. Drug development begins in the laboratory by identifying promising chemicals or compounds; these chemicals and compounds then undergo laboratory and animal testing to answer basic questions about safety (the pre-clinical phase). They are then tested on people to make sure they are safe and effective through the following phases:

- Phase I research, where small doses of a drug candidate are tested in a small number of healthy volunteers. The primary purpose of a Phase I study is to evaluate the safety of a drug candidate before it proceeds to further clinical studies. In addition to safety, researchers usually also measure how much is in the blood after administration, how the drug works in the body, and the side effects associated with increased dosage.
- Phase II research, which uses a relatively larger group of participants with the disease of interest (dozens up to a few hundred) to determine the optimal dose or doses of a drug candidate. The researchers also look at adverse and other biological effects to maximize possible benefits while minimizing risks. These trials are almost always blinded and randomized, and often concern a comparison with a placebo drug. Efficacy is not usually demonstrated convincingly in this phase, as the researchers generally focus on intermediate or surrogate outcomes.

- Phase III research, usually consists of a series of RCTs to ascertain the clinical effects of the dosage selected in Phase II in the populations for which the drug is intended to be used, based on strict protocols and involving far more participants than in Phase II. In Phase III trials, the sample size is selected to demonstrate a clinically relevant effect with sufficient precision. Because Phase III trial results often provide the basis for marketing authorization of drugs, they are sometimes also called pivotal trials. Marketing authorization is the process of reviewing and assessing the evidence to support a medicinal product, such as a drug, in relation to its marketing, finalized by granting a license to be sold.

- Phase IV research comprises the systematic recording of adverse events once the drug has received marketing authorization (post-marketing surveillance). This is often supplemented by research – sometimes imposed on the manufacturer by the regulatory authorities – into certain safety questions that have not yet been sufficiently investigated, the long-term effect of the drug, and its effect in high-risk populations, etc.

10.2.1 The observed effect

Suppose a doctor is consulted by a patient who has been suffering from symptoms suggestive of disease X. The doctor makes a diagnosis and gives the patient treatment Y. If the patient is back to normal one week later, can the doctor conclude that Y is an effective treatment for disease X? Not really. Only if a patient with a chronic disease recovers fully and rapidly after a new treatment (e.g. when a patient with painful osteoarthritis of the hip is given a new hip) can the observed effect be attributed to that treatment with a reasonable degree of certainty. Such cases are rare in practice. If a patient gets better after a treatment, it may be due to the treatment, but there are also usually other explanations, as the treatment is only one of the possible causes of the observed effect.

The observed effect of an intervention consists of five components: effect of the intervention; non-specific effects produced by interaction with the therapist and other aspects of the intervention (the placebo effect); natural course of the disease; effect of the external factors; and measurement errors when measuring the outcomes. The difference in the observed effect between the two groups reflects the true effect of the intervention if the natural course, the external factors, the placebo effect, and the measurement errors are the same for both groups. It is therefore not possible to validly estimate the effect of an intervention without a suitable comparison group.

10.2.1.1   Placebo Effect

In addition to any specific effect, every intervention will also have a non-specific effect, a placebo effect, a phenomenon in which some people experience a benefit after the administration of an inactive substance or treatment. Placebo or sham treatment has no known specific effect; therefore, the effect must be due to the patient's belief in that intervention. Although little is known as yet about the mechanism of the placebo effect, it should be emphasized that its influence on the outcome is just as real as that of the active components in the intervention.

10.2.1.2   Natural Course of the Disease

Although patients and doctors do not always fully realize it, an improvement of a disease can take place without any intervention at all. A person who has thrown his back out, for example, will usually get better in a few days, even without treatment. A common cold will last a week, with or without treatment. Even patients with a chronic disease, such as asthma, experience periods when the symptoms worsen or improve. After a patient has gone to the doctor with severe symptoms, there will often be a phase in which the patient feels better, even if no treatment has been given. This phenomenon is referred to as regression to the mean. It goes without saying that if there is no intervention, the condition can also get worse. It is therefore crucial that participants in the intervention and comparison groups of a trial have the same average prognosis.

10.2.1.3   External Factors that Influence the Observed Effect

An observed treatment effect can be influenced by factors other than the intervention. Some examples of external factors are age, sex, compliance to inter-vention, duration of symptoms, prior treatment, and any medication or therapy being given in addition to the intervention under investigation. These external factors can act as confounders of the effect of the intervention (see Section 5.4.1). Confounders will influence the magnitude of the observed effect, but if they are equally distributed between the groups, they will not distort the contrast in observed effect between the groups. How this can be ensured in the design of the trial or in the data analysis is explained in Sections 10.2.3 and 10.3, respectively.

10.2.1.4   Measurement Errors in Health Outcomes

Random and systematic errors can creep in when measuring the outcomes. If the magnitude and direction of these errors are related to the intervention (differential misclassification: see Section 5.4.1), bias will occur. Participants who are given a new intervention (and are not blinded to the assigned treatment) may, for example, tell the doctor that they are feeling a lot better simply to please the doctor. Information bias of this kind occurs mainly when the outcome measurement is subjective and outcome assessors are not blinded to the intervention (see Section 10.2.4).

10.2.2   Comparing interventions: efficacy or effectiveness?

Intervention studies can be placed on a continuum, with a progression from efficacy trials to effectiveness trials. Efficacy can be defined as the performance of an intervention under ideal and controlled circumstances, whereas effectiveness refers to its performance under "real-world" conditions. An efficacy trial can often over-estimate an intervention's effectiveness when implemented in clinical practice because of poor access, acceptance, utilization, and adherence to the intervention.

To establish efficacy, a new intervention is usually compared with a placebo in an explanatory trial in order to understand the effect of the presumed active ingredient in the intervention under optimal situations – a vital piece of information when it comes to understanding the mechanism involved. A pragmatic trial, on the other hand, is concerned with the question of whether the new intervention is effective when used in routine clinical practice, typically compared with the standard of care. The goal of a pragmatic trial is to inform a clinical or policy decision by providing evidence for adoption of the intervention into real-world clinical practice.

What makes a trial pragmatic? The PRECIS (Pragmatic–Explanatory Continuum Indicator Summary) tool attempts to clarify the concept of pragmatism. The considerations include:

- To what extent are the participants in the trial similar to patients who would receive this intervention if it was part of usual care?
- How much extra effort is made to recruit participants over and above what would be used in the usual care setting to engage with patients?
- How different are the settings of the trial from the usual care setting?
- How different are the resources, provider expertise, and organization of care delivery in the intervention group of the trial from those available in usual care?
- How different is the flexibility in how the intervention is delivered from the flexibility anticipated in usual care?
- How different is the flexibility in how participants are monitored and encouraged to adhere to the intervention from the flexibility anticipated in usual care?
- How different is the intensity of measurement and follow-up of participants in the trial from the typical follow-up in usual care?
- To what extent is the primary outcome of the trial directly relevant to participants?
- To what extent are all data included in the analysis of the primary outcome?

10.2.3 Randomization to create comparability at baseline

Vital to the internal validity of an RCT is how participants are assigned to the interventions being compared in the trial. The allocation procedure needs to ensure that the groups of participants being given different interventions are comparable in terms of natural course and external factors. If allocation is left up to the physicians, the groups will almost certainly not be comparable in terms of prognosis, as physicians will understandably select the intervention that they believe to have the best chance of success for their patients. This is referred to as confounding by indication. Anticipated risks of an intervention for an individual patient could also play a role here, referred to as confounding by contraindication. Either way, differences in effect will not then be due solely to the intervention given but also to differences in prognosis between the participants allocated to different groups. There is confounding by indication whenever the prognosis influences the likelihood of being allocated to a particular intervention.

The solution to this problem is to leave the allocation of interventions to chance, thus bypassing the preferences of patients and their doctors. This is the essence of randomization. The principle of randomization is simple, for example, by tossing an unbiased coin or by referring to a random-digit table each time a participant is eligible to be randomized. In practice, however, it is important to ensure that the sequence is truly random.

Even when the allocation sequence is generated appropriately, knowledge of the next assignment can enable selective enrollment and assignment of participants on the basis of prognostic factors. For example, participants may be directed to the "appropriate" intervention by delaying their entry into the trial until the desired allocation appears. For this reason, successful allocation concealment (not to be confused with blinding) is an essential part of randomization. The random sequence must be concealed such that, at the time of randomization, the intervention being assigned to the next participant is unknown and cannot be changed. This can be achieved, for example, by using sequentially numbered, sealed, opaque envelopes or by calling a coordinating center to randomize a newly enrolled participant in the trial.

Correctly applied, randomization produces study groups comparable with respect to known and unknown confounding factors and prevents confounding by indication or contraindication in the allocation of participants. Randomization cannot of course prevent confounding by external factors that develop later (e.g. due to compliance and co-interventions), possibly influenced by the assigned treatment. Lastly, randomizing provides the possibility of blinding (see Section 10.2.4), which minimizes the influence of measurement errors and placebo effect.

Randomization is regarded as the panacea for preventing confounding and is thus the most essential element in an RCT. It does not guarantee that the various exposures will actually be distributed equally among the intervention groups, however, as unequal distributions can still occur by chance. In studies involving only a small number of participants, an unequal distribution can easily occur, causing major problems when analyzing the data. A check of the distribution of important prognostic factors at baseline is needed; however, statistical tests are of little use since we already know that any differences would have been generated by chance. Such differences in one or more important prognostic factors, if they are associated with the outcome, can be adjusted for during the analysis to improve efficiency of the analysis.

In designing an RCT, when there is a serious concern about unequal distribution on one or more strong prognostic factors despite of randomization (e.g. because of small sample size), the randomization process can be augmented by stratification. In a stratified randomization, randomization is performed separately within each stratum of participants defined by the prognostic factor of interest. This will ensure that that a prognostic factor is distributed evenly among the intervention groups. In theory, we could continue stratifying for combinations of prognostic factors until each stratum has only two individuals available for randomization (individual matching). But in practice, stratified randomization can only be used on a few variables as the strata will otherwise be too small. An alternative is to use minimization: this involves manipulating the likelihood of each new participant being allocated to one group or the other using a computer algorithm so as to achieve an even distribution of important prognostic factors.

Stratified randomization is often combined with block randomization to ensure that the desired ratio of participants (e.g. 2 : 1) in the intervention and comparison groups is achieved. For example, when the randomization ratio is 2 : 1 and the block size is 6, for every six consecutively participants randomized, four would be assigned to the intervention group and two would be assigned to the comparison group (◻ Figure 10.1). When block randomization is used, it is important that only the statistician drawing up the randomization scheme knows the block size, otherwise the researchers will know which treatment the last participant in the block will be allocated to, thus conflicting with the principle of allocation concealment. Block sizes are usually varied to improve allocation concealment. Note that block randomization is also often used in simple randomization without stratification as well to avoid chance imbalance in group size.

◻ **Figure 10.1** Block randomization with a block size of 6 and a randomization ratio of 2 : 1.

For a participant, an intervention study effectively starts at the time of randomization. The principle is that once participants have been randomized, they are members of the study population. An RCT is in effect a cohort study: randomization is the event that defines cohort membership. This has major consequences for the way in which the data, once collected, are analyzed. It is vital for each participant – whatever happens – to be analyzed in the group to which he was originally allocated during randomization (intention-to-treat analysis), regardless of the actual intervention carried out. This point is explained further in Section 10.3.2.

10.2.4 Blinding to maintain comparability right to the end

In order to attribute a difference in outcomes observed between intervention groups to the interventions, the influence of external factors and measurement errors must be comparable between groups. The knowledge about who received which intervention can influence external factors following randomization as well as measurement errors. Think, for instance, of differences in placebo effect or in the use of co-interventions (performance bias). If the participant knows that a sham intervention was given, that person may seek additional care (co-intervention), switch to non-protocol interventions or become non-adherent, distorting the relative effect of the active intervention in comparison with the sham intervention. The results will also be distorted if the outcome assessor has a preconceived belief of the intervention and interprets the outcome measure in a more favorable light in support of personal belief and hypothesis (observer bias).

The solution to minimize these forms of bias is blinding, which implements mechanisms to ensure that participants, care providers, and trial personnel

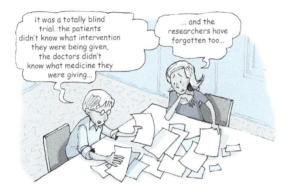

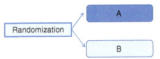

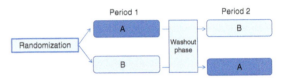

Basic structure of a randomized, parallel group trial

Figure 10.3 Basic structures of a parallel design compared with a crossover design.

Figure 10.2 This is a case of full blinding.

are unaware of the interventions received. Ideally, everyone who could introduce bias – patients, care providers, outcome assessors, and data analysts – should be blinded, but such full blinding is not always possible. With some creativity (sham operations, sham radiotherapy, and even sham psychotherapy), however, a host of credible placebo interventions can be constructed. Blinding the data analyst is not common, yet such blinding has demonstrated added value for bias reduction (**Figure 10.2**). An attempt to blind participants, people delivering the interventions, and outcome assessors does not ensure successful blinding in practice. For many drug trials, the side effects of the drugs allow the possible detection of the intervention being received by some participants.

Blinding should not be confused with allocation concealment. Allocation concealment occurs at the start of the trial, before participants are allocated to their groups or receive any intervention. It ensures strict implementation of the randomly generated sequence to minimize the impact of selection bias and confounding. Blinding occurs after participants are allocated to their groups and is an effective way to minimize information bias. Allocation concealment is almost always possible, even in studies where blinding is impossible.

10.2.5 Crossover design

So far, we have been looking at trial design in which participants are randomized into two or more parallel

groups, for example, intervention A or intervention B, and intervention effect is estimated via comparison of outcome measures between independent groups of participants. In contrast, in a randomized crossover trial, each participant receives multiple interventions. Participants are randomly assigned to a sequence (i.e. the order in which interventions are received, for example, intervention A then intervention B or vice versa), and participants thus serve as their own control (**Figure 10.3**, Case 10.2). As each participant is compared to herself or himself in the statistical analysis, to detect the same effect size, fewer participants will be needed in a crossover design than in a parallel design.

Although the crossover design is very attractive, it can potentially have carryover effects: persistent or residual effects from intervention in one period that may confound the effect in subsequent intervention periods. For example, if the effect of intervention A from period 1 persists to period 2, in which a participant is receiving treatment B, the intervention effect observed in the second period will be a combined effect from both interventions yet, attributed only to treatment B. To minimize a possible carryover effect, investigators use a washout phase that is sufficiently long to eliminate the first intervention's effects.

Another potential issue in crossover trials is the period effect, which occurs when secular changes are present. For example, a period effect may arise if a condition under study is not stable, such that the effects of treatment are not consistent over time and the true effects of each intervention are confounded by the period in which they are received.

Additionally, in terms of missing data, even a small amount of missing data in a crossover trial can result in a compromised study. Finally, the randomized crossover design is inappropriate for conditions in which the intervention in an earlier period permanently alters the course of the condition (e.g. cures the disease), such that, at the entry to the next period, the participant characteristics systematically differ from their initial states at the start of the trial.

Case 10.2 A Randomized Crossover Trial of the Effect of Personalized Incentives on Dietary Quality of Grocery Purchase (Excerpt from the Abstract)

Many factors are associated with food choice. Personalized interventions could help improve dietary intake by using individual purchasing preferences to promote healthier grocery purchases. The trial aimed to test whether a healthy food incentive intervention using an algorithm incorporating customer preferences, purchase history, and baseline diet quality improves grocery purchase dietary quality and spending on healthy foods.

The trial utilized a 9-month crossover design (AB–BA) with a two- to four-week washout period between 3-month intervention periods. Participants included 224 loyalty program members at an independent Rhode Island supermarket who completed baseline questionnaires.

Participants received personalized weekly coupons with nutrition education during the intervention period (A) and occasional generic coupons with nutrition education during the control period (B). An auto-mated study algorithm used customer data to allocate personalized healthy food incentives to participant loyalty cards. The primary outcome was the Grocery Purchase Quality Index–2016 (GPQI-16) scores (range, 0–75, with higher scores denoting healthier purchases) and percentage spending (in terms of dollar amount) on targeted foods were calculated from cumulative purchasing data.

The analytical sample included 209 participants (104 in AB sequence and 105 in BA sequence). Paired t tests showed that the intervention increased GPQI-16 scores (1.06; 95% CI, 0.27–1.86) and percentage spending on targeted foods (1.38%; 95% CI, 0.08–2.69%). In conclusion, this trial demonstrated preliminary evidence for the effectiveness of a novel personalized healthy food incentive algorithm to improve grocery purchase dietary quality.

Trial Registration: ClinicalTrials.gov (NCT0374 8056).

10.2.6 Factorial design

A factorial trial (▢ Table 10.1, Case 10.3) allows researchers to investigate how multiple interventions affect outcomes independently and together. In its simplest form, in a two-by-two factorial design, participants are randomized into four groups. Group 1 receives both interventions, Groups 2 and 3 receive one of the two interventions, and Group 4 receives neither intervention.

Effect modification can be assessed by comparing effect of the combined intervention group (group 1) to the sum of the effects of the one intervention groups (groups 2 and 3). If the combined effect is substantially different (higher or lower) from the sum of the two effects, there is evidence for effect modification. It means that the strength of the effect of one intervention depends on whether the other intervention is also given simultaneously. If the primary aim of the trial is to study effect modification, each intervention group must include enough participants.

▢ **Table 10.1**   Basic structure of a factorial trial.

	Intention B	Placebo (B)	
Intervention A	Group 1	Group 2	Groups 1 + 2
Placebo (A)	Group 3	Group 4	Groups 3 + 4
	Groups 1 + 3	Groups 2 + 4	

Effect of A: (Groups 1 + 2) – (Groups 3 + 4)

Effect of B: (Groups 1 + 3) – (Groups 2 + 4)

Effect of A and B: Group 1 – Group 4

Interaction effect: Group 1 – (Groups 2 + 3)

Case 10.3 A Randomized Factorial Trial of the Effect of Drug Presentation on Asthma Outcomes (Excerpt from the Abstract)

Information that enhances expectations about drug effectiveness improves the response to placebos for pain. Although asthma symptoms often improve with placebo, it is not known whether the response to placebo or active treatment can be augmented by increasing expectation of benefit. The study objective was to determine whether response to placebo or a leukotriene antagonist (montelukast) can be augmented by messages that increase expectation of benefit.

A randomized 20-center controlled trial enrolled 601 asthmatic patients with poor symptom control. Participants were randomly assigned to one of four treatment groups in a factorial design (i.e. placebo with enhanced messages, placebo with neutral messages, montelukast with enhanced messages, or montelukast with neutral messages) or to usual care. The enhanced message aimed to increase expectation of benefit from the drug. The primary outcome was mean change in daily peak flow over four weeks. Secondary outcomes included lung function and asthma symptom control.

Peak flow and other lung function measures were not improved in participants assigned to the enhanced message groups versus the neutral message groups for either montelukast or placebo. Placebo-treated participants had improved asthma control with the enhanced message but not montelukast-treated participants. Headaches were more common in participants who were provided messages that mentioned headache as a montelukast side effect.

In conclusion, optimistic drug presentation augments the placebo effect for patient-reported outcomes (asthma control) but not lung function. However, the effect of montelukast was not enhanced by optimistic messages regarding treatment effectiveness.

Trial registration: http://ClinicalTrials.gov (NCT001 48408).

Table Lung function measures: change from baseline

	Treatment groups				P value[a]		
	Montelukast		Placebo		Message effect	Drug effect	Interaction drug × message
	Enhanced	Neutral	Enhanced	Neutral			
No.	120	117	120	116			
Mean change from baseline (95% CI)							
PEF (l/min)	15 (9 to 20)	14 (8 to 21)	7 (1 to 13)	3 (−3 to 9)	0.42	0.001	0.55
FEV$_1$ before BD (l)	0.09 (0.05 to 0.13)	0.06 (0.01 to 0.10)	0.00 (−0.04 to 0.03)	−0.01 (−0.04 to 0.02)	0.25	<0.001	0.42
FEV$_1$ after BD (l)	0.02 (−0.02 to 0.07)	0.00 (−0.04 to 0.04)	−0.09 (−0.16 to −0.01)	−0.05 (−0.09 to −0.01)	0.66	<0.001	0.16
FVC before BD (l)	0.06 (0.01 to 0.11)	0.05 (0.00 to 0.10)	−0.01 (−0.05 to 0.03)	−0.03 (−0.06 to 0.01)	0.50	0.001	0.93
FVC after BD (l)	0.00 (−0.05 to 0.05)	−0.01 (−0.06 to 0.03)	−0.10 (−0.18 to −0.01)	−0.05 (−0.10 to −0.01)	0.63	0.003	0.25

Message effect, Effect of enhanced message independent of drug; *Drug effect*, effect of montelukast independent of message type; *Enhanced*, enhanced expectancy message for study drug; *Neutral*, neutral message about study drug; *BD*, bronchodilator; *FVC*, forced vital capacity.
[a]P values are adjusted for clinic and visit, and the variance estimates were adjusted for repeated measures. The interaction P value evaluates whether the drug effect is modified by the message effect.

10.2.7 Cluster randomized design

In a cluster randomized trial, a group of individuals, a household, a village, a school, or a clinic, is randomized to an intervention or a control (Case 10.4). Cluster randomized trials differ from individually randomized trials in that the units of randomization are groups, not individual participants. They are commonly used to test educational and public health interventions, policies, service delivery intervention, and the target of the intervention is usually a collective or a system rather than a particular person. For example, cluster randomized trials can be used to evaluate the effects of implementing a new workflow in a hospital or a new vision screening program at primary schools.

Further, cluster randomized trials are particularly suitable when the potential for contamination is high. Contamination occurs when aspects of an intervention are adopted by members of the group that was randomized to *not* receive that intervention. For example, in a trial that compares different smoking cessation strategies, participants seen by the same provider may compare notes in the waiting room. As a result, participants in the comparison group might learn about the experimental intervention and adopt it themselves. Randomization at the provider level, with each provider coaching only one of the strategies, would reduce the risk of contamination. Other practical reasons for adopting a cluster randomized design include administrative convenience, ethical considerations, and cooperation of investigators and participants.

In a cluster randomized trial, observations on individuals within the same cluster are correlated – that is, the outcomes for individuals within clusters are likely to be more similar than those across clusters, creating special challenges for the design and analysis. The statistical measure of this clustering effect is called intracluster correlation coefficient (ICC). Estimates of ICCs are used to inform sample size calculations – standard sample size calculations require to be inflated by a factor: $1 + (n - 1)\rho$, where n is the average cluster size and ρ is the ICC for the desired outcome to accommodate for the lack of independence in the data.

Case 10.4 A Cluster Randomized Trial to Assess the Effectiveness of a Childhood Obesity Prevention Program Delivered through Schools (Excerpt from the Abstract)

A cluster randomized trial was conducted to assess the effectiveness of a school and family based healthy lifestyle program (WAVES intervention) compared with usual practice, in preventing childhood obesity among UK primary schools from the West Midlands. The 12-month intervention encouraged healthy eating and physical activity, including a daily additional 30-minute school time physical activity opportunity, a 6-week interactive skill-based program in conjunction with Aston Villa football club, signposting of local family physical activity opportunities through mail-outs every 6 months, and termly school-led family workshops on healthy cooking skills. Schools allocated to the comparator group continued with ongoing health-related activities. The primary outcomes, assessed blind to allocation, were between arm difference in body mass index (BMI) z score at 15 and 30 months. Secondary outcomes were further anthropometric, dietary, physical activity, and psychological measurements, and difference in BMI z score at 39 months in a subset.

Fifty-four schools were randomized: 26 schools (1,134 pupils) to the intervention group and 28 schools (778 pupils) to the comparator group. Fifty-three schools remained in the trial and data on 1,287 (87.7%) and 1,169 (79.7%) pupils were available at first follow-up (15 month) and second follow-up (30 month), respectively. The mean BMI z score was not significantly lower in the intervention arm compared with the control arm at 15 months (mean difference −0.075 (95% CI −0.183 to 0.033) in the baseline adjusted models. At 30 months the mean difference was −0.027 (−0.137 to 0.083). There was no statistically significant difference between groups for other anthropometric, dietary, physical activity, or psychological measurements (including assessment of harm).

In conclusion, the primary analyses suggest that this intervention had no statistically significant effect on BMI z score or on preventing childhood obesity. Schools are unlikely to impact on the childhood obesity epidemic by incorporating such interventions without wider support across multiple sectors and environments.

Trial registration: Current Controlled Trials ISRCTN97000586.

10.2.8 N-of-1 experiment

Results of RCTs reveal which of the treatments being compared are more effective on average. Sometimes it is desirable and also feasible to test which treatment gives the best result in an individual. If the outcome is reversible and the effects of interventions manifest relatively quickly, we can study the outcome in an individual participant who receives two or more treatment alternatives a number of times in random order. This design has the characteristics of a serial design but with a repeating, random allocation of the intervention, which is similar to a crossover design.

What's different from a crossover design is that it is important to repeat the treatment episodes multiple times to obtain enough measurements on outcomes and eliminate the role of chance, natural course, and external effects. Further, the results concern a single participant. N-of-1 experiment are therefore only possible on participants who have a chronic, stable condition with a treatment effect that comes and goes relatively quickly (◘ Figure 10.4).

The great advantage of an N-of-1 experiment is that the participants are likely to benefit directly from the results. One might wonder what the results of an N-of-1 experiment mean for similar participants. The answer is "not very much," as there is no representative sample of the group to which we would like to extrapolate the results. The question can be answered better if we carry out a number of N-of-1 experiments with the same research question and design. Single N-of-1 experiment can generate hypotheses and prompt larger trials. Several analogous N-of-1 experiments can be combined as a weighted average through a statistical technique called "meta-analysis" (more to come in Chapter 11) and thus produce results that can be generalized.

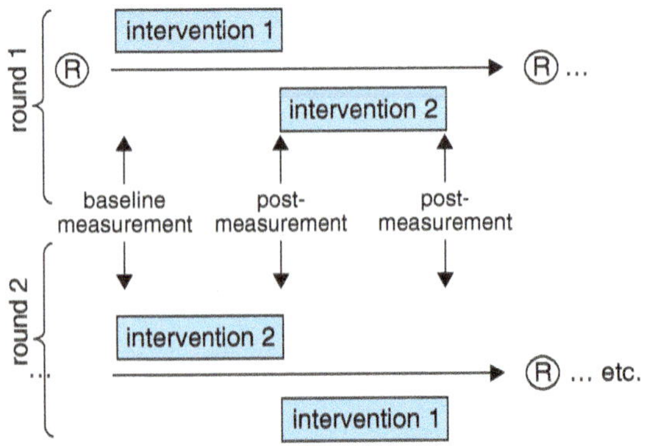

◘ **Figure 10.4** Basic structure of the $N = 1$ experiment.

10.3 Data from RCTs are analyzed to produce a valid estimate of effect

Data from RCTs can be used to arrive at valid estimates of the effect of an intervention. It is important to retain the methodological strengths of an experimental design (the comparability of natural course, external factors, and measurement errors) and even enhance them where possible. Data analysis is once again based on the epidemiological function, which calculates the likelihood of an outcome as a function of the intervention and any other factors influencing the effect.

10.3.1 Successful randomization

On average, randomization creates equal distributions for all factors with the exception of the intervention. Imbalances in baseline variables could arise due to chance. For example, with 250 participants per group and five important prognostic factors each with 20% prevalence, there is a 23% chance that at least one of them will have >7% difference between groups. Baseline imbalance that is clearly beyond what is expected due to chance, may suggest problems with the randomization process, for example, insufficient safeguards of the randomization sequence or unintentional errors occurred in programing. It is a good idea to check the distribution of prognostic factors and participant characteristics at baseline. Should an unequal distribution of important prognostic factors occur, the resulting imbalance can be adjusted for in the data analysis. In the example of Case 10.1, through the play of chance in the unstratified randomization, the mean age was 1.1 years older among participants in the dexamethasone group than among those in the usual care group. To account for this imbalance in an important prognostic factor, estimates of rate ratios were adjusted for the baseline age in three categories (<70 years, 70–79 years, and ≥80 years).

The issue of incomparability of groups on factors other than the intervention (confounding) should not be confused with the issue of subgroup differences in effects. If subgroup differences exist, it implies effect modification (see Section 5.5), reports should show the effects for each subgroup separately with the corresponding CIs. Most intervention trials, however, do not have enough participants to reliably distinguish such subgroup differences in effects. In Case 10.1, pre-specified analyses of the primary outcome (28-day mortality) were performed in five subgroups: age, sex, level of respiratory support, days since symptom onset, and predicted 28-day mortality risk.

10.3.2 Types of analysis

The hallmark of an RCT is random assignment of the interventions to each participant. Yet, some participants will not receive the intervention (or the full intervention) assigned to them. Some may be too ill for surgery, for example, or they may not take their medicine or fail to comply with the rules in some other way. In Case 10.1, in the dexamethasone group, 95% of the participants received at least one dose of the drug. In the usual care group, 8% of the patients received dexamethasone as part of their clinical care. In such situations, there are two options for data analysis:

- In an intention-to-treat analysis, every participant is included in the analysis as originally planned, regardless of whether or not that person actually received the intervention. The advantage of this approach is that it keeps randomization intact, although the intervention effect may be underestimated.
- In a per-protocol analysis, participant groups are compared in the analysis according to the intervention they actually received. This may seem to be a better reflection of what actually happened, but the original comparability of the groups accomplished by the randomization is lost. The randomized experiment then effectively becomes an observational study, with all the disadvantages that entails. Suppose compliance with intervention A is lower than with intervention B because intervention A does relieve patients' symptoms in sufficiently. Not including patients who have discontinued their allocated treatment in the analysis would produce biased results (the effect of intervention A will be overestimated). Modern causal inference methods, which are beyond the level of this book, can be used in some circumstances to

estimate the effect of interventions among participants who received the assigned intervention.

10.3.3 Sequential analyses

It is tempting to analyze the available data while an RCT is in progress, in particular to see whether it is already clear which intervention is superior. If so, the researchers will want to halt the experiment and offer all participants the more effective intervention. It would indeed be unethical to include more participants in an experiment than needed to answer the original research question. This argument is fair, yet it carries a major risk that we will never find out whether this initial positive effect was more than a random fluctuation. Sequential analysis procedures have been developed to deal with this dilemma. These involve prior formulation of the statistical limits that need to be exceeded before a decision is taken to halt the experiment. These limits are set to give chance only a limited role. A variant of this method is to plan in advance that an interim analysis will be done, for example, when outcome has been measured in half of the study population. Part of that prior plan is a decision rule about what results of the interim analysis will lead to the trial being halted in the event of an unexpectedly large (or negligible) effect.

10.4 Assessing harms of interventions

As we have seen in this chapter, RCT is a desirable study design to estimate intended effects of interventions, mainly because it enables the effects of an intervention to be differentiated from the effects of natural course, external factors, and measurement errors. For the study of unintended effects (adverse effects of interventions), RCTs may be unsuitable. A study of rare severe adverse events, for instance, would require a huge number of participants. An RCT of a usual size does not provide much evidence about the safety of the intervention. Research into safety of medical interventions can best be done by large observational studies, as described in Chapter 4. These studies thus obviously have to contend with the same problems as etiological studies (confounding, selection bias, and information bias).

10.4.1 Adverse events come in many shapes and sizes

Drugs are, by definition, chemicals or compounds designed to interfere with particular aspects of metabolism. The whole development of drugs aims, of course, to identify those that act selectively on the pathological process without affecting other vital functions. This is only partly successful: there will always be a risk of unintentional, usually harmful, adverse effects. Adverse effects imply a causal relationship; whereas adverse events refer to medical occurrences associated with the use of an intervention but not necessarily causally related. Although avoiding adverse effects has always been an inherent part of the development and evaluation of drugs, efforts to identify adverse effects were greatly stepped up after the thalidomide scandal, when mothers who took this drug during pregnancy gave birth to children with no limbs.

There are various types of adverse effects:

- Type A reactions are predictable based on the mechanism of the drug. They are generally relatively common, especially at higher doses, and are therefore usually discovered soon, in some cases, even before the drug is tested on trial participants. Hair loss due to chemotherapy is an example of a Type A reaction.
- Type B reactions are unpredictable and rare and are therefore generally only discovered after the drug has been placed on the market. These are the subject of Phase IV studies (post-marketing surveillance). Vaginal cancer in daughters of women who took diethylstilbestrol as a contraction inhibitor at the end of pregnancy is a well-known example that, understandably, took a while to discover.
- Type C reactions are also usually rare but more or less predictable. They are caused by drugs exacerbating rather than reducing the severity of the condition for which they are prescribed. They are very difficult to detect, because it is difficult to distinguish between the effect of the underlying disease and that of the drug. They usually only come to light in large-scale Phase IV studies. An example of a Type C reaction is increased risk of severe asthma and asthma mortality in patients given certain bronchodilators (fenoterol) for their asthma.

In a typical RCT, hundreds of unique adverse events may be recorded. This is because most events are collected non-systematically, which increases their susceptibility to information bias. Non-systematically collected adverse events are recorded only when participants report them to care providers ("spontaneous reporting"), whereas systematically collected adverse events are planned outcomes to be recorded for all participants using consistent procedures in a trial, similarly to efficacy outcomes. Data collection methods directly impact how investigators analyze and present adverse events to patients and the public. It is clear from the foregoing that different approaches are needed to detect and demonstrate the various types of adverse effects. Type A and C reactions can be predicted rationally to a large extent, leading to systematic data collection and testing of specific hypotheses. Detecting Type B reactions is mainly a question of vigilance on the part of patients and their providers, and the untargeted monitoring of patients who have been treated.

Phase IV research, also referred to as post-marketing surveillance, is legally required for every drug in the first few years after its approval. The compliance to this legal requirement is unsatisfactory. Occasionally, a drug is taken off the market as a result of findings from post-marketing surveillance. It is often vigilant patients and their care providers who first express suspicion of a relationship between a drug and the symptoms and signs it has produced. Physicians are expected to report the adverse events to the national pharmacovigilance center and/or the drug manufacturer. These reports are evaluated and compared with other reports worldwide. If there are suspicions regarding possible causal relationships between the use of a particular drug and the occurrence of particular health problems, it makes sense to investigate them further. Because of the rarity of most adverse events, the obvious choice is a case–control study, but a cohort study will sometimes be an option. Some regions in the Netherlands, for instance, keep records of all drugs issued by pharmacies and link these to hospital admission records. This enables testing of particular hypotheses on increased risk for adverse events in patients using particular drugs. As with any observational study, the validity of the results will depend on the availability of data and the possibility of overcoming issues of confounding and effect modification.

Recommended reading

Celentano, D.D., Szklo, M., and Gordis, L. (ed.) (2019). Gordis epidemiology. In: *Epidemiology*, 6e, 1934–2015. Philadelphia, PA: Elsevier. (Chapters 10-11).

Friedman, L.M., Furberg, C.D., and DeMets, D.L. (2010). *Fundamentals of Clinical Trials*, 4e. Springer.

Piantadosi, S. (2017). *Clinical Trials: A Methodologic Perspective*, 3e. New York: Wiley.

Source references (cases)

RECOVERY Collaborative Group, Horby, P., Lim, W.S. et al. (2021). Dexamethasone in hospitalized patients with Covid-19 - preliminary report. *N. Engl. J. Med.* 384: 693, NEJMoa2021436–704. https://doi.org/10.1056/NEJMoa2021436. Epub ahead of print (Case 10.1).

Vadiveloo, M., Guan, X., Parker, H.W. et al. (2021). Effect of personalized incentives on dietary quality of groceries purchased: a randomized crossover trial. *JAMA Netw. Open.* 4 (2): e2030921. https://doi.org/10.1001/jamanetworkopen.2020.30921 (Case 10.2).

Wise, R.A., Bartlett, S.J., Brown, E.D. et al. (2009). Randomized trial of the effect of drug presentation on asthma outcomes: the American Lung Association Asthma Clinical Research Centers. *J. Allergy Clin. Immunol.* 124 (3): 436–444. 444e1-8 (Case 10.3).

Adab, P., Pallan, M.J., Lancashire, E.R. et al. (2018). Effectiveness of a childhood obesity prevention programme delivered through schools, targeting 6 and 7 year olds: cluster randomised controlled trial (WAVES study). *BMJ* 360: k211. https://doi.org/10.1136/bmj.k211 (Case 10.4).

Source references (knowledge assessment questions)

Martin, R.M., Donovan, J.L., Turner, E.L. et al. (2018). Effect of a low-intensity PSA-based screening intervention on prostate cancer mortality: the CAP randomized clinical trial. *JAMA* 319 (9): 883–895. https://doi.org/10.1001/jama.2018.0154. PMID: 29509864. (Question 6)

Knowledge assessment questions

1. Which of the following is NOT a key consideration of designing a randomized trial? (select the one best answer)
   a. The primary outcome must be capable of being assessed in all participants
   b. The question should be specified in advance of the trial, and be as specific as possible
   c. Follow-up should end when a participant stops taking the study medication
   d. The randomization sequence should be concealed from those enrolling and allocating participants

2. Which of the following are threats to internal validity in randomized trials? (select all that apply)
   a. Unblinding of treatment assignment
   b. Drop out and loss to follow up
   c. Participant non-adherence
   d. Protocol deviations/violations
   e. Inadequate sample size
   f. Restrictive eligibility criteria

3. Which of the following is NOT a characteristic of randomized crossover trials? (select the one best answer)
   a. The random assignment is to the order of interventions
   b. There is a higher degree of precision than parallel trials (with the same number of participants)
   c. There is a risk of a "carry-over" effect
   d. They are appropriate for conditions which can be cured in relatively short periods of time
   e. They allow for within-individual comparisons

4. Which is NOT a reason why an investigator might choose to conduct a cluster randomized trial? (select the one best answer)
   a. Ethical considerations
   b. To enhance cooperation of investigators and participants
   c. To minimize contamination
   d. The intervention is naturally applied to the cluster level
   e. It is more efficient than an individually randomized trial because of people within clusters may respond similarly to interventions

5. When trial investigators select composite measures as primary outcomes, they often lump less serious events together with very serious events (e.g. composite outcome of death, myocardial infarction, stroke, and TIA). Why can this be an issue when presenting the results such a trial?

6. To evaluate the effect of a single prostate-specific antigen (PSA) screening and – if positive – standardized diagnostic pathway on prostate cancer–specific mortality, a Cluster Randomized Trial of PSA Testing for Prostate Cancer (CAP) was conducted at 573 primary care practices across the UK. The trial enrolled men aged 50–69 years. The randomization and recruitment of the practices occurred between 2001 and 2009; patient follow-up ended on March 31, 2016. The primary outcome was prostate cancer–specific mortality at a median follow-up of 10 years and all-cause mortality was one of the secondary outcomes.

   Among 4,15,357 randomized men (mean [SD] age, 59.0 [5.6] years), 1,89,386 in the intervention group and 2,19,439 in the control group were included in the analysis (n = 4,08,825; 98%). In the intervention group, 75,707 (40%) attended the PSA testing clinic and 67,313 (36%) underwent PSA testing.

   After a median follow-up of 10 years, 549 (0.30 per 1,000 person-years) died of prostate cancer in the intervention group vs 647 (0.31 per 1,000 person-years) in the control group (incidence rate difference, −0.013 per 1,000 person-years [95% CI, −0.047 to 0.022]; incidence rate ratio [RR], 0.96 [95% CI, 0.85–1.08]). The number diagnosed with prostate cancer was higher in the intervention group (n = 8,054; 4.3%) than in the control group (n = 7,853; 3.6%) (RR, 1.19 [95% CI, 1.14–1.25]). More prostate cancer tumors with a Gleason grade of 6 or lower were identified in the intervention group (n = 3,263/189,386 [1.7%]) than in the control group (n = 2,440/219,439 [1.1%]) (difference per 1,000 men, 6.11 [95% CI, 5.38–6.84]). In the analysis of all-cause mortality, there were 25,459 deaths in the intervention group vs 28 306 deaths in the control group (RR, 0.99 [95% CI, 0.94–1.03]).

a. Is there evidence that PSA screening invitation is effective in reducing the cancer-specific mortality and all-cause mortality?

b. The figure below shows the cumulative risk of all-cause mortality by groups. It appears that mortality differs by attendance. The RR comparing attenders with control is 0.68 (95% CI 0.65, 0.71). Is this analysis comparing the attenders with control appropriate? Why or why not?

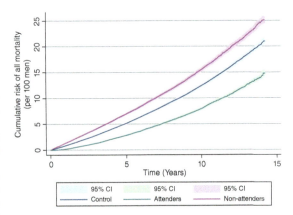

Systematic Review and Meta-Analysis

Textbook of Epidemiology, Second Edition. Lex Bouter, Maurice Zeegers and Tianjing Li.
© 2023 John Wiley & Sons Ltd. Published 2023 by John Wiley & Sons Ltd.
Companion website: www.wiley.com/go/Bouter/TextbookofEpidemiology

11

11.1 Introduction

A systematic review attempts to identify, appraise, and synthesize all relevant studies that fit pre-specified criteria to answer a research question in a transparent, objective, and reproducible way. The research question could be etiologic, diagnostic or prognostic, or concern the effectiveness of a preventive or therapeutic intervention. Some examples include the effects of air pollution on asthma, elevated atmospheric CO_2 concentration on the performance of invasive plants relative to native plants, behavioral strategies to minimize air-pollution exposure, or the effectiveness of indoor air-purification intervention on cardiovascular health. Regardless of the topic, systematic review utilizes a scientific approach to summarizing the existing knowledge and identifies gaps in the literature for future research.

Modern systematic review methods originate in psychology. In 1974, Gene Glass quantitatively summarized the effects of psychotherapy using a statistical technique called "meta-analysis" and the method quickly spread to diverse scientific disciplines such as education, criminal justice, industrial organization, economics, and ecology. The method entered medicine in the 1980s. Peter Elwood, Archibald (Archie) Cochrane, and their colleagues conducted the first randomized trial that assessed whether aspirin could reduce recurrences of heart attack. Although the results were suggestive of a beneficial effect of aspirin, they were not definitive. As additional trials became available, Elwood and Cochrane assembled and synthesized their results using meta-analysis, providing conclusive evidence that aspirin reduces the risk of recurrence of heart attack. The results were published in 1980 in an anonymous *Lancet* editorial, written actually by Sir Richard Peto, a British medical statistician. Peto subsequently provided example using randomized trials of a beta-blocker following a heart attack to encourage clinicians to review randomized trials systematically. The popularity of the method has since then grown exponentially out of a need to ensure that health decisions must be informed by the totality of research evidence instead of reliance on experts' idiosyncratic review and subjective opinion (◘ Figure 11.1; Case 11.1).

Archie Cochrane's call for a collection of randomized trials and systematic reviews led to the creation of Cochrane (previously known as the Cochrane Collaboration) by Sir Iain Chalmers and a group of international colleagues in 1993. Cochrane is an independent, diverse, global organization that collaborates to identify biomedical randomized trials that have been done, produce trusted synthesized evidence, make it accessible to all, and advocate for its use. Cochrane systematic reviews are internationally recognized as the benchmark for high-quality information about healthcare.

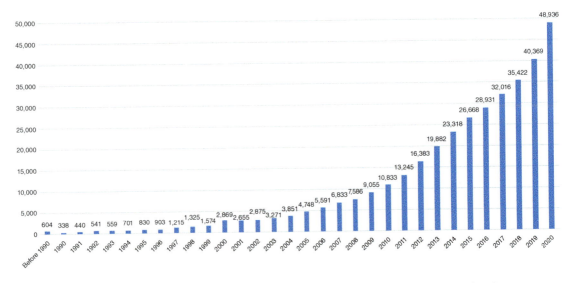

◘ **Figure 11.1** Number of records retrieved by searching "systematic review" or "meta-analysis" in all fields in PubMed.

Evidence summarized and distilled in systematic reviews, together with clinical expertise and patient values, are the three pillars of evidence-based medicine (EBM). David Sacket and a group of clinical epidemiologists at McMaster University in Hamilton, Ontario, Canada started the EBM movement in 1981 when they published a series of articles in the *Canadian Medical Association Journal* advising clinicians how to critically evaluate the medical literature. As readers will learn later in this chapter, critical appraisal is an essential step of conducting a systematic review. Systematic reviews take precedence over other types of research in many hierarchies of evidence because it makes sense for decisions to be based on the *totality* of relevant evidence rather than individual studies or a subset of the evidence. The evidence synthesized in systematic reviews is translated into policy, such as evidence-based clinical practice guidelines.

Case 11.1 The use of intravenous streptokinase as thrombolytic therapy for acute myocardial infarction

Between 1959 and 1988, 33 trials were conducted to evaluate thrombolytic therapy in comparison with placebo in patients who suffered from a heart attack. Were all these trials necessary? If researchers were to combine the results from the first eight trials involving 2,432 participants by 1973 in a meta-analysis, they would have found a consistent, statistically significant reduction in total mortality (combined odds ratio, 0.74; 95% confidence interval, 0.59–0.92). However, this combined odds ratio was not calculated in 1973. Instead, another 25 trials enrolled an additional 34,542 patients through 1988. The results of these trials had little or no effect on the combined odds ratio establishing efficacy of thrombolytic therapy, including the two very large trials, the Gruppo Italiano per lo Studio della Streptochinasi nell'Infarto Miocardico trial published in 1986 (11,712 patients) and the Second International Study of Infarct Survival trial published in 1988 (17,187 patients). This example demonstrates the importance of keeping track of the evidence systematically while it was accumulating – benefits and harms of interventions could have been identified earlier than they were, and effective treatments could have been recommended and used in practice sooner.

11.2 Steps in completing a systematic review

Unlike a narrative review, a systematic review follows highly structured, rigorous, and reproducible methods established in a protocol to minimize bias and errors. Review authors should follow widely adopted methodological standards in performing reviews. For example, *The Cochrane Handbook for Systematic Reviews of Interventions* is the "go-to" reference for conducting a systematic review, and the Institute of Medicine in the US has recommended standards for conducting high-quality systematic reviews.

Protocols of systematic reviews should be registered, for example, at the International Prospective Register of Systematic Reviews (PROSPERO). In addition, it is critical to gather an appropriate team that involves members with relevant and complementary expertise, perspectives, and experience. At a minimum, the team should include healthcare professionals with expertise in the topic area of the review, methodologists (e.g. statisticians, epidemiologists) with expertise in evidence synthesis methodology, and information specialists (librarians).

The key steps in conducting a systematic review include (i) define the research question; (ii) identify all potentially relevant studies; (iii) collect data from, and assess the risk of bias in included studies; (iv) analyze and synthesize data; (v) interpret the findings and write the report. The next few sections elaborate on each of these steps.

11.2.1 Frame the research question and decide on the eligibility criteria

As described in Section 4.1.1, the research questions for any type of epidemiological research need to be formulated in specific, measurable terms; the same principle and the PICO (Population, Interventions, Comparators, and Outcomes) framework applies to systematic reviews. In the context of non-interventional exposures (e.g. air pollution), the interventions (I) element is replaced by exposure factors (E). Within each element, systematic reviewers specify study characteristics that would determine the eligibility of a review. Additionally, systematic reviewers specify the types of study designs that would be eligible for the systematic review, such as randomized trials, cohort studies, and case–control studies. An example of specifying PICO in a review of intervention effectiveness, a review of association, and a review of diagnostic test accuracy is presented in Case 11.2, Case 11.3, and Case 11.4, respectively. Note that, in the case of diagnostic test accuracy, "I" refers to "index test," "C" is replaced by "reference standard(s)" or "comparison test," and "O" is replaced by "target condition" of interest.

Case 11.2 Effect of early versus late initiation of epidural analgesia on birth outcomes for women in labor

Participants: pregnant term women requesting epidural analgesia in labor, regardless of whether the labor was spontaneous or induced.
Intervention: early initiation of epidural analgesia. Early initiation is typically defined as cervical dilatation of less than 4–5 cm, as defined by the authors of the trials.
Comparison: late initiation of epidural analgesia. Late initiation is typically defined as cervical dilatation of 4–5 cm or more, as defined by the authors of the trials.

Outcomes*:
- Incidence of cesarean section
- Incidence of instrumental birth
- Duration of first stage of labor from randomization
- Duration of second stage of labor.

*Only primary outcomes are shown.
Type of studies: randomized controlled trials.

Case 11.3 Patterns of red and processed meat consumption and risk of cardiometabolic and cancer outcomes

Participants: adults older than 18 years of age with or without cardiometabolic conditions but without cancer or any infectious or chronic noncardiometabolic conditions.
Exposure: dietary patterns higher* in red and processed meat intake across categories of dietary habits. Red meat was defined as mammalian meat, and processed meat was defined as white or red meat preserved by smoking, curing, salting, or adding preservatives.

Comparison: dietary patterns lower* in red and processed meat intake (replacement with fish, white meats, or vegetarian and vegan dietary patterns).

Outcomes:
- All-cause mortality
- Risk of cardiovascular outcomes including cardiovascular mortality; fatal and nonfatal stroke, myocardial infarction, and other cardiovascular diseases
- Risk of type 2 diabetes
- Overall cancer incidence and mortality.

Type of studies: cohort studies with 1,000 or more participants
*The highest category (for example, tertiles or quartiles) was compared with the lowest category as a proxy.

Case 11.4 Computed tomography for diagnosis of acute appendicitis in adults

Participants: adolescents and adults (>14 years of age) with suspected appendicitis based on history, physical examination, and/or blood testing.
Index test: a sequential or helical abdominopelvic computed tomography (CT)-scan whereby the interpreter was assessing the appendix and its surroundings for signs of appendicitis.
Reference standards: histological examination of the removed appendix as well as clinical follow-up of participants who did not have surgery; or laparoscopic assessment of the appendix by the surgeon as inflamed or normal, as well as clinical follow-up of participants who did not have surgery.
Target condition: acute appendicitis.

11.2.2 Search for and select studies

Develop a comprehensive search strategy

Because systematic reviews attempt to identify *all* eligible studies to answer a research question, it is imperative that the search for literature is comprehensive and reproducible. Many systematic reviews fail to meet the minimal quality criteria because the searches are non-comprehensive. Involving information specialists who have expertise in designing and running searches for systematic reviews can help mitigate this problem.

In designing a search strategy, elements of the PICO and eligible study design(s) are translated into concepts. In Case 11.2, the concepts are pregnant women, early or late initiation of epidural analgesia, and randomized trials. Note that systematic reviews of interventions would rarely limit their searches by outcomes. This is because not all outcomes may appear in the titles and abstracts of a report. There is a good chance that only positive outcomes make it into the abstract, creating potential bias. When outcomes make it to the titles and abstracts, outcomes may be less well described or indexed with controlled vocabulary terms. A controlled vocabulary is an organized arrangement of words and phrases used to index content and/or to retrieve content through browsing or searching. As an example, the Medical Subject Headings (MeSH) is a controlled and hierarchically organized vocabulary produced by the US National Library of Medicine (NLM). Trained professionals assign MeSH terms to each record in MEDLINE.

The structure of a search strategy should be considered on a question-by-question basis. The three concepts for building a search strategy for systematic reviews of interventions include the population, intervention(s), and the study design. Search filters can be used for study designs (e.g. randomized controlled trials). Unlike systematic reviews of effects of interventions, for systematic reviews on etiological research questions, the concepts would include both the risk factor and the outcome, as well as eligible study designs when applicable.

Search terms for each concept should include both free-text words that might appear in a title, abstract, or keywords of a record in a database, as well as controlled vocabulary terms. Terms within each concept are combined using a Boolean operator "OR" to achieve sensitivity within concepts. The results for each concept are then joined together using the Boolean operator "AND" to ensure that all concepts are represented in the search strategy. Interested readers can find examples of full search strategies in any Cochrane systematic review.

For health-related topics, review authors typically start building a MEDLINE search. MEDLINE is the NLM journal citation database started in the 1960s. MEDLINE contains more than 28 million references

(as of August 2021) to journal articles in life sciences with a concentration on biomedicine. PubMed is a searchable portal for accessing MEDLINE. PubMed contains additional contents, including references to books and chapters, in-process and ahead-of-print citations, old citations, and some articles which lie slightly outside of the subject scope of MEDLINE.

No single electronic database is comprehensive enough to merit being the only database to be searched in a systematic review. Therefore, multiple electronic databases, including topic area-specific databases, if available should be searched. Once a search strategy is developed for one database, the next step is to translate it into search terms and syntax suitable for other databases.

In addition to searching bibliographic databases, review authors should also look for ongoing studies, unpublished studies, and other data sources. Ongoing clinical trials can be identified from searching trial registries such as http://clinicaltrialg.gov and the WHO International Clinical Trials Registry Platform. Awareness of ongoing studies allows review authors to better assess the evidence gaps and future research needs. When the results from the ongoing studies become available, they can be incorporated into updates of the systematic review. In addition, examining registration records enable review authors to identify outcomes that may have been prespecified but were changed or not reported in any of the publications associated with a given study, a sign of outcome-reporting bias. Other data sources for systematic reviews include materials from the regulatory agencies (e.g. the US Food and Drug Administration, the European Medicines Agency), clinical study reports, dissertations, conference abstracts, among others. Finally, review authors should read the reference lists of included studies and of other relevant systematic reviews to find studies that might have been missed. Review authors may also reach out to researchers and experts in the field who may know of additional studies.

Searches for systematic reviews should capture as many eligible studies as possible without restrictions by time periods, language, or publication status. Review authors should justify the use of any restrictions in the search strategy. For example, it's legitimate to impose a publication date limit when a new device or drug was not in development or available before a certain date. Finally, there is a tradeoff between being comprehensive (i.e. high sensitivity) and making the searching and screening process manageable within the constraints of time, financial and human resources available to the team (i.e. high specificity). Systematic review teams must balance these to ensure that the review is both comprehensive and manageable.

Select studies

Once the searches have been run, all records retrieved from different databases and sources are downloaded and managed by bibliographic software (e.g. EndNote®, Zotero, or Mendeley). Duplicates are removed at this stage. The next step is to conduct title and abstract screening (citation screening) to determine the potential relevance of each record assessed against the eligibility criteria. This is typically performed by two persons independently, preferably a topic-area expert and a methodologist. Discrepancies should be resolved through discussion or by a third person. Software platforms such as AbstrackR, DistillerSR®, and Covidence® can facilitate citation screening. Some of these platforms employ machine-learning algorithms to learn from assessments by humans and predict the likelihood of relevance of new records.

Titles and abstracts considered as definitely or maybe relevant during citation screening are then advanced to the stage of full-text screening. In this stage, which is also typically completed independently and in duplicate, review authors apply the same eligibility criteria to the full-text reports to confirm their final eligibility. Discrepancies between two reviewers are usually resolved through discussion or in consultation with a third review author. Reasons for excluding full-text reports are documented and reported.

For both citation screening and full-text screening, the level of agreement between two review authors can be quantified using intra observer reliability measures, although this is not often done in practice.

Document the search

Review authors should document search strategies and the search process in enough detail to ensure that it can be reproduced, following the Preferred Reporting Items for Systematic reviews and Meta-Analyses literature search extension (PRISMA-S).

11.2.3   Extract data and assess risk of bias

The unit of interest for systematic reviews is studies rather than reports, therefore, multiple reports of the same study, once deemed eligible for inclusion, need to be linked together for data abstraction. Data that are relevant for extraction for each study relate minimally to the following aspects:

- Study identification information, e.g. citation, link to other reports of the same study;
- Study design, e.g. randomized design, observational design, recruitment and sampling procedures, participants follow-up, methods used to prevent and minimize biases, statistical methods, sources of funding, and potential conflict of interest;
- Study characteristics, e.g. participant characteristics, interventions (risk factors), and outcomes;
- Results, e.g. estimates and precision (standard errors or confidence intervals) for each of the systematic review outcomes;
- Miscellaneous, e.g. key conclusions by the study authors, comments by review authors.

Many elements extracted from a study facilitate critical appraisal of the validity of a study's result. This process is called the risk of bias assessment. Depending on the study design, the most appropriate tool should be chosen for assessing the risk of bias of each included study. Examples are the revised Cochrane Risk of Bias tool for randomized trials (RoB 2), the Risk of Bias in Nonrandomized Studies of Interventions (ROBINS-I), and the Newcastle-Ottawa Scale (NOS) for observational studies of exposure-outcome associations.

To briefly describe RoB 2 for individually randomized, parallel group trials, the tool requires review authors to select a single numerical result for which the risk of bias will be assessed. Next, RoB 2 requires review authors to answer a set of signaling questions under five domains:

1. Risk of bias arising from the randomization process;
2. Risk of bias due to deviations from the intended interventions;
3. Risk of bias due to missing outcome data;
4. Risk of bias in measurement of the outcome; and
5. Risk of bias in selection of the reported result.

For each of the five domains, an algorithm maps answers to signaling questions to arrive at a judgment regarding the risk of bias (low risk of bias, some concerns, and high risk of bias). Finally, the tool guides review authors in summarizing the five domain-specific judgments of risk bias into an overall risk of bias judgment for the chosen result for the trial.

Many features of ROBINS-I are shared with the RoB 2 tool. ROBINS-I covers the risk of bias due to lack of randomization. The tool specifically asks the users to imagine a hypothetical "target" randomized trial. Then, the evaluation of risk of bias in the results of nonrandomized studies of interventions are facilitated by examining the strengths of the design features of studies in terms of how well they emulate the target trial.

NOS has been developed to assess case–control and cohort studies of exposure-outcome associations. A study is judged on three broad perspectives: the selection of the study groups; the comparability of the groups; and the ascertainment of either the exposure or outcome of interest for case–control or cohort studies respectively.

It has traditionally been recommended that data extraction and risk of bias assessment should be completed by two individuals independently with discrepancies adjudicated. A recent study has shown that independent dual abstraction is necessary for outcomes and results data and a verification approach is sufficient for other data. Tools and software to facilitate data extraction and risk of bias assessment vary from word processing software to spreadsheets, relational databases and online cloud-based data systems. Online cloud-based data systems, such as the Systematic Review Data Repository (SRDR), DistillerSR, Covidence, and EPPiReviewer offer advantages in terms of specific development for systematic reviews, flexibility, online collaborative ability, in-built risk of bias assessment tools, and, in the case of SRDR, a public, free, open-access platform for sharing data.

11.2.4 Analyze and synthesize data

Synthesis is the process of bringing together data from a set of included studies with the aim of drawing conclusions about the review question based on the body of evidence. Results of a systematic review can be very misleading if suitable attention has not been given to the review question, the eligibility criteria, identification and selection of studies, assessment of risk bias, and collection of appropriate data.

◻ Figure 11.2 presents a general framework for synthesis. Importantly, synthesis needs to be carefully planned out during the protocol stage (stage 1). When the goal is to compare a pair of interventions or an exposure-outcome relationship, a pairwise meta-analysis (i.e. the statistical combination of the results of several independent studies) should be considered. Whereas, when the goal is to compare multiple interventions for the same condition, a network meta-analysis

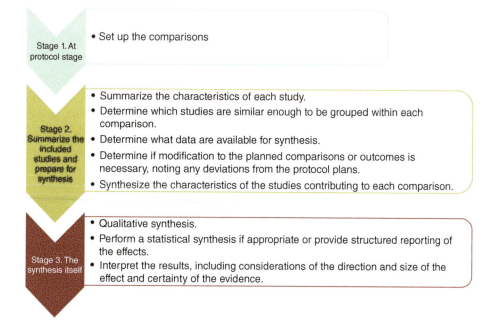

Stage 1. At protocol stage
• Set up the comparisons

Stage 2. Summarize the included studies and prepare for synthesis
• Summarize the characteristics of each study.
• Determine which studies are similar enough to be grouped within each comparison.
• Determine what data are available for synthesis.
• Determine if modification to the planned comparisons or outcomes is necessary, noting any deviations from the protocol plans.
• Synthesize the characteristics of the studies contributing to each comparison.

Stage 3. The synthesis itself
• Qualitative synthesis.
• Perform a statistical synthesis if appropriate or provide structured reporting of the effects.
• Interpret the results, including considerations of the direction and size of the effect and certainty of the evidence.

◻ **Figure 11.2** A general framework for synthesis.

(i.e. a statistical technique for comparing three or more interventions simultaneously in a single analysis by combining evidence within and across a network of studies) should be planned.

Before exploring the potential for conducting a quantitative synthesis, review authors summarize the existing evidence to determine which studies are similar enough to be grouped within each comparison, whether data are available for quantitative synthesis (recalculations are often needed to make the study estimates more comparable), and if modification to the planned comparisons or outcomes is necessary (documenting any deviations from the protocol plans) (stage 2).

Review authors then conduct what is known as a "qualitative synthesis" (stage 3). It should be clarified that this is a distinct concept from "qualitative research." According to the Institute of Medicine, a qualitative synthesis is a "structured summary, description and discussion of the studies' characteristics that may affect the cumulative evidence". It is an "assessment of the body of evidence that goes beyond factual descriptions or tables that, for example, simply detail how many studies were assessed, the reasons for excluding other studies, the range of study sizes and treatments compared, or quality of each study as measured by a risk of bias tool." The purpose of the qualitative synthesis is "to develop and convey a deeper understanding of the diversity of questions addressed, designs, strength of evidence, methods used in the underlying literature and the combinability of the studies." Qualitative synthesis also informs quantitative synthesis, including subgroup analysis and meta-regression (introduced later in this chapter).

Meta-analysis

A systematic review should always include a qualitative synthesis regardless of whether a meta-analysis is feasible or sensible. To decide whether to combine results in a meta-analysis, review authors should justify whether studies are estimating – in whole or in part – a common effect, and whether studies are addressing the same fundamental biological, clinical, or mechanistic research question. This qualitative analysis (before any statistical synthesis) is critical as it explores the clinical and methodological diversity. Clinical diversity refers to the variability in the participants, interventions, outcomes, and settings studied; and variability in study design and risk of bias can be described as methodological diversity.

Meta-analysis adds value to a systematic review in several ways. Given that individual studies can be underpowered to estimate the difference in effect between two interventions or associations between a risk factor and an outcome, meta-analyses are advantageous because they may generate estimates with increased precision by combining data from multiple studies. Meta-analysis can also be used to explore reasons for different and sometimes contradictory findings among individual studies (see subgroup analysis and meta-regression below).

To perform a meta-analysis, a relative or additive effect measure (e.g. risk ratio, odds ratio, hazard ratio, mean difference, risk difference) and its associated uncertainty (e.g. standard error, variance, confidence interval[CI]) are needed from each study. The overall measure of effect or association is a weighted average of results from individual studies. More weights are given to studies that carry more information. Weights are usually chosen to reflect of the precision of the estimate.

$$\frac{\sum W_i * Y_i}{\sum W_i}$$

where W_i is the weight assigned to each study and Y_i is the estimate from each study. Note that when working with ratios (e.g. odds ratios, risk ratios), the Y_i is the natural logarithm of the estimate.

When combing the data using a fixed-effects model, it is assumed that each study is estimating the same quantity. The W_i equals to the inverse of the within study variance because there is only one source variance.

$$W_i \ fixed \ effect \ model = \frac{1}{Variance_i}$$

The combination of estimates across studies may also depart from the assumption that the studies are all estimating the same effect; instead, the studies may estimate effects that follow a distribution across studies. This is the basis of a random-effects meta-analysis. The W_i is modified by adding an estimate of between study variance τ^2. τ^2 is an estimate of the variance of the effect-size parameters across the population of studies, reflecting random differences of the true effect sizes.

$$W_i \ random \ effects \ model = \frac{1}{Variance_i + \tau^2}$$

Readers interested in methods for estimating between study variance and for calculating the standard error for the combined effect should consult the meta-analysis literature.

Heterogeneity

For most meta-analyses, the assumption for a random-effects meta-analysis is more plausible because studies are inherently different. This is because the variability in the participants, interventions (or exposures), outcomes, as well as variability in the study design, execution, and risk of bias across studies is inevitable. These clinical and methodological diversities may introduce inconsistency in the results across studies. We call the variability in the effects evaluated in different studies statistical heterogeneity. Statistical heterogeneity can be detected by inspecting the degree of overlap of CIs of studies in a meta-analysis. When CIs do not overlap with each other, it is suggestive that there is greater variations between the results of the studies than is compatible with the play of chance.

The between study variance τ^2 is a direct measure of the amount of statistical heterogeneity and τ is on the same scale as the outcome itself. Another commonly used measure to quantify the proportion of the variability in effect estimates due to heterogeneity rather than sampling error is called I^2 statistics. Thresholds for the interpretation of I^2 can be misleading because the importance of inconsistency depends on several factors: (i) magnitude and direction of effects and (ii) strength of evidence for heterogeneity (e.g. P value from the chi-squared test, or a CI for I^2).

A rough guide to the interpretation of I^2 in the context of meta-analyses of randomized trials is as follows:
- 0–40%: might not be important;
- 30–60%: may represent moderate heterogeneity;
- 50–90%: may represent substantial heterogeneity;
- 75–100%: considerable heterogeneity.

Of note, although I^2 can inform whether a meta-analysis is sensible, the most important assessment of whether to combine the results across studies relies on a thorough and thoughtful qualitative synthesis taking into consideration the magnitude and direction of effects and the risk of bias assessment. A combined estimate of several biased studies is worse than the studies themselves as it may reach a precise but invalid answer to the research question.

Heterogeneity may also be present because of the choice of effect measures. Empirical evidence suggests that risk differences are unlikely to give consistent estimates of intervention effect compared with relative risk because the baseline risks may vary substantially between studies. The opposite can also be true (there is more consistency on the additive scale and less on the multiplicative scale). Heterogeneity observed in a meta-analysis is therefore specific to the choice of summary statistic for each study and that the choice needs to fit the research question. For decisions in clinical care and public health, risk difference (and the reciprocal of risk difference – the number needed to treat) matters more to patients and clinicians.

If there are plausible reasons for heterogeneity, review authors could explore it in subgroup analysis or meta-regression; both methods answer the question how the specific differences between studies might impact on the results of those studies. In subgroup analysis, studies are divided into subsets and separate meta-analysis is performed within each subset. This may be viewed as an investigation of how a categorical study characteristic is associated with the effects in meta-analysis. An inference that the effects or associations differ between subgroups should be based on a formal statistical test. Meta-regression is an extension of subgroup analysis that allows both categorical and continuous characteristics to be investigated. In essence, meta-regressions resemble simple linear regressions. In meta-regression, the outcome variable is the effect estimate (e.g. a mean difference, a log relative risk) and explanatory variables are characteristics of studies that might influence the size of effect. The unit of analysis in meta-regression is the individual study.

Almost all statistical software (e.g. STATA, R, SAS) can perform a meta-analysis. The output is usually presented in a "forest plot" (□ Figure 11.3). □ Figure 11.3 is extracted from a systematic review on the efficacy and safety of low and very low carbohydrate diets for type 2 diabetes remission. It shows that participants on low carbohydrate diets achieved greater weight loss compared with control (mean difference –3.46, 95% CI –5.25 to –1.67; 18 studies, n = 882; τ^2 = 6.20; I^2 = 63%). On the basis of subgroup by risk of bias, the authors found that in studies at low risk of bias, low carbohydrate diets achieved 7.41 kg greater weight loss compared with controls (mean difference –7.41, 95% CI –9.75 to –5.08; 6 studies, n = 171; τ^2 = 0.00; I^2 = 0%). The subgroup difference is statistically significant. The study contributing the most relative weight to the overall meta-analysis is Daly 2006 (12.3%), whereas the study given the least relative weight is Sato 2017 (0.8%).

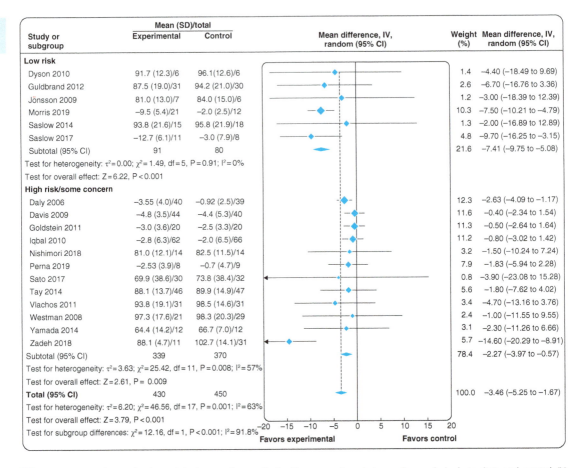

Figure 11.3 A forest plot for weight loss at six months for the comparison between low carbohydrate diets and control. IV, Inverse variance.

11.2.5 Interpret the findings and write the report

After conducting the synthesis, review authors sometimes also grade the certainty of the body of evidence. One widely adopted framework has been developed by the Grades of Recommendation, Assessment, Development, and Evaluation Working Group (GRADE). The five considerations to assess the certainty of evidence are risk of bias, consistency of effect, imprecision, indirectness, and publication bias (see paragraph below). Depending on the judgment of these five considerations, the body of evidence would be placed at one of the four levels: high, moderate, low, and very low.

Reporting of clinical trials is biased when it is influenced by the nature, size, and direction of its results. Reporting biases in clinical trials may manifest in different ways, including results not being reported at all (publication bias), or reported in part and selectively (outcome-reporting bias). Biased reporting of clinical trials in turn can introduce bias into research syntheses, with the eventual consequence being misinformed healthcare decisions.

Review authors interpret the certainty of evidence, discuss the limitations of the included studies and of the systematic review methods, the implications for research and practice, and then draw appropriate conclusions. In preparing the report of a systematic review, review authors should follow the reporting guideline appropriate for review type. The Preferred Reporting Items for Systematic Reviews and Meta-Analyses (PRISMA) and its extensions are available from the Enhancing the QUAlity and Transparency Of health Research (EQUATOR) Network.

11.3 Where can systematic reviews be found?

One should not underestimate the time and resources required to conduct a high-quality systematic review. Before embarking on a new systematic review, it makes sense to assess whether a relevant systematic review already exists or is underway. In addition to searching bibliographic databases such as MEDLINE and Embase, Box 11.1 below lists searchable databases for identifying systematic reviews.

11.4 Other review types

Emerging technological advances, such as increased use of artificial intelligence (AI), for the systematic review tasks of informational retrieval, screening, data extraction, and risk of bias assessment can revolutionize the efficiency of systematic review production and updating. Recent years have seen the development and advancement of methodology and tools for living systematic reviews. These types of reviews incorporate findings from clinical trials and other types of studies

soon after they become available. A rapid review is a form of knowledge synthesis that accelerates the process of conducting a traditional systematic review through streamlining or omitting specific methods to produce evidence for stakeholders in a resource-efficient manner. Rapid reviews, for instance, answered time-sensitive needs during the COVID-19 pandemic covering topics such as digital contact-tracing technologies in epidemics, rapid point-of-care tests for diagnosis of SARS-CoV-2 infection, and travel-related control measures to contain the COVID-19 pandemic. Scoping reviews are a relatively new approach to evidence synthesis. Researchers may conduct scoping reviews instead of systematic reviews where the objective is to scope a body of literature, identify the main sources and types of evidence available, identify knowledge gaps, clarify concepts, or to investigate research conduct. While useful in their own right, scoping reviews may also be helpful precursors to systematic reviews and can be used to confirm the relevance of topics, the eligibility criteria, and the size of the literature. Overviews of reviews use explicit and systematic methods to search for and identify multiple systematic reviews on related research questions in the same topic area for the purpose of extracting and analyzing their results across

Box 11.1 Searchable Databases for Identifying Systematic Reviews

Resource/Database	URL	Type of systematic review
Agency for Healthcare Research and Quality Effective Health-care Program	https://www.ahrq.gov/research/findings/evidence-based-reports/search.html	Health interventions, diagnostic tests, etiologic associations
Cochrane Library	https://www.cochranelibrary.com	Health interventions and diagnostic tests
Campbell Collaboration Library	https://campbellcollaboration.org/library.html	Crime and justice, education, international development, knowledge translation and implementation, nutrition, and social welfare
Epistemonikos	https://www.epistemonikos.org	Health interventions, diagnostic tests, etiologic associations
KSR Evidence	https://ksrevidence.com	Health-related systematic reviews published since 2015
Joanna Briggs Institute EBP Database	http://know.lww.com/JBI-resources.html	Health-related systematic reviews, specifically targeted for allied healthcare professionals
SYRCLE	https://www.radboudumc.nl/en/research/departments/health-evidence/systematic-review-center-for-laboratory-animal-experimentation	Animal research

important outcomes. In an overview of reviews, the unit of searching, inclusion and data analysis is the systematic review rather than the primary study.

11.5   Using a systematic review

A variety of stakeholders may use systematic reviews for a range of different purposes. Patients and doctors refer to systematic reviews and clinical practice guidelines based on systematic reviews for healthcare decisions. Researchers use systematic reviews to stay up-to-date with literature and to justify future research needs. The National Institute of Health Research, a major public funder of clinical trials in the UK, explicitly requires justification for new research both in terms of time and relevance, and emphasizes that it "will only fund primary research where the proposed research is informed by a review of the existing evidence." It is not uncommon that reviews are commissioned by organizations seeking to set evidence-based policy or clinical guidelines. The review presented in Case 11.3, for example, was done to inform recommendations on red- and processed-meat intake from the NutriRECS (Nutritional Recommendations) consortium. Government agencies and private health insurers rely on systematic reviews to gauge the safety and effectiveness of treatments and make coverage and other decisions.

However, users should not accept the findings of systematic reviews uncritically. When there are multiple systematic reviews on the same topic, findings may be inconsistent. This is because the conduct and reporting of systematic reviews are variable and often poor, despite the sharp increase in number. When Page and colleagues examined all systematic reviews indexed in MEDLINE in one month (February 2014), they found important methodology was either not used or not reported: unpublished data were rarely sought, risk of bias assessment was not performed or rarely incorporated into analysis, and at least one third of the reviews used statistical methods discouraged by leading organizations.

Systematic reviews considered to be reliable in methods should have *at minimal* (i) defined eligibility criteria, (ii) conducted comprehensive literature search, (iii) assessed risk of bias of included studies, (iv) used appropriate methods for meta-analysis, and (v) drawn conclusions that are consistent with findings. Users of systematic reviews can undertake formal critical appraisal of the methodological rigor of systematic reviews using tools developed for this

purpose. The 2017 revision to "A MeaSurement Tool to Assess systematic Reviews" (AMSTAR 2) and Risk Of Bias In Systematic reviews (ROBIS) tool are among the most recent tools.

In summary, systematic reviews have become a standard approach for summarizing the existing scientific evidence in many fields. In health, they can be used to answer questions about effects of intervention, accuracy of diagnostic tests, etiology and prognosis of a condition, disease burden, among others. The methods for producing systematic reviews are highly structured and, in theory, reproducible. Review authors are urged to follow the recommended methodology while users of the evidence should be critical. Our confidence in the findings of systematic reviews rests on the soundness of the methods used.

Recommended reading

Higgins, J.P.T., Thomas, J., Chandler, J. et al. (ed.) (2019). *Cochrane Handbook for Systematic Reviews of Interventions*, 2e. Chichester, UK: Wiley.

IOM (2011). Committee on Standards for Systematic Reviews of Comparative Effectiveness Research, Board on Health Care Services. In: *Finding What Works in Health Care: Standards for Systematic Reviews* (ed. J. Eden, L. Levit, A. Berg and S. Morton). Washington, D.C.: National Academies Press.

Borenstein, M., Hedges, L.V., Higgins, J.P.T., and Rothstein, H.R. (2021). *Introduction to Meta-Analysis*, 2e. Wiley.

Source references (cases)

Lau, J., Antman, E.M., Jimenez-Silva, J. et al. (1992). Cumulative meta-analysis of therapeutic trials for myocardial infarction. *N. Engl. J. Med.* 327 (4): 248–254. (Case 11.1).

Sng, B.L., Leong, W.L., Zeng, Y. et al. (2014). Early versus late initiation of epidural analgesia for labour. *Cochrane Database Syst. Rev.* (10): CD007238. https://doi.org/10.1002/14651858 .CD007238.pub2 accessed 28 July 2021 (Case 11.2).

Goldenberg, J.Z., Day, A., Brinkworth, G.D. et al. (2021). Efficacy and safety of low and very low carbohydrate diets for type 2 diabetes remission: systematic review and meta-analysis of published and unpublished randomized trial data. *BMJ* 372: m4743. https://doi.org/10.1136/bmj.m4743. PMID: 33441384 (Figure 11.3).

Vernooij, R.W.M., Zeraatkar, D., Han, M.A. et al. (2019). Patterns of red and processed meat consumption and risk for cardiometabolic and cancer outcomes: a systematic review and meta-analysis of cohort studies. *Ann. Intern. Med.* 171 (10): 732–741. https://doi.org/10.7326/M19-1583. Epub 2019 Oct 1. PMID: 31569217 (Case 11.3).

Rud, B., Vejborg, T.S., Rappeport, E.D. et al. (2019). Computed tomography for diagnosis of acute appendicitis in adults. *Cochrane Database Syst. Rev.* (11): CD009977. https://doi.org/10.1002/14651858.CD009977.pub2 accessed 22 September 2021 (Case 11.4).

Source references (knowledge assessment questions)

Schumacher, M., Rücker, G., and Schwarzer, G. (2014). Meta-analysis and the surgeon general's report on smoking and health. *N. Engl. J. Med.* 370 (2): 186–188. https://doi.org/10.1056/NEJMc1315315. PMID: 24401072. (Question 6)

Knowledge assessment questions

1. What is NOT true about systematic reviews? (select the one best answer)
   A. Ideally, clinical and public health practice guidelines should be based on systematic reviews.
   B. Systematic reviews are comprehensive reviews of existing literature/knowledge that use explicit and scientific methods.
   C. Systematic reviews must include at least one study.
   D. Systematic reviews should be conducted by a team of reviewers that includes both content (e.g. clinical) and methods experts.
2. Which of the following is/are important strategies for identifying randomized controlled trials in a systematic review of a drug intervention? (select all that apply)
   A. Searches of electronic bibliographic databases (e.g. MEDLINE).
   B. Searches of clinical trial registers (e.g. http://clinicaltrials.gov).
   C. Hand-searches of reference lists of included trials.
   D. Contact with experts in the field and in industry who may have knowledge of unpublished data.

3. Which of the following are challenges to obtaining data for systematic reviews? (select all that apply)
   A. Primary studies are sometimes not published at all.
   B. Data that are reported lead to conflicting conclusions.
   C. Published data may be incomplete.
   D. None of the above
4. Which of the following is a legitimate reason to NOT do a meta-analysis? (select the one best answer)
   A. The outcome data needed for the meta-analysis are not available from 9 out of the 15 studies included in the systematic review.
   B. There are only two studies included in the systematic review.
   C. The studies included in the systematic review enrolled between 127 to 756 patients.
   D. The studies included in the systematic review do not address the same research question.
5. Which of the following is NOT true about meta-analysis? (select the one best answer)
   A. When there is little heterogeneity, the meta-analytic effect estimate usually has greater precision than individual study effect estimates.
   B. Meta-analysis allows the statistical evaluation of homogeneity/heterogeneity of results.
   C. A high-quality meta-analysis gets rid of heterogeneity that might be observed across individual studies.
   D. Meta-analysis can help generate new hypotheses.
6. Below is a forest plot showing the incidence rate ratio between smoking and all-cause mortality.

A   Death from Any Cause

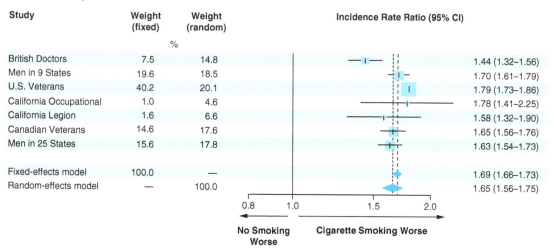

Study	Weight (fixed)	Weight (random) %	Incidence Rate Ratio (95% CI)
British Doctors	7.5	14.8	1.44 (1.32–1.56)
Men in 9 States	19.6	18.5	1.70 (1.61–1.79)
U.S. Veterans	40.2	20.1	1.79 (1.73–1.86)
California Occupational	1.0	4.6	1.78 (1.41–2.25)
California Legion	1.6	6.6	1.58 (1.32–1.90)
Canadian Veterans	14.6	17.6	1.65 (1.56–1.76)
Men in 25 States	15.6	17.8	1.63 (1.54–1.73)
Fixed-effects model	100.0	—	1.69 (1.66–1.73)
Random-effects model	—	100.0	1.65 (1.56–1.75)

No Smoking Worse   Cigarette Smoking Worse

6.1 What is the combined incidence rate ratio based on the random-effects model?
6.2 Why is the confidence interval based on the random-effects model wider than the confidence interval based on the fixed-effect model?

6.3 The studies included in the meta-analysis are all observational. Can you think of potential threats to the internal validity of included studies?
6.4 Is there sufficient evidence to conclude that smoking kills (think of criteria for causal inference)?

Answers to knowledge assessment questions

Chapter 1 Answers to knowledge assessment questions

1 Are the following statements true or false?
   1.1 Health outcomes are always binary (i.e. diseased or non-diseased).
      False
   1.2 Prevalence is a proportion.
      True
   1.3 Incidence is calculated using the number of new cases in the numerator.
      True
   1.4 All explanatory factors can be modified.
      False
   1.5 Deduction is the process by which one goes from theory to one or more hypotheses for testing.
      True

2 Epidemiology, as defined in this chapter, would include which of the following activities? (select all that apply)
   A. Describe the demographic characteristics of persons with colorectal cancer in Denver, Colorado
   B. Prescribe anti-hypertensive drugs to treat a patient with high blood pressure
   C. Compare the demographic characteristics, family history, and environmental exposures of those with and without newly diagnosed glaucoma
   D. Conduct a randomized study to compare two different surgical procedures for hip fractures
      A, C, D

3 John Snow's investigation of cholera is considered a model for epidemiologic field investigations because it included a: (select all that apply)
   A. Biologically plausible hypothesis
   B. Comparison of a health outcome among exposed and unexposed groups
   C. Multivariate statistical modeling
   D. Known biological mechanism
   E. Recommendation for public health action
      A, B, E

Chapter 2 Answers to knowledge assessment questions

1 The figure below shows the number of COVID-19 deaths in Sweden, by age groups (as of February 2, 2021). (Source: https://www.statista.com/statistics/1107913/number-of-coronavirus-deaths-in-sweden-by-age-groups)

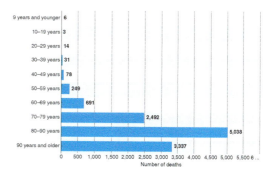

1.1 Which age group has the highest number of deaths?
     The 80-90 years age group.
1.2 Based on this figure, can you tell which group has the highest mortality?
     No, because mortality is the incidence of death; in this example, we do not know the number of people at risk in each age group.
1.3 What additional piece(s) of information you will need in order to calculate age-specific mortality?
     We will need the number of people at risk in each age group.
1.4 What additional piece(s) of information you will need in order to calculate age-specific case fatality?
     We will need number of COVID-19 cases in each age group.

2 Which of the following is NOT a proportion? (select the one best answer)
   A. Prevalence
   B. Incidence density
   C. Proportional mortality
   D. Case fatality
      B

3 A South Korean university releases a report that they have seen a dramatic rise in depressive symptoms among students in recent years. They have observed a total of 1800 students reporting depressive symptoms in 2019, with 780 students reporting newly developed symptoms in 2020. If the enrollment at the start 2019 was 35007 (and there is no drop out or new admission), what was the cumulative incidence of new cases reporting depressive symptoms in 2020?
     Cumulative incidence = 780/(35007-1800) = 0.0234 (or 23.4 cases per 1000 students)

4 Investigators successfully recruited 35 individuals at risk for flu into their study but lost 5 individuals to follow up after two weeks and 4 more at week 4. Five cases of flu have been reported at the end of week 6. Calculate the incidence density (also known as incidence rate) of the flu outbreak using appropriate person-time measures.
     For the 5 individuals who lost to follow-up at week 2, the total follow-up person-week = 5*2 = 10.

Textbook of Epidemiology, Second Edition. Lex Bouter, Maurice Zeegers and Tianjing Li.
© 2023 John Wiley & Sons Ltd. Published 2023 by John Wiley & Sons Ltd.
Companion website: www.wiley.com/go/Bouter/TextbookofEpidemiology

For the 4 individuals who lost to follow-up at week 4, the total follow-up person-week = 4*4 = 16.

For those who made it to the end of week 6, the total follow-up person-week = (35−5−4)*6 = 156.

Incidence density = number of new cases/total person-time at risk = 5/(10 + 16 + 156) = 0.027 cases per person-week

5 The figure below shows the age distribution of disabilities in the United States (US) in 2016. Which of the following statement(s) is/are correct? (select all that apply)

(Figure source: https://disabilitycompendium.org/sites/default/files/user-uploads/2017_AnnualReport_2017_FINAL.pdf.)

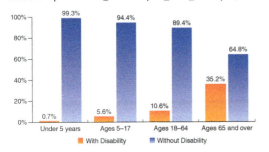

A. The percentage of people with disabilities is highest among those ages 65 and over
B. There is an age-related increase in the risk of disabilities
C. The percentage of people with disabilities increases with age

D. Most individuals with disabilities are in the ages of 65 and over

A, C

B is incorrect because the figure presents the prevalence of disability, not the risk. D is incorrect because the composition of the population is unknown. As a matter of fact, of the US population in 2016 with disabilities, over half were people in the working-ages of 18–64.

6 The table below gives information on two towns – Dragonstone and Winterfell – in the year 10 000 BCE.

Age Group (years)	Dragonstone		Winterfell	
	Population	# of deaths	Population	# of deaths
0–20	4000	350	6000	400
21–40	5000	500	10 000	700
41+	3000	150	12 000	1000

6.1 What is the crude mortality in Dragonstone in 10 000 BCE?
(350 + 500 + 150)/(4000 + 5000 + 3000) = 0.083

6.2 Using the direct adjustment method and the combined populations of Dragonstone and Winterfell as the standard population, what is the age-adjusted mortality in Dragonstone in 10 000 BCE?

Age Group (years)	Dragonstone		Winterfell		Combined population
	Population	# of deaths	Population	# of deaths	
0–20	4000	350	6000	400	10 000
21–40	5000	500	10 000	700	15 000
41+	3000	150	12 000	1000	15 000

The expected number of deaths based on the age-specific mortality in Dragonstone is:
350/4000*10 000 + 500/5000*15 000 + 150/3000* 15 000 = 3125
The age-adjusted mortality in Dragonstone is: 3125/ (10 000 + 15 000 + 15 000) = 0.078

6.3 There were 40 deaths observed among the silversmiths at King's Landing. Using the indirect method and the data below, calculate the standardized mortality ratio (SMR) for silversmiths with the combined population as the comparison population.

Age Group (years)	Combined population		Age-specific number of silversmiths	Number of expected deaths
	Population	# of deaths		
0–20	10 000	750	100	100*(750/10 000) = 7.5
21–40	15 000	1200	200	200*(1200/15 000) = 16
41+	15 000	1150	150	150*(1150/15 000) = 11.5

SMR = 40/(7.5 + 16 + 11.5) = 1.14

Chapter 3 Answers to knowledge assessment questions

A researcher in rural Ethiopia was investigating if exposure to guinea worm increases the risk for sepsis in children. He enrolled and followed a cohort of children from age 0 to 10, and documents their hospital visits and conditions. At the end of 10 years, of 1298 children in the cohort, 370 were exposed to guinea worm and 25 experienced sepsis, while 3 children not exposed to guinea worm experienced sepsis.

1   Create a contingency table to model this relationship.

	Sepsis +	Sepsis -	Totals
Guinea worm +	22	348	370
Guinea worm -	3	925	928
Totals	25	1273	1298

2   What is the attributable risk of sepsis among those exposed to guinea worm in this study?
AR = 22/370 − 3/928 = 0.056 (or 5.6%)

3   How many individuals would you have to treat for guinea worm to prevent one cases of sepsis (NNT)? (hint: round up for whole numbers of people)
NNT = 1/0.056 = 18

4   Calculate the relative risk of sepsis for children exposed to guinea worm compared with children not exposure to guinea worm.
RR = (22/370)/(3/928)=18.39

5   Which of the following is a correct interpretation of the relative risk calculated above? (select the one best answer)
   a.   Individuals with guinea worm are (100-answer 4) times more likely to have sepsis as compared to individuals without guinea worm.
   b.   The population was (answer 4) times more likely to develop guinea worm over the course of 10 years.
   c.   Individuals with guinea worm have (answer 4) times the risk of developing sepsis as compared to individuals without guinea worm.
   d.   (answer 4) percent of the risk for sepsis in the population can be attributed to guinea worm

   c

Investigators at the University of Paris wanted to look at the effect of passive smoking on hospitalization due to asthma symptoms. They recruited 1025 restaurant workers with asthma in the city and ask them to report if their restaurant allows individuals to smoke in their facilities. They then ask for participants to report whether in the past 6 months they have been hospitalized because of their asthma symptoms. Of 1025 participants, 700 report they work in restaurants that permit smoking. Sixty-four of these individuals report hospitalization in the past 6 months due to asthma symptoms, compared with 25 in the control group.

6   Fill in the contingency table below. What is the odds for hospitalization due to asthma for restaurant workers exposed to passive smoking?

	Hospitalized +	Hospitalized -	Totals
Passive smoking +	64	654	700
Passive smoking -	25	300	325
Totals	71	954	1025

Odds = 46/654 = 0.07

7   Calculate the odds ratio and 95% confidence interval of hospitalization due to asthma symptoms comparing those exposed to passive smoking with those not exposed to passive smoking.
OR = (64*300)/(654*25) = 1.17
lnOR = 0.16
SE(ln(OR)) = sqrt(1/64 + 1/654 + 1/25 + 1/300) = 0.25
95% CI for lnOR = 0.16±1.96*0.25 = (-0.33 to 0.65)
95% CI for OR = exp(-0.33 to 0.65) = (0.72 to 1.92)

8   What is the correct interpretation of the confidence interval above?
   a.   The interval includes 1, thus the result is not statistically significant. There is insufficient evidence to conclude that passive smoking increases the odds of hospitalization due to asthma in this study.
   b.   The interval does not include 0, thus the result is statistically significant. There is sufficient evidence to conclude that passive smoking increases the asthma risk in this study odds of hospitalization due to asthma in this study
   c.   The interval includes 1, thus the result is not statistically significant. Passive smoking reduces the odds of hospitalization due to asthma in this study.
   d.   The interval does not include 0, thus the result is not statistically significant.

   a

Chapter 4 Answers to knowledge assessment questions

1   The local department of public health in Mumbai has been alerted of a recent outbreak of Botulism. One hundred and forty-five people have been reported as cases in the last six days — the largest outbreak of the century. Researchers quickly mobilized to determine the source. Enrolling all cases and 145 controls without Botulism, researchers collect a detailed food intake history to try to determine the source of the outbreak. This study would best be described as: (select the one best answer)
   a.   Analytical, observational, case-control study
   b.   Descriptive, ecological, cross-sectional study

c.   Analytical, observational, cohort study
d.   Analytical, ecological, time trend study
a

2   You are designing a study you hope to generalize to the citizens of Lithuania. Which of the following would you deem to be a suitable study sample? (select all that apply)
a.   A cross section of staff and students at Vilnius University in Lithuania
b.   All members of a random sample of 500 households from the last census
c.   A group of individuals who regularly participate in food pantry distribution at a local elementary school
d.   A new mother's support group
e.   A random sample of phone numbers of residents throughout the country
f.   A cross section of the largest metropolitan hospital patients on a given day
g.   Respondents to a food assistance government-offered program
b, e

3   Which of the following is NOT an advantage of a cohort study? (select the one best answer)
a.   Incidence and incidence rates can be calculated
b.   Information bias in the measurement and ascertainment of exposure is minimized compared with a case-control study
c.   Many health outcomes can be studied simultaneously
d.   Rare outcomes can be studied easily
e.   Clarity of temporal sequence

4   Which of the following is NOT an advantage of a case control study? (select the one best answer)
a.   Efficient for rare diseases or diseases with a long latency period between exposure and disease manifestation
b.   Less costly and less time-consuming compared with a cohort study
c.   Suitable when exposure data are expensive or hard to obtain
d.   Suitable when studying dynamic populations in which follow-up is difficult
e.   Exposures can be measured with little information bias
e

5   To study whether psoriasis is associated with an increased risk of depression, researchers in Denmark looked at all individuals aged ≥18 years from 2001 to 2011 from national registries. They excluded individuals with prevalence for depression and/or psoriasis at baseline. The outcome of interest was the initiation of antidepressants or hospitalization for depression. The researchers compared the incidence rates of outcome in those with psoriasis and those without psoriasis. This study can be best described as a: (select the one best answer)
a.   Cross-sectional study
b.   Case-control study
c.   Cohort study
d.   Randomized controlled trial
e.   Time trend study
c

6   To study antibiotic resistance in isolates of *Propionibacterium acnes*, researchers in India recruited 80 patients with acne vulgaris in a tertiary care hospital in India. They collected specimens from study participants. These specimens were then cultured, the growth identified, and antibiotic susceptibility and resistance were assessed. They isolated *P. acnes* in 52% of the cases. In these isolates, resistance for erythromycin, clindamycin, and azithromycin was observed in 98, 90, and 100% of the isolates, respectively. This study can be best described as a: (select the one best answer)
a.   Cross-sectional study
b.   Case-control study
c.   Cohort study
d.   Randomized controlled trial
a

7   To study tobacco use and risk of myocardial infarction, researchers identified 12 461 cases of first acute myocardial infarction and 14 820 age-matched and sex-matched controls from 52 countries. Trained staff administered a structured questionnaire and did physical examinations for all participants in the same manner. Participants were asked if they regularly used tobacco products. This study can be best described as a: (select the one best answer)
a.   Cross-sectional study
b.   Case-control study
c.   Cohort study
d.   Randomized controlled trial
e.   Geographic correlation study
a

Chapter 5 Answers to knowledge assessment questions

1   Researchers are three weeks into their study when they realize that their scale has been wrongly calibrated and adds an extra 5 lb to every participant's weight. Explain whether this would lead to differential or non-differential misclassification and how you reached that conclusion.
This is an example of non-differential misclassification: a systematic error that leads to a consistent bias of always the same size and in always the same direction.

2   In each example, determine which of the following sources of error could cause the point estimate to differ from the population parameter: selection bias, information bias, confounding, sampling error.
a.   An uncalibrated heart monitor consistently measures all participants with a heartbeat 10 beats per minute too fast [information bias]
b.   In an Argentinian study, researchers prefer to speak English over Spanish, and opt to only thoroughly interview those participants that are English-speaking [selection bias]
c.   In an exercise study, a miscommunication among team members results in all children who are positive for thyroid disease being excluded from a study that did not to include them from being eligible for participation [confounding]
d.   Researchers struggle to recruit participants and their resulting sample has confidence intervals that are too wide to draw meaningful conclusions from their data [sampling error]

3   Selecting the controls is an important part of a patient control examination. Name 3 differences between a so-called "hospital-based-case control study" and a "population-based-case control study." Briefly explain your answers and explain whether the difference you describe has to do with validity or reliability.

Population based case control studies will have controls selected from the general population, whereas hospital-based case control studies will have controls selected from the hospital population. This can decrease the external validity of the study; comparisons cannot be made between hospital populations and the general population. Moreover, the study results may be biased if the controls from hospital-based case control studies differ systematically from the controls from general population and this is not accounted for.

4   In a cohort study the association was studied between frequent music festival attendance and the occurrence of hearing damage. The frequency of festival visits was divided into 3 categories. The results are shown below.

	Hearing damage (+)	Hearing damage (−)	
>6 times per year	80	20	100
1–6 times per year	60	50	110
Never	60	40	100
	200	110	310

a. Calculate the relative risk of visiting a music festival >6 times a month compared to "never" of developing hearing damage.

RR = (80/100)/(60/100) = 1.33

In the next step of the analysis, the researcher wants to examine whether there is effect modification or confounding by gender when comparing visiting a music festival >6 times a year compared to never. To this end, he performs a stratified analysis. Out of a total of 100, 40 men visit a festival >6 times a year and have suffered hearing damage. In total there were 70 men with hearing damage at the follow-up measurement. 50 men never attended a festival. Of the 50 women who attended a festival >6 times a year, 10 did not suffer any hearing damage. Even though they never attended a festival, 30 women still suffered hearing damage.

b. construct the corresponding 2×2 tables and calculate the relative risks for both men and women

male

	Hearing damage (+)	Hearing damage (−)	
>6 times per year	40	10	50
Never	30	20	50
	70	30	100

female

	Hearing damage (+)	Hearing damage (−)	
>6 times per year	40	10	50
Never	30	20	50
	70	30	100

c. According to these results, is gender an effect modifier or a confounder? Briefly explain your answer.

RR the same in both strata, so no effect modification. Sex-adjusted RR same as "raw" RR, so no confounding either.

Chapter 6 Answers to knowledge assessment questions

1   Which of the following best describes the main difference between association and causation?
a. Association is a relationship while causation is a model
b. Association reflects an underlying relationship while causation reflects an outcome
c. Association quantifies relationship between an explanatory variable and an outcome, while causation concludes that this relationship is causal
d. Association can only be determined by determining temporality of the underlying relationship

c

2   Researchers at Edinburgh University are conducting a study on respiratory disease and air pollution exposure. In a sample of 547 hospitalized individuals, they found a relationship between exposure to high levels of air pollution and incidence of respiratory disease in the past year (odds ratio 9.61). This association made sense – exposure to high levels of pollution may irritate the lining of the lungs and increase susceptibility to respiratory disease. However, when researchers repeated their analysis in the general population with a sample of 5000 individuals, the association was not detected (odds ratio 1.07). Upon conducting a stratified analysis, researchers concluded that both respiratory disease and exposure to high levels of pollutants caused individuals to be hospitalized.

Draw and label the variables and relationships in the study described using a directed acyclic graph. Describe what type of bias explains the different findings in the hospital and the general population samples. Which of these two provides the more valid odds ratio?

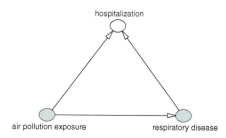

225

3 Match these Hill criteria for causation with its description. The names of the criteria are: strength, consistency, temporality, biological gradient, plausibility, coherence, experimentation

Criterion	Description
Temporality	This criterion requires that exposure precede the onset of disease by a reasonable amount of time.
Experimentation	This criterion suggests evidence from clinical trials, in vitro experiments, animal models, and so on support for the theory.
Biological gradient	This criterion says increase in the level, intensity, duration, or total level of exposure to the factor leads to progressive increases in risk. This is in keeping with the general dose-response relationship seen with many biologic phenomena.
Strength	This criterion holds that large associations provide firmer evidence of causality than do small ones, and that the most direct measure of association is found in the form of ratio measures of association such as the risk ratio.
Consistency	This criterion holds that diverse methods of study carried out in different populations under a variety of circumstances by different investigators providing non-contradictory results.
Coherence	This criterion suggests that all available evidence concerning the natural history and biology of the disease "sticks together" as a whole. By that, the proposed causal relationship should not conflict or contradict information from experimental, laboratory, epidemiologic, theory, or other knowledge sources.
Plausibility	This criterion suggests that it is helpful for an association to be based on known biological fact. This, of course, is contingent on the state of the biological knowledge of the day.

Chapter 7 Answers to knowledge assessment questions

1 **Genetic Terminology**
   What is a phenotype?
   A. the genetic make-up (code)
   B. the physical trait
   B
2 The passing of genetic traits from parents to offspring can also be called
   A. gene
   B. trait

C. heredity
D. allele
C
An alternative form of a gene can also be called
A. marker
B. heterozygous
C. DNA
D. allele
D
The minor allele variant of a polymorphism has a frequency of
A. at least 1% in the population
B. at least 5% in the population
C. maximum 1% in the population
D. maximum 5% in the population
A
If two alleles are in linkage disequilibrium. This means that
A. the DNA variants of two loci are equal
B. the DNA variants of two loci are not equal
C. the DNA variants of two loci are correlated
D. the DNA variants of two loci are not correlated
C

2 Describe how a GWAS Manhattan plot looks like and what do the peaks on this plot represent?
   In GWAS Manhattan plots, genomic coordinates are displayed along the X-axis, with the negative logarithm of the association P-value for each single nucleotide polymorphism (SNP) displayed on the Y-axis, meaning that each dot on the Manhattan plot signifies a SNP. Because the strongest associations have the smallest P-values (e.g. 10–15), their negative logarithms will be the greatest (e.g. 15). It gains its name from the similarity of such a plot to the Manhattan skyline: a profile of skyscrapers towering above the lower level "buildings" which vary around a lower height

3 Previous twin studies have estimated that the heritability of endometriosis is 51%, 75%, and 87%. Do you interpret these three estimates as consistent with each other? If so, explain why. If not, explain possible reasons for this inconsistency. What additional pieces of information could help you jointly interpret these results?
   A classical twin analysis aims to break down the variance of a certain trait into three components: genetic, shared environment and unique environment. Heritability is calculated as the genetic variance divided by the total variance. As the symptoms of endometriosis are variable and vague, healthcare workers do not easily diagnose it. This, in turn, is one of the factors that the (total) variance of endometriosis varies from population to population, altering its population-specific heritability. Also, the shared environmental factors (e.g. cultural) can vary from population to population influencing population-specific heritability.

4. Genomic data were used to determine genetic ancestry, and only samples of 95% or more European ancestry were included in statistical analysis. Why did the investigators do this?
   Genetic ancestry goes back many generations and may not be easy for researchers to trace. However, genetic ancestry is, by definition, related to differing allele frequencies across races. If one of those alleles are related to the outcome confounding is introduced. This phenomenon is also called population stratification and needs to be prevented in genetic epidemiologic studies.

Chapter 8 Answers to knowledge assessment questions

1 An outbreak of diarrheal illness occurred following a birthday party held at a petting zoo in Aurora, Colorado on June 10. One person has tested positive for Salmonella indicating that this outbreak was likely caused by *Salmonella*. There were cows, goats, sheep, and llamas present at the petting zoo. Most ill people reported petting the llamas.

   a. Construct a case definition for the outbreak. Assume you are constructing an outbreak case definition early in the outbreak investigation.

   A case defined as a person with diarrhea, fever, or stomach cramps with onset between June 10 and June 16 who had physical contact with animals at the Denver Zoo in Aurora, Colorado on June 10th, 2021.

   b. How might your outbreak case definition change later in the outbreak? Give 1–2 examples of how the case definition might change.

   The outbreak case definition would likely change moving forward if it were confirmed that llamas were the source of the outbreak or if a specific strain of Salmonella were identified. This would help to limit the case definition to exclude people who did not test positive for that strain, or who did not have contact with the specific species causing the outbreak.

2 Health workers reported an increased number of diarrhea cases at Hapsvil village beginning on June 17. They notified the local Ministry of Health (MOH) Office on June 19. Hapsvil is a remote village in rural southern India. Many villagers lack access to electricity, toilets, and potable water.

   a. Do you think this could be an outbreak? Why or why not?

   This could be classified as an outbreak if the diseases are due to a single pathogen. It would first have to be determined that this is an actual increase in the number of diarrheal diseases as compared to baseline. If there is more disease than previous years and individuals have the same or a similar set of symptoms such that we can form a case definition, this could be considered an outbreak.

   b. What additional information would help you in making this determination?

   As stated above, we would want to know if the sick individuals had a shared etiology and/or a similar set of symptoms. We would also want to look at data to see if more diseases have in fact been reported since June 17th than what is typical for this village.

   c. What other explanations might explain the increase in cases (other than an outbreak)?

   Other explanations that do not include an outbreak might be contamination in the water sources of the village with hard metals or pesticides, etc. seasonal flare-up of parasites that persist commonly in the village or increased alcohol consumption among villagers (for example, during a holiday season).

3 Health workers reported an increased number of diarrhea cases at Hapsvil village beginning on June 17. They notified the local Ministry of Health (MOH) Office on June 19. Hapsvil is a remote village in rural southern India. Many villagers lack access to electricity, toilets, and potable water.

MOH staff visited the local clinic and reviewed health clinic records for diarrhea cases over the past three years. The number of cases reported on June 17–19 was three-times that reported during the same week in the previous two years. There were no reported changes in the composition of the village population, health care seeking behaviors, or the case definition used; therefore, you consider this to be a real outbreak.

   a. How would you define a case? Provide a case definition.

   Since we lack much information on the outbreak, we would define a case as follows: An individual who spent time in Hapsvil village who developed diarrhea on or after June 17th, 2021. This would likely change if many individuals were found who had symptom onset before June 17th or if other symptoms are identified.

   b. How would you find additional cases? Describe two ways in which you would do this.

   It is necessary to search for additional cases in the village to determine the scope of the outbreak. (i) Firstly, we would contact other local doctors, hospitals and nurses in the area to ask if any patients meeting the case definition had been seen in the clinic for medical attention. (ii) We would also question the initial cases if they knew of anyone (family members, friends, party guests, etc.) who were experiencing similar symptoms and request they provide names and contact information of those people.

   c. Name one other thing you would do at this early stage in the outbreak investigation.

   Early in this outbreak, we would probably gather fecal and blood samples from all known cases to see if we could begin identifying the cause of the outbreak with laboratory testing.

4 Health workers reported an increased number of diarrhea cases at Hapsvil village beginning on June 17. They notified the local Ministry of Health (MOH) Office on June 19. Hapsvil is a remote village in rural southern India. Many villagers lack access to electricity, toilets, and potable water.

MOH staff visited the local clinic and reviewed health clinic records for diarrhea cases over the past three years. The number of cases reported on June 17–19 was three-times that reported during the same week in the previous two years. There were no reported changes in the composition of the village population, health care seeking behaviors, or the case definition used; therefore, you consider this to be a real outbreak.

Laboratory tests confirmed cholera in 3 villagers. Cholera is an acute, diarrheal illness caused by infection of the intestine with the bacterium *Vibrio cholerae*. Symptoms can include profuse watery diarrhea, vomiting, and leg cramps. It can take anywhere from a few hours to five days for symptoms to appear after infection. Symptoms typically appear in two to three days. It is typically spread by water or food that has been contaminated with human feces containing the bacteria.

After interviewing some villagers, you hypothesize that contaminated surface water from the local pond was the source of the outbreak. Villagers use pond water for washing utensil and garments, bathing, and preparation of foods.

   a. What type of epidemiological study would you conduct to test the hypothesis that contaminated pond water was the cause of the outbreak? Why?

We would conduct a case control study, identifying cases and matched controls and asking about exposures. We would test the odds that individuals exposed to pond water developed diarrhea.

b. Explain how you would go about identifying people for your epidemiological study?

We would identify controls by matching cases with individuals of similar sex and age in the village who did not develop diarrhea. Ideally there would be some kind of list or registry from which we could identify both cases and controls from.

c. What exposure period would you ask about?

We would ask about exposure from June 10th to June 17th to cover the incubation period plus two days.

5. Health workers reported an increased number of diarrhea cases at Hapsvil village beginning on June 17. They notified the local Ministry of Health (MOH) Office on June 19. Hapsvil is a remote village in rural southern India. Many villagers lack access to electricity, toilets, and potable water.

MOH staff visited the local clinic and reviewed health clinic records for diarrhea cases over the past three years. The number of cases reported on June 17–19 was three-times that reported during the same week in the previous two years. There were no reported changes in the composition of the village population, health care seeking behaviors, or the case definition used; therefore, you consider this to be a real outbreak.

Laboratory tests confirmed cholera in 3 villagers. Cholera is an acute, diarrheal illness caused by infection of the intestine with the bacterium *V. cholerae*. Symptoms can include profuse watery diarrhea, vomiting, and leg cramps. It can take anywhere from a few hours to five days for symptoms to appear after infection. Symptoms typically appear in two to three days. It is typically spread by water or food that has been contaminated with human feces containing the bacteria.

After interviewing some villagers, you hypothesize that contaminated surface water from the local pond was the source of the outbreak. Villagers use pond water for washing utensil and garments, bathing, and preparation of foods.

The investigators decided to undertake a case-control study. In the case-control study, 30 of 41 cases reported the pond water used for fermented rice preparation, compare with 15 of 41 controls.

a. Based on the data provided above, calculate the appropriate measure of association for using the pond water for fermented rice preparation.

OR = ad/bc = (13*26)/(15*11) = 4.73

Exposure	Case	Control
+	30	15
–	11	26

b. Interpret what the measure of association means.

An odds ratio of 4.73 suggests that cases had 4.73 times the odds of being exposed to pond water as compared to controls.

c. Is this finding statistically significant?

This finding is statistically significant (95%CI: 1.85, 12.09). The 95% confidence interval does not include 1, so this finding is statistically significant. We reject the null hypothesis that there is no association between pond water exposure and cholera.

SE(log(OR)) = sqrt(1/a + 1/b + 1/c + 1/d) = SE(log(OR)) = sqrt(1/30 + 1/15 + 1/11 + 1/26)

95%CI = 1.96+/− SE(log(OR)) = (1.85, 12.09)

Chapter 9 Answers to knowledge assessment questions

1 From the local health authorities, you have received data of 800 participants of a study on the validity of an at-home rapid COVID-19 test kit. Participants with complaints of COVID-19 presenting at a drive-through testing site were asked to read the test kit manual and perform the at-home test in addition to the standard polymerase chain reaction (PCR) test performed by a healthcare professional. Of all participants, 187 had a positive PCR test, 128 had a positive at-home test. Only 4 participants had a positive at-home test, but a negative PCR test.

a. Construct a 2 × 2 table and compute sensitivity and specificity of the at-home test using the PCR test as reference test. Interpret sensitivity and specificity in your own words.

	PCR$^+$	PCR$^-$	
At-home$^+$	124	4	128
At-home$^-$	63	609	672
	187	613	800

Sensitivity = 124/187 ≈ 0.66 or 66%. In words: "The probability that someone has a positive at-home test, given that their PCR test was positive (i.e., that they have COVID-19, as the PCR test is regarded as reference)."

Specificity = 609/613 ≈ 0.99 or 99%. In words: "The probability that someone has a negative at-home test, given that their PCR test was negative (i.e., that they are free of COVID-19)."

b. Compute PV$^+$ and PV$^-$. How much do the posterior probabilities (i.e. PV$^+$ and PV$^-$) differ from the prior probability (prevalence)?

PV$^+$ = 124/128 ≈ 0.97, or 97%

PV$^-$ = 609/672 ≈ 0.91, or 91%

The posterior probability of having COVID-19 (to be more precise: of having a positive PCR test) is 97% for those with a positive at-home test, and 9% (i.e. 100–91%) for those with a negative at-home test. The prevalence is 187/800 ≈ 0.23, or 23%. Hence, a positive at-home test increases someone's probability from 23 to 97%.

c. Given the sensitivity and specificity computed for 1a., how would PV$^+$ and PV$^-$ change if the at-home test were applied in a population with a prior probability (prevalence) of COVID-19 of 1%? Verify your answer by calculating PV$^+$ and PV$^-$ for a hypothetical sample of, e.g. 10 000 participants by constructing another 2x2 table given a prevalence of 1%.

	PCR⁺	PCR⁻	
At-home⁺	66	99	165
At-home⁻	34	9801	9835
	100	9900	10000

$PV^+ = 66/165 \approx 0.40$, or 40%
$PV^- = 9801/9835 \approx 1.00$, or 100%

d. Compute the likelihood ratio of a positive and a negative test result using the 2×2 table of 1a. How would these change if the at-home test were applied in a population with a prior probability of COVID-19 of 1%?

$LR^+ = \text{sensitivity}/1 - \text{specificity} = 0.66/(1-0.99) = 66$
$LR^- = 1 - \text{sensitivity}/\text{specificity} = (1-0.66)/0.99 \approx 0.34$

Both sensitivity and specificity remain the same, regardless of the prior probability. Hence, the likelihood ratios do not change.

2 To test reproducibility of axillary ultrasound to detect advanced axillary nodal disease in breast cancer patients, two observers rated 100 ultrasound images independent from each other. The following 2×2 table resulted from the study:

		Observer 1		
		Positive	Negative	
Observer 2	positive	40	10	50
	negative	17	33	50
		57	43	100

a. Compute the agreement rate for the two observers and interpret it in your own words.
Agreement rate = (40+33)/100 = 0.73, or 73%. Of all images scored by the two observers, they agreed in 73% of cases.

b. Compute Cohen's kappa. What was the expected agreement based on chance alone?
Expected agreement = ((57/100)*50 + (43/100)*50)/100 = 0.50, or 50%
Cohen's kappa = (73−50%)/(100%−50%) = 0.46

c. Compute the specific agreement for both positive and negative test results. Why are some cells counted twice in the computation?
Specific agreement⁺ = (2*40)/(2*40+10+17) ≈ 0.75, or 75%
Specific agreement⁻ = (2*33)/(2*33+17+10) ≈ 0.71, or 71%
Some cells are counted twice as they are positive (or negative in the second computation) results scored by both observers separately, so they need to be counted once for each observer.

3 As an obstetrician, you are interested in applying the prediction model for successful vaginal delivery in women with a previous caesarian section (see Table 9.9).
a. Compute the probability of a successful vaginal delivery for a 28-year-old Hispanic woman with a body mass index of 21, who has never had a previous vaginal delivery, with no recurrent indication for a caesarian section.
P(success) = 1/(1+exp(−[3.766−0.039*28−0.060*21−0.671*0−0.680*1+0.888*0+0.632*0])) ≈ 0.68 ≈ 68%

b. Would her probability of a successful vaginal delivery be lower or higher if she had a body mass index of 32 instead of 21? How can you know this using the information from Table 9.9?
Her probability of a successful vaginal delivery would be lower, the regression coefficient is negative.

c. Using the regression coefficient for body mass index from Table 9.9, what is the odds ratio for each increase of 1 BMI-point? Interpret the odds ratio in your own words.
Odds ratio = exp.(regression coefficient) = exp.(−0.060) ≈ 0.94. For each increase in 1 point BMI, the odds of a successful vaginal delivery is multiplied by 0.94 (or decreases by 6%).

Chapter 10 Answers to knowledge assessment questions

1 Which of the following is NOT a key consideration of designing a randomized trial? (select the one best answer)
a. The primary outcome must be capable of being assessed in all participants
b. The question should be specified in advance of the trial, and be as specific as possible
c. Follow-up should end when a participant stopped taking the study medication
d. The randomization sequence should be concealed from those enrolling and allocating participants
c

2 Which of the following are threats to internal validity in randomized trials? (select all that apply)
a. Unblinding of treatment assignment
b. Drop out and loss to follow up
c. Participant non-adherence
d. Protocol deviations/violations
e. Inadequate sample size
f. Restrictive eligibility criteria
a, b, c, d

3 Which of the following is NOT a characteristic of randomized crossover trials? (select the one best answer)
a. The random assignment is to the order of interventions.
b. There is a higher degree of precision than parallel trials (with the same number of participants).
c. There is a risk of a "carry-over" effect.
d. They are appropriate for conditions which can be cured in relatively short periods of time.
e. They allow for within-individual comparisons.
d

4 Which is NOT a reason why an investigator might choose to conduct a cluster randomized trial? (select the one best answer)
a. Ethical considerations
b. To enhance cooperation of investigators and participants
c. To minimize contamination
d. The intervention is naturally applied to the cluster level
e. It is more efficient than an individually randomized trial because of people within clusters may respond similarly to interventions.
e

5   When trial investigators select composite measures as primary outcomes, they often lump less serious events together with very serious events (e.g. composite outcome of death, myocardial infarction, stroke, and TIA). Why can this be an issue when presenting the results such a trial?

When the components of a composite outcome are very different in their frequency, severity, and importance to patients, it can make the results of trial misleading because the significance of an intervention's effect, and its size, will often be exaggerated by the inclusion of the components that occur more frequently than others. For example, an intervention may drastically reduce the incidence of TIA, but not of stroke, MI, or mortality. In cases such as this, the composite results make it appear as though the intervention has a greater effect on patient-important outcomes than the intervention actually does. Furthermore, when the components of a composite outcome are poorly correlated, the composite outcome may be impossible to interpret.

6   To evaluate the effect of a single prostate-specific antigen (PSA) screening and – if positive – standardized diagnostic pathway on prostate cancer–specific mortality, a Cluster Randomized Trial of PSA Testing for Prostate Cancer (CAP) was conducted at 573 primary care practices across the United Kingdom. The trial enrolled men aged 50–69 years. The randomization and recruitment of the practices occurred between 2001 and 2009; patient follow-up ended on March 31, 2016. The primary outcome was prostate cancer–specific mortality at a median follow-up of 10 years and all-cause mortality was one of the secondary outcomes.

Among 415 357 randomized men (mean [SD] age, 59.0 [5.6] years), 189 386 in the intervention group and 219 439 in the control group were included in the analysis (n = 408 825; 98%). In the intervention group, 75 707 (40%) attended the PSA testing clinic and 67 313 (36%) underwent PSA testing.

After a median follow-up of 10 years, 549 (0.30 per 1000 person-years) died of prostate cancer in the intervention group vs 647 (0.31 per 1000 person-years) in the control group (rate difference, −0.013 per 1000 person-years [95% CI, −0.047 to 0.022]; incidence rate ratio [RR], 0.96 [95% CI, 0.85–1.08]; P = 0.50). The number diagnosed with prostate cancer was higher in the intervention group (n = 8054; 4.3%) than in the control group (n = 7853; 3.6%) (RR, 1.19 [95% CI, 1.14–1.25]; P < 0.001). More prostate cancer tumors with a Gleason grade of 6 or lower were identified in the intervention group (n = 3263/189386 [1.7%]) than in the control group (n = 2440/219439 [1.1%]) (difference per 1000 men, 6.11 [95% CI, 5.38–6.84]; P < 0.001). In the analysis of all-cause mortality, there were 25459 deaths in the intervention group vs 28306 deaths in the control group (RR, 0.99 [95% CI, 0.94–1.03]; P = 0.49).

a.   Is there evidence that PSA screening invitation is effective in reducing the cancer-specific mortality and all-cause mortality?

After a median follow-up of 10 years, 549 (0.30 per 1000 person-years) died of prostate cancer in the intervention group vs 647 (0.31 per 1000 person-years) in the control group (incidence rate ratio [RR], 0.96 [95% CI, 0.85–1.08]; P = 0.50). In the analysis of all-cause mortality, there were 25 459 deaths in

the intervention group vs 28 306 deaths in the control group (RR, 0.99 [95% CI, 0.94–1.03]; P = 0.49).
Because the RRs cover the null value of 1, there is no evidence that PSA screening invitation is effective in reducing the cancer-specific mortality or all-cause mortality.

b.   The figure below shows the cumulative risk of all-cause mortality by groups. It appears that mortality differs by attendance. The RR comparing attenders with control is 0.68 (95% CI 0.65, 0.71); p < 0.001. Is this analysis comparing the attenders with control appropriate? Why or why not?

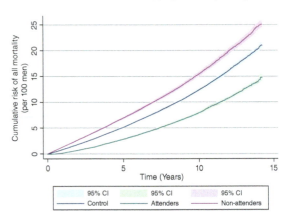

	95% CI		95% CI		95% CI
	Control		Attenders		Non-attenders

The analysis that compares the attenders with control is inappropriate. Randomization ensures comparability of prognostic factors at baseline. Following the principle of intention-to-treat analysis, participants in randomized trials should be analyzed in the intervention groups to which they were randomized, regardless of the intervention they actually received. Many individuals (64%) in the CAP trial did not receive PSA screening and therefore deviated from the assigned intervention. This deviation was unlikely to be "random", in the sense that attenders and non-attenders were different in the distribution of their prognostic factors. A naïve analysis that compares the attenders with control is therefore biased.

Chapter 11 Answers to knowledge assessment questions

1   What is NOT true about systematic reviews? (select the one best answer)
a.   Ideally, clinical and public health practice guidelines should be based on systematic reviews.
b.   Systematic reviews are comprehensive reviews of existing literature/knowledge that use explicit and scientific methods.
c.   Systematic reviews must include at least one study.
d.   Systematic reviews should be conducted by a team of reviewers that includes both content (e.g. clinical) and methods experts.

c

2 Which of the following is/are important strategies for identifying randomized controlled trials in a systematic review of a drug intervention? (select all that apply)
   a. Searches of electronic bibliographic databases (e.g. MEDLINE)
   b. Searches of clinical trial registers (e.g. clinicaltrials.gov)
   c. Hand-searches of reference lists of included trials
   d. Contact with experts in the field and in industry who may have knowledge of unpublished data
   a, b, c, d

3 Which of the following are challenges to obtaining data for systematic reviews? (select all that apply)
   a. Primary studies are sometimes not published at all.
   b. Data that are reported lead to conflicting conclusions.
   c. Published data may be incomplete.
   d. None of the above
   a, b, c

4 Which of the following is a legitimate reason to NOT do a meta-analysis? (select the one best answer)
   a. The outcome data needed for the meta-analysis are not available from 9 out of the 15 studies included in the systematic review.

   b. There are only two studies included in the systematic review.
   c. The studies included in the systematic review enrolled between 127 and 756 patients.
   d. The studies included in the systematic review do not address the same research question.
   d

5 Which of the following is NOT true about meta-analysis? (select the one best answer)
   a. When there is little heterogeneity, the meta-analytic effect estimate usually has greater precision than individual study effect estimates.
   b. Meta-analysis allows the statistical evaluation of homogeneity/heterogeneity of results.
   c. A high-quality meta-analysis gets rid of heterogeneity that might be observed across individual studies.
   d. Meta-analysis can help generate new hypotheses.
   c

6 Below is a forest plot showing the incidence rate ratio between smoking and all-cause mortality.

A   Death from Any Cause

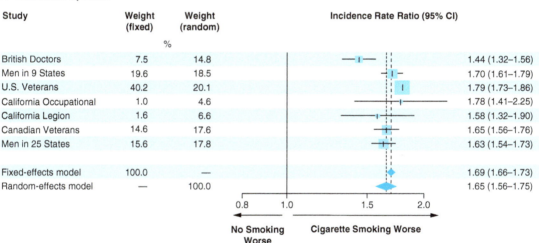

Study	Weight (fixed)	Weight (random) %	Incidence Rate Ratio (95% CI)
British Doctors	7.5	14.8	1.44 (1.32–1.56)
Men in 9 States	19.6	18.5	1.70 (1.61–1.79)
U.S. Veterans	40.2	20.1	1.79 (1.73–1.86)
California Occupational	1.0	4.6	1.78 (1.41–2.25)
California Legion	1.6	6.6	1.58 (1.32–1.90)
Canadian Veterans	14.6	17.6	1.65 (1.56–1.76)
Men in 25 States	15.6	17.8	1.63 (1.54–1.73)
Fixed-effects model	100.0	—	1.69 (1.66–1.73)
Random-effects model	—	100.0	1.65 (1.56–1.75)

0.8   1.0   1.5   2.0

No Smoking Worse   Cigarette Smoking Worse

6.1 What is the combined incidence rate ratio based on the random-effects model?
   1.65 (95% CI: 1.56–1.75)

6.2 Why is the confidence interval based on the random-effects model wider than the confidence interval based on the fixed-effect model?
   Under the fixed-effect model the only source of uncertainty is the within-study (sampling or estimation) error. Under the random-effects model there is this same source of uncertainty plus an additional source (between-studies variance). It follows that the variance, standard error, and confidence interval for the summary effect will always be larger (or wider) under the random-effects model than under the fixed-effect model (unless the between study variance is zero, in which case the two models are the same).

6.3 The studies included in the meta-analysis are all observational. Can you think of potential threats to the internal validity of included studies?
   Selection bias, information bias, and confounding.

6.4 Is there sufficient evidence to conclude that smoking kills (think of criteria for causal inference)?
   Yes, there is sufficient evidence to conclude that smoking kills. The association has been consistently and coherently observed across many studies, across different populations and population subgroups. The strength of the association is strong and any residual confounding is unlikely to change the direction of the association. There is a temporal relationship between exposure and outcome, as well as a dose–response relationship. Lastly, the etiology is biologically plausible.

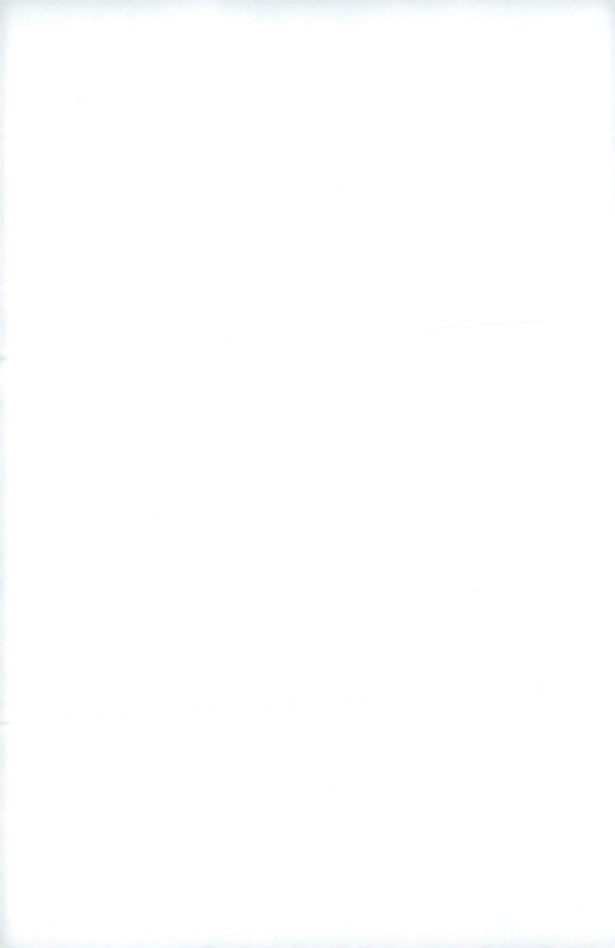

Index

Textbook of Epidemiology, Second Edition. Lex Bouter, Maurice Zeegers and Tianjing Li.
© 2023 John Wiley & Sons Ltd. Published 2023 by John Wiley & Sons Ltd.
Companion website: www.wiley.com/go/Bouter/TextbookofEpidemiology